FEMINIST, QUEE

FEMINIST, QUEER, CRIP

Alison Kafer

Indiana University Press

Bloomington and Indianapolis

This book is a publication of

Indiana University Press
601 North Morton Street
Bloomington, Indiana 47404-3797 USA

iupress.indiana.edu

Telephone orders   800-842-6796
Fax orders   812-855-7931

A shorter version of chapter 3 was published as "Debating Feminist
Futures: Slippery Slopes, Cultural Anxiety, and the Case of the Deaf
Lesbians," in *Feminist Disability Studies*, ed. Kim Q. Hall (Bloomington:
Indiana University Press, 2011), 218–41, and is reprinted with permission.
Portions of chapter 6 appeared in much earlier form as "Hiking Boots
and Wheelchairs: Ecofeminism, the Body, and Physical Disability,"
in *Feminist Interventions in Ethics and Politics*, ed. Barbara Andrew,
Jean Keller, and Lisa H. Schwartzman (Lanham, MD: Rowman and
Littlefield, 2005), 131–50, and are also reprinted with permission.

♾ The paper used in this publication meets the minimum requirements
of the American National Standard for Information Sciences—
Permanence of Paper for Printed Library Materials, ANSI Z39.48–1992.

Manufactured in the United States of America

Cataloging-in-Publication Data is available
from the Library of Congress.

ISBN: 978-0-253-00922-7 (cloth)
ISBN: 978-0-253-00934-0 (paper)
ISBN: 978-0-253-00941-8 (ebook)

1 2 3 4 5 18 17 16 15 14 13

For Dana

Contents

Acknowledgments

I CANNOT BEGIN TO thank Katherine Sherwood enough for letting me use her magnificent painting, *Vesalius's Pump*, for the cover of this book. (A description of the painting immediately follows these acknowledgments.) I first saw this painting during a 2007 show of Sherwood's work at the University of California, Berkeley, and I began at that moment to hope that it might one day grace the cover of this book. I am deeply grateful that Katherine gave me permission to use it; her work has been and continues to be an inspiration to me, in all the best senses of that word.

This book began as a dissertation at Claremont Graduate University, and I hope my early mentors can still see their influences on it and on me; I continue to feel the benefits of their guidance. Thanks to Rosemarie Garland-Thomson, Ranu Samantrai, Karen Jo Torjesen, and Peggy Waller for pushing me to think more critically and more carefully; I am equally grateful for their willingness to help me imagine an academic career for myself. May all graduate students be so lucky. I was lucky as well in having a solid group of graduate school writing buddies: Dana Newlove, Sara Patterson, and Zandra Wagoner. That stage of this project would have been much more difficult, and much less enjoyable, without them.

It is no exaggeration to say that I could not have written this book without the generous support of the women's studies department at the University of California, Santa Barbara. By bringing me to UCSB for a dissertation fellowship, they provided me with the time and space to think through the early stages of this project. More importantly, they introduced me to a staggeringly smart and insightful group of graduate students who embodied exactly the kind of engaged scholarship I describe in these pages. For helping me to see, think, and feel differently, thanks to Karl Bryant, Ted Burnes, Simone Chess, Sharon Doetsch, Dana Collins, Beth Currans, Laura Hill-Bonnet, Jessi Quizar, Matt Richardson, Jeanne Scheper, Molly Talcott, and Tiffany Willoughby-Herard. For building the kind of academic programs and spaces in which such students could thrive, thanks to Jacqueline Bobo, Sharon Hoshida, Eileen Boris, Lou Anne Lockwood, Laury Oaks, and Leila Rupp.

My postdoctoral year at UC Berkeley was equally transformative; I cannot heap enough praise on the people and ideas behind the Ed Roberts Postdoctoral Fellowship in Disability Studies. Being able to think and talk through this project with the extended Ed Roberts group (Fred Collignon, Anne Finger, Lakshmi Fjord, Laura Hershey, Devva Kasnitz, Corbett O'Toole, Sue Schweik, and Russell Shuttleworth) was a dream come true, as was having the fellowship at the same time as Ellen Samuels and Robin Stephens. I am equally grateful to the fellowship for providing me the opportunity to expand my circle of disability comrades. Getting to work, think, and play with

Patty Berne, Mel Chen, Michele Friedner, Sujatha Jesudason, Cathy Kudlick, Jessica Lehman, Anna Mollow, Leroy Moore, Alice Sheppard, Katherine Sherwood, Bethany Stevens, Jean Stewart, and Sunaura Taylor has made my world a more beautiful place; each of these fine folks has helped make this book better. Thanks to Zona Roberts for opening her house to me and for doing it with such easy generosity.

I am immensely grateful to be teaching feminist studies to undergraduates at a small liberal arts college, and that gratitude only multiplies when I think of my fiercely smart students and colleagues. I owe many thanks to all of my colleagues in feminist studies at Southwestern, most especially those who have served on the feminist studies committee over the years; for supporting me in and through the program, thanks to Elaine Craddock, Lysane Fauvel, Elizabeth Green-Musselman, Julia Johnson, Kathleen Juhl, Helene Meyers, and Sandi Nenga. Double thanks to Helene, Julia, and Sandi for talking through parts of this project with me, and to Elaine for reading so much of it. Thanks are due as well to Melissa Johnson, Maria Lowe, Brenda Sendejo, and all the other folks on the hall who fill my days with raucous laughter. I feel incredibly fortunate to have been able to teach—and to learn from—all of the students I have had at Southwestern; being in and out of the classroom with them is a gift. Special thanks to those students who have said just the right thing at just the right time, making this project richer than it would have been otherwise: Chelsey Clammer, Siobhan Cooke, Marie Draz, Jordan Johnson, Alex Lannon, and Danielle Roberts; thanks as well to Michelle Redden for research assistance. I also want to thank Lynne Brody, Dana Hendrix, and all of the librarians at the Smith Library Center; thanks, too, to Lisa Anderson for her quick help with interlibrary loans. Although she is no longer at Southwestern, I also want to thank Suzy Pukys for our many conversations about community engagement.

Austin has felt like home from the moment we arrived, in no small part because of the warm embrace of friends we found here. Writing this book was made easier by this sense of grounding. Thanks to Jo and John Dwyer, Kris Hogan and Milly Gleckler, Maria Lowe and Emily Niemeyer, Allison Orr and Blake Trabulsi, Shannon Winnubst and Jenny Suchland, and all of their children, dogs, cats, and chickens. When I needed more than all of these animals could give, the cold waters of Barton Springs kept me going.

My other home, intellectual and otherwise, is more virtual but no less sustaining: A hearty thank you to all of my colleagues in the Society for Disability Studies and the community of disability studies scholars and activists more broadly. For being great friends, colleagues, and dance partners, thanks to Liat Ben-Moshe, Nirmala Erevelles, Anne Finger, Michele Friedner, Lezlie Frye, Rosemarie Garland-Thomson, Elaine Gerber, Michelle Jarman, Kate Kaul, Petra Kuppers, Simi and David Linton, Riva Lehrer, Samuel Lurie, Robert McRuer, Anna Mollow, Joan Ostrove, Corbett O'Toole, Katherine Ott, Margaret Price, Carrie Sandahl, Sami Schalk, Alice Sheppard, Sue Schweik, Cindy Wu, and many, many more. Lots of these folks read drafts or partial drafts of chapters, offered feedback on conference papers, talked through ideas, and generously shared their critical responses to this work; I thank each and every one of them for their full and rich collegiality. Thanks are due as well to Jackie Cuevas, Judith Plaskow, and Judy Rohrer for knowing what I needed to hear, and to Eunjung Kim, Sunaura Taylor, and Shannon Winnubst for cheering me on. Susan Burch, Mel Chen, Eli Clare, Cathy Kudlick, and Ellen Samuels generously read versions of the manuscript over the years, and I am still learning from their insights. Stacy Alaimo, Licia Carlson, and Kim Q. Hall read the entire manuscript, and both I and the book benefited immensely from their readings; I want to thank them for their careful, sharp, and incisive feedback. I am fortunate to be in such an intellectually generous community of scholars.

Thanks to all the PISSAR Patrol members, who work tirelessly to improve the restrooms of the world, especially Simone Chess, Jessi Quizar, and Matt Richardson; thanks, too, to all those who created and attended the 2002 Queer Disability Conference, in particular Eli Clare, Laura Hershey, Samuel Lurie, Corbett O'Toole, Ellen Samuels, Robin Stephens, and Jen Williams. My understandings of the promise of queer, crip space owes much to all of them. I am thankful that I got to witness the founding and development of Generations Ahead, where I learned a great deal about being fully in the world from my fellow board members: Le'a Malia Kanehe, Jackie Payne, Crystal Plati, Dorothy Roberts, Silvia Yee, Miriam Yeung, and our fearless leader, Sujatha Jesudason. I am grateful, too, for the opportunity to work with Patty Berne, Jessica Lehman, and Marina Ortega.

My work has been made better by the conversations, ideas, projects, and moments I was lucky enough to share with Chris Bell, Tanis Doe, Laura Hershey, and Paul Longmore. They are, and will continue to be, missed by all of us working in disability studies and beyond.

Deep thanks to Dee Mortensen at Indiana University Press for her steady and enthusiastic support of me and this project. She and Sarah Jacobi have made every step of this process easy and enjoyable. Thanks as well to Tim Roberts and Kerrie Maynes for their keen assistance through the production stages.

I have been helped in this project by the generous support of several institutions. I am deeply appreciative for long-term support from Southwestern University through its Cullen fellowships, sabbatical funding, competitive faculty development funds, and a Brown Junior Faculty Research Fellowship. Thanks are due as well to the University of California, Berkeley, for an Ed Roberts Postdoctoral Fellowship in Disability Studies. For support through the dissertation stage, I owe thanks to Claremont Graduate University for a Dissertation Grant; to the Women's Studies Department at the University of California, Santa Barbara, for a Dissertation Scholars Teaching Fellowship; and to the Woodrow Wilson Foundation for a Women's Studies Dissertation Fellowship.

Thanks to the Kafer, Melton, Newlove, and Cotton families for nurturing and supporting me throughout this work and all that led up to it. I am still uncertain that they fully understand what it is I do, which makes it all the more noteworthy that they continue to support me in it. I am grateful for being part of their warm hearts and homes, and for having them in mine.

Finally, and happily, to the two beloved creatures who share my everyday life: I want to thank Maya for all the meows and keyboard interruptions, but she is already fully aware of her importance. Thanks to Dana Newlove for the first word, the last word, and all the spaces in between; this book is for her.

Textual Description of the Cover Art

THE IMAGE ON the front cover is of a mixed-media painting by Katherine Sherwood titled *Vesalius's Pump* (2006, 36 x 36 inches). The painting takes up the bottom two-thirds of the book's cover and consists mostly of large, looping swirls of paint over an ivory-colored background. Some of the paint on the right edge of the painting is so thick that it has cracked, creating a branching network of brown lines. In the center of the painting, Sherwood has affixed several anatomical drawings of brains taken from Andreas Vesalius's sixteenth-century anatomy text *On the Structure of the Human Body*. Rendered in oranges and yellows, the brains are placed alongside images of the arterial system from Sherwood's own brain scans. The brains are jumbled together, with the loops of paint moving around and over them; the overall effect is of a slow-moving organic machine.

FEMINIST, QUEER, CRIP

Introduction

Imagined Futures

I dream of more inclusive spaces.
 —Kavitha Koshy, "Feels Like Carving Bone"

I HAVE NEVER CONSULTED a seer or psychic; I have never asked a fortune-teller for her crystal ball. No one has searched my tea leaves for answers or my stars for omens, and my palms remain unread. But people have been telling my future for years. Of fortune cookies and tarot cards they have no need: my wheelchair, burn scars, and gnarled hands apparently tell them all they need to know. My future is written on my body.

In 1995, six months after the fire, my doctor suggested that my thoughts of graduate school were premature, if not misguided. He felt that I would need to spend the next three or four years living at home, under my parents' care, and only then would it be appropriate to think about starting school. His tone made it clear, however, that he thought graduate school would remain out of reach; it was simply not in my future. What my future did hold, according to my rehabilitation psychologist and my recreation therapist, was long-term psychological therapy. My friends were likely to abandon me, alcoholism and drug addiction loomed on my horizon, and I needed to prepare myself for the futures of pain and isolation brought on by disability. Fellow rehab patients, most of whom were elderly people recovering from strokes or broken hips, saw equally bleak horizons before me. One stopped me in the hallway to recommend suicide, explaining that life in a wheelchair was not a life worth living (his son, he noted offhandedly, knew to "let him go" if he was eventually unable to walk).

My future prospects did not improve much after leaving the rehabilitation facility, at least not according to strangers I encountered, and continue to encounter, out in the world. A common response is for people to assume they know my needs better than I do, going so far as to question my judgment when I refuse their offers of help. They can apparently see into my immediate future, forecasting an inability to perform specific tasks and predicting the accidents and additional injuries that will result. Or, taking a longer view, they imagine a future that is both banal and pathetic: rather than involving dramatic falls from my wheelchair, their visions assume a future of relentless pain, isolation, and bitterness, a representation that leads them to bless me, pity me, or refuse to see me altogether. Although I may believe I am leading an engaging and satisfying life, they can see clearly the grim future that awaits me: with no hope of a cure in sight, my future cannot be anything but bleak. Not even the ivory tower of academia protected me from these dismal projections of my future: once I made it to graduate school, I had a professor reject a paper proposal about cultural approaches to disability; she cast the topic as inappropriate because insufficiently academic. As I prepared to leave her office, she patted me on the arm and urged me to "heal," suggesting that my desire to study disability resulted not from intellectual curiosity but from a displaced need for therapy and recovery. My future, she felt, should be spent not researching disability but overcoming it.

These grim imagined futures, these suggestions that a better life would of necessity require the absence of impairment, have not gone unchallenged. My friends, family, and colleagues have consistently conjured other futures for me, refusing to accept ableist suggestions that disability is a fate worse than death or that disability prohibits a full life. Those who have been most vocal in imagining my future as ripe with opportunities have been other disabled people, who are themselves resisting negative interpretations of their futures. They tell stories of lives lived fully, and my future, according to them, involves not isolation and pathos but community and possibility: I could write books, teach, travel, love and be loved; I might raise children or become a community organizer or make art; I could engage in activist struggles for the rights of disabled people or get involved in other movements for social justice.

At first glance, these contradictory imagined futures have nothing in common: the first casts disability as pitiable misfortune, a tragedy that effectively prevents one from leading a good life, while the second refuses such inevitability, positioning ableism—not disability—as the obstacle to a good life. What these two representations of the future share, however, is a strong link to the present. How one understands disability in the present determines how one imagines disability in the future; one's assumptions about the experience of disability create one's conception of a better future.

If disability is conceptualized as a terrible unending tragedy, then any future that includes disability can only be a future to avoid. A better future, in other words, is one that excludes disability and disabled bodies; indeed, it is the very *absence* of disability that signals this better future. The *presence* of disability, then, signals something else: a future that bears too many traces of the ills of the present to be desirable. In this framework, a future with disability is a future no one wants, and the figure of the disabled person, especially the disabled fetus or child, becomes the symbol of this undesired future. As James Watson—a geneticist involved in the discovery of DNA and the development of the Human Genome Project—puts it, "We already accept that most couples don't want a Down child. You would have to be crazy to say you wanted one, because that child has no future."[1] Although Watson is infamous for making claims about who should and shouldn't inhabit the world, he's not alone in expressing this kind of sentiment.[2] Watson's version simply makes clear some of the assumptions underlying this discourse, and they are assumptions that cut to the heart of this project. The first is that disability is seen as the sign of no future, or at least of no good future. The second, and related, assumption is that we all agree; not only do we accept that couples don't want a child with Down syndrome, we know that anyone who feels otherwise is "crazy."[3] To want a disabled child, to desire or even to accept disability in this way, is to be disordered, unbalanced, sick. "We" all know this, and there is no room for "you" to think differently.

It is this presumption of agreement, this belief that we all desire the same futures, that I take up in this book. I am particularly interested in uncovering the ways the disabled body is put to use in these future visions, attending to both metaphorical and "corporeal presence and absence."[4] I argue that disability is disavowed in these futures in two ways: first, the value of a future that includes disabled people goes unrecognized, while the value of a disability-free future is seen as self-evident; and second, the political nature of disability, namely its position as a category to be contested and debated, goes unacknowledged. The second failure of recognition makes possible the first; casting disability as monolithic fact of the body, as beyond the realm of the political and therefore beyond the realm of debate or dissent, makes it impossible to imagine disability and disability futures differently. Challenging the rhetoric of naturalness and inevitability that underlies these discussions, I argue that decisions about the future of disability and disabled people are political decisions and should be recognized and treated as such. Rather than assume that a "good" future naturally and obviously depends upon the eradication of disability, we must recognize this perspective as colored by histories of ableism and disability oppression. Thus, in tracing these two failures of recognition—the disavowal of disability from "our" futures—I imagine futures otherwise, arguing for a cripped politics of access and engagement based on the work of disability activists and theorists.

What *Feminist, Queer, Crip* offers is a politics of crip futurity, an insistence on thinking these imagined futures—and hence, these lived presents—differently. Throughout the course of the book, I hold on to an idea of politics as a framework for thinking through how to get "elsewhere," to other ways of being that might be more just and sustainable. In imagining more accessible futures, I am yearning for an elsewhere—and, perhaps, an "elsewhen"—in which disability is understood otherwise: as political, as valuable, as integral.

Before going any further, I admit to treading tricky ground here. "A future with disability is a future no one wants": while I find it absolutely essential to dismantle the purported self-evidence of that claim, I can't deny that there is truth to it. Not only is there abstract truth to it, there's personal, embodied truth: it is a sentiment I myself hold. As much joy as I find in communities of disabled people, and as much as I value my experiences as a disabled person, I am not interested in becoming more disabled than I already am. I realize that position is itself marked by an ableist failure of imagination, but I can't deny holding it. Nor am I opposed to prenatal care and public health initiatives aimed at preventing illness and impairment, and futures in which the majority of people continue to lack access to such basic needs are not futures I want.[5] But there is a difference between denying necessary health care, condoning dangerous working conditions, or ignoring public health concerns (thereby causing illness and impairment) and recognizing illness and disability as part of what makes us human.[6] While definitively mapping that difference is beyond the scope of this book—and, I would argue, neither fully possible nor desirable—sketching out some of the potential differences is exactly the work we need to be doing.

Defining Disability: A Political/Relational Model

The meaning of disability, like the meaning of illness, is presumed to be self-evident; we all know it when we see it. But the meanings of illness and disability are not nearly so fixed or monolithic; multiple understandings of disability exist. Like other disability studies scholars, I am critical of the medical model of disability, but I am equally wary of a complete rejection of medical intervention. In the pages that follow, I offer a hybrid political/relational model of disability, one that builds on social and minority model frameworks but reads them through feminist and queer critiques of identity. My concern with imagining disability futures differently frames my overview of each model; thinking about the kinds of futures imagined or implicit in each definition provides a useful lens for examining the assumptions and implications of these frameworks.

Despite the rise of disability studies in the United States, and decades of disability rights activism, disability continues to be seen primarily as a personal problem afflicting individual people, a problem best solved through strength of character and resolve. This individual model of disability is embodied in the disability simulation exercises that are a favored activity during "disability awareness" and diversity events on college campuses (including, in years past, my own). For these kinds of events, students are asked to spend a few hours using a wheelchair or wearing a blindfold so that they can "understand" what it means to be blind or mobility-impaired.[7] Not only do these kinds of exercises focus on the alleged failures and hardships of disabled bodies (an inability to see, an inability to walk), they also present disability as a knowable fact of the body. There is no accounting for how a disabled person's response to impairment shifts over time or by context, or how the nature of one's impairment changes, or, especially, how one's experience of disability is affected by one's culture and environment. Wearing a blindfold to "experience blindness" is going to do little to teach someone about ableism, for example, and suggests that the only thing there is to learn about blindness is what it feels like to move around in the dark. The meaning of blindness, in other words, is completely encapsulated in the experience of wearing a blindfold; there is simply nothing else to discuss. Although these kinds of exercises are intended to reduce fears and misperceptions about disabled people, the voices and experiences of disabled people are absent. Absent also are discussions about disability rights and social justice; disability is depoliticized, presented more as nature than culture. As Tobin Siebers notes, these are exercises in "personal imagination" rather than "cultural imagination," and a limited imagination at that.[8]

This individual model of disability is very closely aligned with what is commonly termed the medical model of disability; both form the framework for dominant understandings of disability and disabled people. The medical model of disability frames atypical bodies and minds as deviant, pathological, and defective, best understood and addressed in medical terms. In this framework, the proper approach to disability is to "'treat' the condition and the person with the condition rather than 'treating' the social processes and policies that constrict disabled people's lives."[9] Although this framing of disability is called the "medical" model, it's important to note that its use isn't limited to doctors and other service providers; what characterizes the medical model isn't the position of the person (or institution) using it, but the positioning of disability as an exclusively medical problem and, especially, the conceptualization of such positioning as both objective fact and common sense.[10]

Indeed, some of the most passionate defenses of the medical model of disability occur outside the hospital or clinic. Literary critic Denis Dutton exemplifies this pattern of thought, condemning a writing manual for its attempt to describe disability in social rather than medical terms. Dutton refutes the need for such attention to disability language, countering that "*it is the medical condition that is the problem, not the words that describe it.*"[11] Because disability is a purely medical problem, Dutton finds no need to engage with disability as a category of analysis; concepts such as able-bodiedness, healthiness, and the normal body, or conditions such as "blindness, wheelchairs, polio, and cretinism" do not require or merit critical attention for they are merely facts of life.[12] For Dutton, disability is a self-evident, unchanging, and purely medical phenomenon, and the meanings, histories, and implications of "cretinism," for example, are not available for debate or dissent.

Thus, in both the individual and medical models, disability is cast as a problematic characteristic inherent in particular bodies and minds. Solving the problem of disability, then, means correcting, normalizing, or eliminating the pathological individual, rendering a medical approach to disability the only appropriate approach. The future of disability is understood more in terms of medical research, individual treatments, and familial assistance than increased social supports or widespread social change.

Disability studies scholars and disability activists, however, refute the premises of the medical/individual framework. Rather than casting disability as a natural, self-evident sign of pathology, we recast disability in social terms. The category of "disabled" can only be understood in relation to "able-bodied" or "able-minded," a binary in which each term forms the borders of the other. As Rosemarie Garland-Thomson explains, this hierarchical division of bodies and minds is then used to "legitimat[e] an unequal distribution of resources, status, and power within a biased social and architectural environment."[13] In this construction, disability is seen less as an objective fact of the body or mind and more as a product of social relations.

Thus, the definitional shift away from the medical/individual model makes room for new understandings of how best to solve the "problem" of disability. In the alternative perspective, which I call the political/relational model, the problem of disability no longer resides in the minds or bodies of individuals but in built environments and social patterns that exclude or stigmatize particular kinds of bodies, minds, and ways of being. For example, under the medical/individual model, wheelchair users suffer from impairments that restrict their mobility. These impairments are best addressed through medical interventions and cures; failing that, individuals must make the best of a bad situation, relying on friends and family members to negotiate inaccessible spaces for them. Under a political/relational model of disability, however, the problem of disability is located in inaccessible buildings, discriminatory attitudes, and ideological systems that attribute normalcy and deviance to particular minds and bodies. The problem of disability is solved not through medical intervention or surgical normalization but through social change and political transformation.

This is not to say that medical intervention has no place in my political/relational model. By my reckoning, the political/relational model neither opposes nor valorizes medical intervention; rather than simply take such intervention for granted, it recognizes instead that medical representations, diagnoses, and treatments of bodily variation are imbued with ideological biases about what constitutes normalcy and deviance. In so doing, it recognizes the possibility of simultaneously desiring to be cured of chronic pain and to be identified and allied with disabled people.[14] I want to make room for people to acknowledge—even mourn—a change in form or function while also acknowledging that such changes cannot be understood apart from the context in which they occur.

In juxtaposing a medical model with a political one, I am not suggesting that the medical model is not itself political. On the contrary, I am arguing for increased recognition of the political nature of a medical framing of disability. As Jim Swan argues, recognizing that a medical model is political allows for important questions about health care and social justice: "How good is the care? Who has access to it? For how long? Do they have choices? Who pays for it?"[15] Swan's questions remind us that medical framings of disability are embedded in economic realities and relations, and the current furor over health care reform underscores the political nature of these questions. Moreover, as scholars of feminist science studies, reproductive justice, and public health continue to make clear, medical beliefs and practices are not immune to or separate from cultural practices and ideologies. Thus, in offering a political/relational model of disability, I am arguing not so much for a rejection of medical approaches to disability as for a renewed interrogation of them. Insisting upon the political dimension of disability includes thinking through the assumptions of medical/individual models, seeing the whole terrain of "disability" as up for debate.[16]

My framing of disability as political/relational is intended as a friendly departure from the more common social model of disability. Like Margrit Shildrick and Janet Price, my intent is to "demand an unsettling of its certainties, of the fixed identities of which it is bound up" and to pluralize the ways we understand bodily instability.[17] Although both the social and political/relational models share a critique of the medical model, the social model often relies on a distinction between impairment and disability that I don't find useful. In that framework, impairment refers to any physical or mental limitation, while disability signals the social exclusions based on, and social meanings attributed to, that impairment.[18] People with impairments are disabled by their environments; or, to put it differently, impairments aren't disabling, social and architectural barriers are. Although I agree that we need to attend to the social, asserting a sharp divide between impairment and disability fails to recognize that *both* impairment and disability are social; simply trying to determine what constitutes impairment makes clear that impairment doesn't exist apart from social meanings and understandings. Susan Wendell illustrates this problem when she queries how far one must be able to walk to be considered able-bodied; the answer to that question, she explains, has much to do with the economic and geographic context in which it is addressed.[19] What we understand as impairing conditions—socially, physically, mentally, or otherwise—shifts across time and place, and presenting impairment as purely physical obscures the effects of such shifts. As feminist theorists have long noted, there is no mention of "the" body that is not a further articulation of a very particular body.[20]

At the same time, the social model with its impairment/disability distinction erases the lived realities of impairment; in its well-intentioned focus on the disabling effects of society, it overlooks the often-disabling effects of our bodies. People with chronic illness, pain, and fatigue have been among the most critical of this aspect of the social model, rightly noting that social and structural changes will do little to make one's joints stop aching or to alleviate back pain. Nor will changes in architecture and attitude heal diabetes or cancer or fatigue. Focusing exclusively on disabling barriers, as a strict social model seems to do, renders pain and fatigue irrelevant to the project of disability politics.[21]

As a result, the social model can marginalize those disabled people who are interested in medical interventions or cures. In a complete reversal of the individual/medical model, which imagines individual cure as the desired future for disability, a strict social model completely casts cure out of our imagined futures; cure becomes the future no self-respecting disability activist or scholar wants. In other words, because we are so often confronted with the medical framing of disability as unending burden, or as a permanent drag on one's quality of life, disability rights activists and scholars tend to deny our own feelings of pain or depression; admitting to struggling with our impairments or to wanting a cure for them is seen as accepting the very framings we are fighting against, giving fodder to the enemy, so to speak. But by positioning ourselves only in opposition to the futures imagined through the medical model, and shutting down communication and critique around vital issues, we limit the discourses at our disposal. As Liz Crow warns, in refusing to acknowledge pain, fatigue, or depression, "our collective ability to conceive of, and achieve, a world which does not disable is diminished."[22]

Finally, drawing a hard line between impairment and disability, and having this distinction serve as the foundation for theorizing disability, makes it difficult to explore the ways in which notions of disability and able-bodiedness affect everyone, not just people with impairments.[23] Anxiety about aging, for example, can be seen as a symptom of compulsory able-bodiedness/able-mindedness, as can attempts to "treat" children who are slightly shorter than average with growth hormones; in neither case are the people involved necessarily disabled, but they are certainly affected by cultural ideals of normalcy and ideal form and function. Or, to take this idea in a different direction, friends and family members of disabled people are often affected by ableist attitudes and barriers, even if they are not themselves disabled. Their social lives may shrink, for example, because others are uncomfortable or embarrassed by their stories of illness and adaptation, or friends may feel guilty inviting them to inaccessible houses; difficulty accessing reliable and affordable attendant care or finding appropriate housing certainly affects entire families, not only the disabled person herself or himself. Moreover, not only does disability exist in relation to able-bodiedness/able-mindedness, such that disabled and abled form a constitutive binary, but also, to move to a different register of analysis, disability is experienced in and through relationships; it does not occur in isolation. My choice of a *relational* model of disability is intended to speak to this reality.

Similarly, my articulation of a *political* framing of disability is a direct refusal of the widespread depoliticization of disability. Dutton's medicalized description of disability assumes that "cretinism" is a natural category, derived purely from objective medical study and irrelevant to discussions of politics or prejudice; proclaiming the naturalness of disability, he goes on to ridicule attempts to discuss disability in terms of language or identification.[24] By asserting that we cannot (or should not) resignify disability identities and categories, refusing to recognize the impact disability rhetoric and terminology might have on understandings of disability (and thus on the lives of disabled people), and insisting that medical approaches to disability are completely objective and devoid of prejudice or cultural bias, Dutton completely removes disability from the realm of the political. In doing so, he forecloses on the possibility of understanding disability differently; divorcing disability and disabled people from understandings of the political prohibits incorporating disability into programs of social change and transformation or, in other words, into visions of a better future. Once disability has been placed solely in the medical framework, and both disability and the medical world are portrayed as apolitical, then disability has no place in radical politics or social movements—except as a problem to be eradicated.

A political/relational model of disability, on the other hand, makes room for more activist responses, seeing "disability" as a potential site for collective reimagining. Under this kind of framework, "disability awareness" simulations can be reframed to focus less on the individual experience of disability—or imagined experience of disability—and more on the political experience of disablement. For example, rather than placing nondisabled students in wheelchairs, the Santa Barbara-based organization People in Search of Safe and Accessible Restrooms (PISSAR) places them in bathrooms, armed with measuring tapes and clipboards, to track the failures and omissions of the built environment. As my fellow restroom revolutionaries explain in our manifesto, "This switch in focus from the inability of the body to the inaccessibility of the space makes room for activism and change in ways that 'awareness exercises' may not."[25] In creating and disseminating a "restroom checklist," PISSAR imagines a future of disability activism, one with disability rights activists demanding accessible spaces; contrast that approach with the simulation exercises, in which "awareness" is the future goal, rather than structural or systemic change.

In reading disability futures and imagined disability through a political/relational model, I situate disability squarely within the realm of the political. My goal is to contextualize, historically and politically, the meanings typically attributed to disability, thereby positioning "disability" as a set of practices and associations that can be critiqued, contested, and transformed. Integral to this project is an awareness that ableist discourses circulate widely, and not only in sites marked explicitly as about disability; thus, thinking about disability as political necessitates exploring everything from reproductive practices to environmental philosophy, from bathroom activism to cyberculture. I am influenced here by Chantal Mouffe, who argues that "the political cannot be restricted to a certain type of institution, or envisaged as constituting a specific sphere or level of society. It must be conceived as a dimension that is inherent to every human society and that determines our very ontological condition."[26] To say that something is "political" in this sense means that it is implicated in relations of power and that those relations, their assumptions, and their effects are contested and contestable, open to dissent and debate.

In other words, I'm concerned here with what Jodi Dean calls "the *how* of politics, the ways concepts and issues come to be political common sense and the processes through which locations and populations are rendered as in need of intervention, regulation, or quarantine."[27] This focus on the *how* of politics parallels the first set of questions that motivate my project: Is disability political? How is it political? How is the category of disability used to justify the classification, supervision, segregation, and oppression of certain people, bodies, and practices? Addressing these questions requires a recognition of the central role that ideas about disability and ability play in contemporary culture, particularly in imagined and projected futures.

After stressing the importance of the "how" of politics, Dean insists on the need "to take *depoliticization* seriously, to address the means through which spaces, issues, identities, and events are taken out of political circulation or are blocked from the agenda—or are presumed to have already been solved."[28] Attending to the ways in which disability is political leads to my second set of motivating questions: How has disability been depoliticized, removed from the realm of the political? Which definitions of and assumptions about disability facilitate this removal? What are the effects of such depoliticization? I'm not so much arguing for or positing a chronology here—"disability used to be political and now it's not"—as highlighting the need for disability studies to attend to the specific ways in which ableist understandings of disability are taken as common sense.[29] Such attention is vital in a context in which, as Susan Schweik notes, disability-based discrimination and prejudice are often condemned not as markers of structural inequality but of cruelty or insensitivity; this kind of rhetoric "sidesteps the reality of social injustice, reducing it to a question of compassion and charitable feelings."[30]

These questions—of politicization and of depoliticization—lie at the root of my interest in political frameworks of the future: Do the futures I examine in these chapters assume and perpetuate the depoliticization of disability, and if so, how? What is it about disability that makes it a defining element of our imagined futures, such that a "good" future is one without disability, while a "bad" future is overrun by it? Why is disability in the present constantly deferred, such that disability often enters critical discourse only as the marker of what must be eliminated in our futures or what was unquestioningly eliminated in our pasts? And, most importantly, why are these characterizations taken for granted, recognized as neither partial nor political?

Identifying Disability: Bodies, Identities, Politics

Seeing disability as political, and therefore contested and contestable, entails departing from the social model's assumption that "disabled" and "nondisabled" are discrete, self-evident categories, choosing instead to explore the creation of such categories and the moments in which they fail to hold. Recognizing such moments of excess or failure is key to imagining disability, and disability futures, differently. Thus I understand the very meanings of "disability," "impairment," and "disabled" as contested terrain.[31] Disability can then be understood, in Jasbir Puar's framework, as an *assemblage*, where "[c]ategories—race, gender, sexuality [and, I would add, disability]—are considered as events, actions, and encounters between bodies, rather than as simply entities and attributes of subjects."[32]

Thus, a political/relational framework recognizes the difficulty in determining who is included in the term "disabled," refusing any assumption that it refers to a discrete group of particular people with certain similar essential qualities. On the contrary, the political/relational model of disability sees disability as a site of questions rather than firm definitions: Can it encompass all kinds of impairments—cognitive, psychiatric, sensory, and physical? Do people with chronic illnesses fit under the rubric of disability? Is someone who had cancer years ago but is now in remission disabled? What about people with some forms of multiple sclerosis (MS) who experience different temporary impairments—from vision loss to mobility difficulties—during each recurrence of the disease, but are without functional limitations once the MS moves back into remission? What about people with large birthmarks or other visible differences that have no bearing on their physical capabilities, but that often prompt discriminatory treatment?

Government and nongovernmental organizations alike frequently issue guidelines for determining who is disabled and thus eligible for certain programs and protections. Such groups, ranging from the World Health Organization to the US Social Security Administration, would not have to be so precise in defining "disability" if such definitions were without controversy; the very fact that so much energy is funneled into defining disability and impairment suggests the fundamental instability of the terms. Moreover, the desire for fixed definitions cannot be divorced from the economic effects of such fixing. The Social Security Administration uses its definitions of disability to determine who qualifies for benefits and at what level; the US Supreme Court has continued to revisit the Americans with Disabilities Act in order to determine who merits protection under its provisions and who does not. Both entities rule as if there were bright lines between disabled and non-, even though the need for such rulings suggests otherwise. But there is clearly a notion that there are people whose claims do not rise to the level of disability, and who therefore are undeserving of such protections.

In contrast, the disability theory and politics that I develop in these pages do not rely on a fixed definition of "disability" and "disabled person" but recognize the parameters of both terms as always open to debate. I am concerned here with disability not as a category inherent in certain minds and bodies but as what historian Joan W. Scott calls a "collective affinity." Drawing on the cyborg theory of Donna Haraway, Scott describes collective affinities as "play[ing] on identifications that have been attributed to individuals by their societies, and that have served to exclude them or subordinate them."[33] Collective affinities in terms of disability could encompass everyone from people with learning disabilities to those with chronic illness, from people with mobility impairments to those with HIV/AIDS, from people with sensory impairments to those with mental illness. People within each of these categories can all be discussed in terms of disability politics, not because of any essential similarities among them, but because all have been labeled as disabled or sick and have faced discrimination as a result. Simi Linton illustrates this fundamental diversity of the disability community when she writes,

> We are everywhere these days, wheeling and loping down the street, tapping our canes, sucking on our breathing tubes, following our guide dogs, puffing and

sipping on the mouth sticks that propel our motorized chairs. We may drool, hear voices, speak in staccato syllables, wear catheters to collect our urine, or live with a compromised immune system. We are all bound together, not by this list of our collective symptoms but by the *social and political circumstances that have forged us as a group.*[34]

Linton's formulation strikes me as a fitting place to begin this exploration of accessible futures, primarily because it reads more as promise than fact. Both disability studies and disability movements have been slow to recognize potential linkages among people who hear voices, people with compromised immune systems, and people using wheelchairs. Although there have been notable exceptions, disability studies, especially in the humanities, has focused little attention on cognitive disabilities, focusing more often on visible physical impairments and sensory impairments.[35] Chronic illness has become more common in these discussions, but only in particular forms; discussion of chronic fatigue syndrome and mental disability has increased thanks to the work of scholars such as Susan Wendell, Ellen Samuels, and Margaret Price, but diabetes, asthma, and lupus remain largely unexplored by disability studies scholars.[36] (This oversight is all the more troubling given the fact that diabetes occurs disproportionately among "members of racial and ethnic minority groups in the United States," and asthma is a common side-effect of living in heavily polluted neighborhoods, which, unsurprisingly, are more likely to be populated by poor people.)[37] I repeat Linton's formulation then in an effort to call it into being, to invoke it as a possibility for thinking disability differently. I want to hold on to the possibility of a disability studies and a disability movement that does take all of these locations seriously, that feels accountable to these bodies and identities and locations.

One of the arguments I will make in this book, however, is that part of the work of imagining this kind of expansive disability movement is to simultaneously engage in a critical reading of these very identities, locations, and bodies. We must trace the ways in which we have been forged as a group, to use Linton's terminology, but also trace the ways in which those forgings have been incomplete, or contested, or refused. We need to recognize that these forgings have always already been inflected by histories of race, gender, sexuality, class, and nation; failing to attend to such relations will ensure that disability studies remains, as Chris Bell puts it, "white disability studies."[38] We must, in other words, think through the assumptions and erasures of "disabled" and "disability," reckoning with the ways in which such words have been used and to what effect.

Doing so might mean imagining a "we" that includes folks who identify as or with disabled people but don't themselves "have" a disability. Scholars of chronic illness have started this work, arguing for the necessity of including within disability communities those who lack a "proper" (read: medically acceptable, doctor-provided, and insurer-approved) diagnosis for their symptoms. Doing so not only provides such people with the social supports they need (everything from access to social services to recognition from friends and family), it also presents disability less as diagnostic category and more as collective affinity; moving away from a medical/individual model of disability means that disability identification can't be solely linked to diagnosis.

Less familiar, and potentially more complicated, would be people identifying with disability and lacking not only a diagnosis but any "symptoms" of impairment. How might we understand the forging of a group that includes, in Carrie Sandahl's and Robert McRuer's framings, a "nondisabled claim to be crip?"[39] Hearing Children of Deaf Adults, or CODAs, would be a clear example of this kind of identification, as CODAs consider themselves part of Deaf communities, and some even claim Deaf identity, but are not themselves deaf or hard-of-hearing.[40] But does claiming crip require this kind of blood or kinship tie? What might it mean for lovers or friends to claim crip, or to understand themselves as "culturally disabled"? Or for theorists and activists committed to rethinking disability and able-bodiedness/able-mindedness to make such claims? Can claiming crip be a method of imagining multiple futures, positioning "crip" as a desired and desirable location regardless of one's own embodiment or mental/psychological processes? As McRuer notes, these practices run the risk of appropriation, but they also offer a vital refusal of simplistic binaries like disabled/nondisabled and sick/healthy.[41] Claiming crip, then, can be a way of acknowledging that we all have bodies and minds with shifting abilities, and wrestling with the political meanings and histories of such shifts. Thus, to circle back to the notion of "we" as more promise than fact: thinking through what nondisabled claims to crip might entail will require exploring whether such claims might be more available, or more imaginable, to some people than others (and on what basis).

Attention to these kinds of questions—the histories and effects of disability claims, the different availability and viability of disability identification—distinguishes this kind of "nondisabled claim to crip" from the well-intentioned but deeply ableist declaration that "we are *all* disabled." The latter obscures the specificities I call for here, conflating all experiences of physical, mental, or sensory limitation without regard to structural inequality or patterns of exclusion and discrimination. It is for this reason that Linton cautions against "erasing the line between disabled and nondisabled people," explaining that "naming the category" of disabled remains necessary because it effectively "call[s] attention to" disability-based discrimination. But I suggest that exploring the possibilities of nondisabled claims, as well as attending to the promises and dangers of the category's flexibility, can facilitate exactly this kind of critical attentiveness.[42] To claim crip critically is to recognize the ethical, epistemic, and political responsibilities behind such claims; deconstructing the binary between disabled and able-bodied/able-minded requires *more* attention to how different bodies/minds are treated differently, not less.

Attending to the epistemological challenges raised by disability claims introduces yet another set of questions about claiming crip. Thinking through this collective "we," this forging of crip communities, means accounting for those who do "have" illnesses or impairments, and who might be recognized by others as part of this "disabled we," but who do not recognize themselves as such. This group would include the largest proportion of disabled people: those folks with hearing impairments, or low vision, or "bum knees," or asthma, or diabetes who, for a whole host of reasons, would claim neither crip identity nor disability. Even though most people with impairments might fall into this camp, it is actually the hardest group for me to address in this book; indeed, I think it is the hardest group for disability studies and disability rights activism to address.[43] Given my (our) focus on disability rights and justice, on radical queercrip activism, on finding disability desirable, how am I (how are we) to deal with those who want no part of such names?

One answer to these questions is that it doesn't matter whether such people claim crip or not: rethinking our cultural assumptions about disability, imagining our disability futures differently, will benefit all of us, regardless of our identities. As Ladelle McWhorter notes, "The practices and institutions that divide, for example, the 'able-bodied,' 'sane,' and 'whole' from the 'impaired,' 'mentally ill,' and 'deficient' create the conditions under which all of us live; they structure the situation within which each one of us comes to terms with ourselves and creates a way of life."[44] As someone writing and teaching disability studies, as someone imagining readers and students with a whole range of bodies and minds, I find hope in McWhorter's prediction, in her articulation of a better future. Much as feminist activism benefits people who want no part of feminism, disability studies and activism ideally benefit people who are not interested or invested in either.[45] At the same time, I'm certain this is not the only, or not the full, answer. As I embark on this journey into accessible futures, I want to highlight the question of crip affiliation, what it means, what it entails, what it excludes.

Feminist, Crip, Queer: A Note on Terms, Methods, and Affiliations

I became disabled before I began reading feminist theory, yet it was feminist theory that led me to disability studies. It was through reading feminist theoretical approaches to the body that I came intellectually to understand disability as a political category rather than as an individual pathology or personal tragedy. Feminist theory gave me the tools to think through disability and the ways in which assumptions about disability and disabled bodies lead to resource inequalities and social discrimination. Just as feminist theorists had questioned the naturalness of femininity, challenging essentialist assumptions about "the" female body, I could question the naturalness of disability, challenging essentialist assumptions about "the" disabled body. My understanding of the political/relational model of disability has been made possible by my engagement with the work of feminist theorists, an engagement that I hope will become clear in the following pages. Simply put, feminism has given me the theoretical tools to think critically about disability, the stigmatization of bodily variation, and various modes and strategies of resistance, dissent, and collective action.

I locate this project, then, within the larger field of feminist theory and politics. Although I examine a range of radical political visions, some explicitly feminist and others less so, I understand my investment in radical politics as a feminist investment. As many historians of feminism and women's studies have noted, feminism has long been interested in bridging theory with practice. Activists and scholars alike continue to explore the ways in which theory can inform political practice; conversely, feminists often theorize from practice, developing concepts and frameworks based on the strategies, conversations, conflicts, and achievements of feminist activists. My interest in radical politics derives in part from my theoretical and activist commitment to blending theory with practice, a commitment that I associate with feminism. I think it only appropriate to make this indebtedness explicit as I begin my exploration of possible futures, given recent disability studies texts that have downplayed or dismissed any connections to feminism; my readings and my imaginings are resolutely feminist.[46]

They also are undeniably crip, a term that has much currency in disability activism and culture but still might seem harsh to those outside those communities. Indeed, that harshness is a large part of its appeal, as suggested by essayist Nancy Mairs: "People—crippled or not—wince at the word 'crippled' as they do not at 'handicapped' or 'disabled.' Perhaps I want them to wince."[47] This desire to make people wince suggests an urge to shake things up, to jolt people out of their everyday understandings of bodies and minds, of normalcy and deviance. It recognizes the common response of nondisabled people to disabled people, of the normative to the deviant—furtive yet relentless staring, aggressive questioning, and/or a turning away from difference, a refusal to see.[48] This wincing is familiar to many disabled people, but here Mairs turns it back on itself, almost wincing back. Like "queer," "crip" and "cripple" are, in Eli Clare's formulation, "words to help forge a politics."[49]

Two related examples of such forging, of crafting an inducement to wince, would be Carrie Sandahl's preference for "crip studies" and "crip theory" over "disability studies" and Robert McRuer's decision to name his theoretical project *Crip Theory*. According to both Sandahl and McRuer, disability studies and crip theory differ in orientation and aim: crip theory is more contestatory than disability studies, more willing to explore the potential risks and exclusions of identity politics while simultaneously and "perhaps paradoxically" recognizing "the generative role identity has played in the disability rights movement."[50] I see *Feminist, Queer, Crip* as engaging in exactly this kind of contradictory crip theory, and I use both "crip" and "crip theory" as a way to stake my claim alongside the activists and cultural workers engaged in these multiple sites of radical politics.[51]

One of the most productive and provocative elements of crip theory, and of crip in general, is the potential expansiveness of the term. As Sandahl notes, "cripple, like queer, is fluid and ever-changing, claimed by those whom it did not originally define. . . . The term crip has expanded to include not only those with physical impairments but those with sensory or mental impairments as well."[52] I agree with Sandahl, and this potential flexibility is precisely what excites me about crip theory, but, as with Linton's "we are everywhere," this inclusiveness is often more hope than reality. Many expressions of crip pride or crip politics often explicitly address only physical impairments, thereby ignoring or marginalizing the experiences of those with sensory or mental impairments. Others position crip as a way of naming opposition to cure, potentially making it difficult for "crip theory" to encompass the perspectives and practices of those who both claim disability identity and desire an end to their own impairments. Thus, I move back and forth between naming this project one of "feminist and queer disability studies" and one of "crip theory," raising the possibility that the two can be, and often are, intertwined in practice; indeed, given the rich analyses of identity that circulate within feminist and queer studies, a "feminist and queer disability studies" may very well engage in the "paradoxical" approach to identity practiced in crip theory while making room for those who do not or cannot recognize themselves in crip.[53]

Similarly, throughout *Feminist, Queer, Crip,* I combine references to bodies with references to minds and pair "compulsory able-bodiedness" with "compulsory able-mindedness."[54] If disability studies is going to take seriously the criticism that we have focused on physical disabilities to the exclusion of all else, then we need to start experimenting with different ways of talking about and conceptualizing our projects.[55] At the same time, I'm well aware that my use of such terms is partial in both senses of the word: I am invested in shifting the terrain of disability studies even as my own performances of it bear the marks of its current terrain, and I have only just begun to scratch the surface of what able-mindedness might mean in relation to able-bodiedness. Thus, as with Linton's "we" and Sandahl's "crip," I use "mind" alongside "body" in the hope that writing and reading "bodies and minds" or "compulsory able-bodiedness/able-mindedness" makes me think disability differently. Rather than assuming that the mere use of such language is sufficient in and of itself, I'm calling for an engagement with the hard work of actually making such coalitions happen. As I suggest in the last chapter of the book, such expansiveness—mind and body, a crip of us all—can never be fully or finally achieved, but serves as a kind of hopeful horizon, "fluid and ever-changing," as Sandahl notes, and used in ways unimagined in advance.

Queer (theory) readers will likely recognize this talk of fluidity, ever-changing horizons, and paradoxical treatments of identity as kin to queer projects, and, like Sandahl and McRuer, I position crip theory in general, and this project in particular, as such. "Queer" also remains contested terrain, with theorists and activists continuing to debate what (and whom) the term encompasses or excludes; it is this kind of contestation I welcome for disability. Indeed, Butler argues for queer as a "site of collective contestation" to be "always and only redeployed, twisted, queered."[56] The circularity of that definition—queerness is something always to be queered—serves only to support this desire for dissent and debate. In naming my project "queer," then, I am wanting both to twist "queer" into encompassing "crip" (and "crip," "queer") and to highlight the risks of such twisted inclusion. Critical examinations of compulsory able-bodiedness and compulsory able-mindedness are queer and crip projects, and they can potentially be enacted without necessarily flattening out or stabilizing "crip" and "queer."[57] What is needed, then, are critical attempts to trace the ways in which compulsory able-bodiedness/able-mindedness and compulsory heterosexuality intertwine in the service of normativity; to examine how terms such as "defective," "deviant," and "sick" have been used to justify discrimination against people whose bodies, minds, desires, and practices differ from the unmarked norm; to speculate how norms of gendered behavior—proper masculinity and femininity—are based on nondisabled bodies; and to map potential points of connection among, and departure between, queer (and) disability activists. As we shall see, one productive site for such explorations is the imagined future invoked in popular culture, academic theory, and political movements; *Feminist, Queer, Crip* begins to trace some of these queer/crip connections.

I want, then, to position this book as a fundamentally coalitional text. The "feminist, queer, crip" named in the title signals methodology as much as content. This work quite obviously, and necessarily, involves bringing disability identities and experiences to bear on existing feminist and queer theoretical frameworks. It is not simply, or not only, an additive intervention, however. While I am indeed arguing that disability needs to be recognized as a category of analysis alongside gender, race, class, and sexuality, my larger goal is to address how disability is figured in and through these other categories of difference.[58] What work does able-bodiedness do, for example, in feminist appropriations of the cyborg, or queer uses of reproductive technologies, or ecofeminist imaginings of a better life? How does reckoning with histories and experiences of disability, in other words, critique or transform feminist environmental philosophy or queer approaches to assisted reproductive technologies? I want to explore the theoretical terrain opened up by reading disability into those queer narratives and feminist analyses that never use the word "disability." How might such readings shift our understandings of terms like "disabled," or "queer," or "feminist"? Or how might they expand our understanding of what it means to do cross-movement work, both in terms of theoretical development and activist practice? *Feminist, Queer, Crip* argues that a coalitional politics requires thinking disability, and disabled bodies, differently—recognizing the work done by disability and able-bodiedness/able-mindedness in different political visions, for example, or acknowledging the exclusions enacted in the desire for a unified disability community.

I know that in carefully delineating my affiliations here—feminist, queer, crip—I run the risk of further reifying these categories, thereby presenting them as discrete, separable identities. This kind of personal and theoretical positioning has long been a mainstay of feminist intersectional scholarship, and, as Puar warns, too easily requires the "stabilizing of identity across space and time."[59] But taking such risks feels necessary because we are operating in a theoretical and activist context in which this combination of analytics and practices too rarely appears. It feels important at this particular moment to identify explicitly as feminist, queer, crip—even as I want to trouble such identifications—and to explicitly practice feminist, queer, crip work. I'm calling attention to these shifting positions not to fix them in place, but to get them moving on the questions that face those of us committed to and invested in such positions.

I'm writing out of a concern, for example, about the silence of disability studies scholars and disability activists in response to how our movements have often (been) publicly aligned with the right. Where were the public feminist/queer/crip responses to Sarah Palin? How might we have intervened in the representation of her as a disability rights advocate, questioning the blurring of antichoice ideologies and disability critiques of prenatal testing? Or how might a feminist/queer/crip–informed analysis expand or complicate queer theoretical texts that rely on a trope of mobility for their analyses or that tend to allegorize rather than analyze disability and disabled bodies? Or, when only a small handful of papers and presentations at the annual Society for Disability Studies conference make explicit use of feminist and queer theories in their analyses, does it not become essential to name and inhabit these very intersections?[60] And, importantly, how can we do this kind of naming, demand these kinds of analytic and political practices, without stabilizing feminist/queer/crip or gender/sexuality/disability, without treating these very categories, nodes, and positions as themselves self-evident? I'm wanting this particular imagining of accessible futures—my imagining of accessible futures—to carve out a place on the theoretical/political map where feminist/queer/crip can feed and inform each other, even as they are always already bound up in each other. More, I'm wanting this imagining to generate more such imaginings, such that the nodes on the map and the map itself multiply, proliferate, regenerate. We need multiple iterations of crip theory, ones that its practitioners might not always recognize, ones that contest and exceed its very parameters, and ones that take this particular iteration to task.

In the hopes of such proliferations, questions take center stage throughout *Feminist, Queer, Crip*. Part of this focus is stylistic, aesthetic; I like the cadence of a question. But it is also, and primarily, methodological. If one of my goals with this project is to get us to think disability differently, to begin to see both the category and the experience of disability as contested and contestable, then what better way to do that then to ask questions? (I've started already.) Rhetorical questions are common in conclusions as authors hint at their next projects, or discover new problems, or point toward the need for more research. I'm including such questions in the introduction as a reminder that I should imagine readers talking back, taking these ideas in new directions, turning my own questions back on me in different contexts or to different effects. The format of the question insists on seeing these complex subjects—the future of the child with Down syndrome or the desirability of disability—as debatable, contestable: as *in question*. It also opens up the possibilities of new answers, shifting answers, unforeseen answers. As I explain in the final chapter, I am interested in a crip politics of access and engagement that is resolutely a work in progress, open-ended, aiming for but never reaching the horizon. Questions keep me focused on the inconclusiveness of my conclusion, of the desire to think otherwise.

This book contains not only unanswered questions but also contradictions and logical inconsistencies. In chapter 3, for example, I am much more critical about dese-lecting disability (i.e., terminating a pregnancy because tests reveal potential "genetic anomalies") than I am about selecting for disability (i.e., using a sperm donor who car-ries a desired genetic trait), even though both practices involve parents wanting to have a child like themselves. Such contradictions are inevitable in a project like this one, reflecting our convoluted approaches to disability; I am writing in a culture in which inconsistency about disability is commonplace. Might it be logically inconsistent, for example, that we claim to value the lives of disabled people even as we create (and man-date) more and more prenatal tests to screen out "undesirable" fetuses? Glossing over these inconsistencies, or pretending that they can be easily and definitively resolved, simplifies the complexities inherent in questions of social justice. The desire for clear answers, free of contradiction and inconsistency, is understandable, but I want to sug-gest that accessible futures require such ambiguities. Following Puar, I believe that "contradictions and discrepancies . . . are not to be reconciled or synthesized but held together in tension. They are less a sign of wavering intellectual commitment than symptoms of the political impossibility to *be on one side or the other*."[61] Indeed, part of the problem I'm tracing in these pages is the assumption that there is only one side to the question of disability and that we're all already on it.

In this spirit, my use of "we" and "they," "them" and "us," shifts throughout this book. To always use the third person in discussing disabled people would be to impose a distancing between myself and my subject that rings false. It also would run coun-ter to this notion of "claiming crip," denying the possibility of a deep and abiding connection to the identities, bodies, minds, and practices discussed here. At the same time, to always use the first person would be to answer in advance the question of a unified community of disabled people, to presume not only that we all share the same positions but also that one person—and in this case, I—can accurately represent the whole. In other words, when it comes to the vexed issue of personal pronouns, I will occasionally use "we/us" even when I am not an obvious member of the group being discussed, and, by the same token, will occasionally use "they/them" even when I am obviously included in the category. I do this to trouble the very notion of "obvious" identifications as well as the disabled/able-bodied and disabled/nondisabled binaries.[62] Even though I am a disabled person, I do not exist apart from the ableist discourses circulating through US society; to act as if my impairments render me immune to, or incapable of, ableist rhetoric and ideology would be to deny the insidiousness of com-pulsory able-bodiedness and able-mindedness.[63] "I," Sedgwick reminds us, can be a powerful heuristic, and so can "we," "they," "you," and "them."[64]

Overview of the Book

Whenever I tell people I have been working on a book about the role of disability in imagined futures, they almost always assume I'm writing about science fiction. I understand their response: science fiction is full of "imagined futures," and disabled characters are common in such novels (even if they aren't referred to as "disabled" within the narratives themselves). I do indeed focus on stories in this book, but they are more the stories we tell ourselves as a culture—disability is a tragedy, children are our future—than the stories of literature or film.

Over the course of the book, I examine uses and representations of disability and able-bodiedness/able-mindedness across a range of sites in the contemporary United States. Given my future focus, and the ways in which the figure of the child often serves as a sign of the future, I pay particular attention to issues of reproduction, even as I work to unpack this elision between reproduction and futurity. Notions of space also play a key role here; disability rights activists have long worked to make more and more spaces accessible to disabled people, describing both flights of stairs and discriminatory hiring practices as barriers to access. As will become clear in the chapters that follow, spaces get imagined differently in different futures; creating accessible futures requires attention to space, both metaphorical and material.

Chapter 1, "Time for Disability Studies and a Future for Crips," extends the theoretical frameworks established in this introduction, focusing primarily on the lenses of time and futurity. I begin to specify what I mean by "crip time," positioning the project of *Feminist, Queer, Crip* alongside other work on queer temporality and critical futurity. Although rhetoric about futures—from warnings of slippery slopes to fears of deformity—pervades current discourses about disability, disability studies has yet to take up crip temporalities and futures as sites of extended analysis. In this chapter, then, I sketch out what is at stake in these frameworks, distinguishing "crip time" from "curative time" and working through what it means to project disability into the future.

The next two chapters focus on the question of medical intervention, addressing the ways in which the "future" is portrayed as a time of cures, genetic and otherwise. The cases under discussion here are characterized by a debate over the appropriate use of technology: technological attempts to eliminate disability are met with widespread praise and support because they are assumed to mark progress toward a better future, while refusals of such "healing" technology are condemned as backward and dystopic. Challenging the rhetoric of naturalness and inevitability that underlies these discussions, I argue that decisions about the future of disability and disabled people are *political* decisions and should be recognized and treated as such. Rather than assume that a "good" future naturally and obviously depends upon the eradication of disability, we must recognize this perspective as colored by histories of ableism and disability oppression. The first part of *Feminist, Queer, Crip* also zeroes in on the assumption that this kind of "elsewhere," one without disability, is one "we" all want. Each of the chapters in this part of the book maps the ways in which disability is removed from debate, taken only as self-evident and given; these chapters unpack what it means to assume that we all want the same things.

In chapter 2, I analyze the case of Ashley X, a young disabled girl "frozen in time" through a growth attenuation regimen, hysterectomy, and bilateral mastectomy. These procedures, known as "the Ashley Treatment," were seen as necessary by her parents and doctors to protect Ashley from future harms. According to this logic, Ashley's body required intervention because her body was growing apart from her mind; physically, her body was developing rapidly, but mentally, her mind was failing to develop at all. As a result, she was embodied asynchrony; her mind and body were out of sync. By arresting the growth of Ashley's body, the Treatment could stop this gap between mind and body from growing any wider. In order to make this argument, Ashley's parents and doctors had to hold her future body—her *imagined* future body—against her, using it as a justification for the Treatment. Adding to the future framing of the case is the fact that both parents and doctors have offered the Treatment as a template for other children; they have expressed the hope that the Treatment will, in the future, become more widespread. The Ashley case, in other words, is shot through with temporal framings of the body/mind, especially the disabled body/mind, and with rhetoric about the future. As this case makes painfully clear, not all disability futures are desirable.

Using a popular example of feminist utopian fiction as an impetus for my continued exploration of cultural attitudes about disability, technology, and cure, chapter 3 begins with a description of Marge Piercy's 1976 novel *Woman on the Edge of Time* and its evocation of a feminist utopia. While Piercy's future is populated by peoples of all skin colors, genders, and sexualities, it is almost completely devoid of people with disabilities: advances in medicine have led to the elimination of most illnesses, and genetic "aberrations" have been eradicated or can easily be corrected. It is a utopia made possible by advances in reproductive technologies, and one frequently featured on women's studies syllabi to discuss feminist futures. Inspired—and troubled—by Piercy's novel, I speculate on the place of disability in the future, questioning whether "utopia," by definition, excludes disability and illness. I focus on the use of reproductive technologies to screen out disability, highlighting the ways in which the expansion of such tests presumes the desire for futures without disability. In this context, parents who refuse such tests or, especially, who use them to select *for* disability, are portrayed as leading the nation down a slippery slope. The 2002 story of Sharon Duchesneau and Candace McCullough, a Deaf lesbian couple who used a deaf sperm donor to conceive their children, anchors my reflection on what it might mean to choose futures of disability.

Chapter 4 maintains a focus on reproduction, but looks more broadly at the reproduction of "community values" and the place of disability in such constructions. In this chapter, I offer a close reading of a widespread public service campaign in the United States, one that has reached billboards, bus shelters, movie theaters, and television stations all over the country. In the years since 9/11, the philanthropic organization Foundation for a Better Life (FBL) has funded a campaign touting "community values" and "character development," arguing that these values will result in a "better life" and future for the United States. Positioning itself as nonpartisan, the FBL's mission is to foster individual and collective betterment through values education and engagement. It is this positioning that I want to examine here: this attempt to depoliticize notions of community, this assumption of shared values, and this articulation of what a better life entails. By presenting these concepts as apolitical, the FBL renders them natural, accepted, common sense, and therefore beyond the scope of debate or discussion. Representations of disability and illness play a large role in this campaign, with a majority of billboards praising individuals with disabilities for having the strength of character to "overcome" their disabilities. The depoliticization mandated by these billboards and the FBL itself is made possible through reference to the disabled body. Indeed, the presence of the disabled body is used to render this campaign not as ideology but as common sense. The billboards seem to promise a future that includes disability—disabled people are a highly visible presence in the campaign—but disability appears here only as the site for personal triumph and overcoming.

In the next section of the book, I turn to two existing frameworks for thinking disability futures: cyborg theory and environmentalism. Both of these bodies of theory have explicitly imagined what a better future might look like, and, in doing so, have relied on tropes of disability, illness, and hyper-ability in their constructions. After making this figuration of ability/disability apparent, I explore the ways in which these same bodies of knowledge can be reimagined from feminist, queer, crip perspectives.

Chapter 5 examines the figure of the cyborg, focusing on its appearance in feminist theories of politics, a use that began with Donna Haraway and continues in the work of theorists such as Malini Johar Schueller, Anne Balsamo, and Jennifer Gonzalez. In her "cyborg manifesto," Haraway positions the cyborg figure as an intervention in feminist theory and politics, using it to critique the reductionist approaches to technology and the exclusionary definitions of "women" that pervaded feminist thought in the 1970s and 1980s. She argues that the cyborg can offer a model for how to do feminist politics, suggesting that the figure can be useful in imagining a feminist "elsewhere." But what is the place of disability in her imagining? Can the cyborg figure offer an effective model for a feminist disability theory and politics? Does it facilitate the articulation and creation of an anti-ableist "elsewhere"? As I argue, cyborg theories, because of their focus on cybertechnologies and human/machine interfaces, tend to represent disability exclusively as an individual, medical problem, a positioning that depoliticizes disability and disabled people. This contemporary understanding of disability, evident in the frequent use of disabled bodies as illustrations of cyborgism, presents a future vision of technological and medical intervention—not social transformation or political action—as the only proper response to disability. However, the practices and identifications of queer disability activists begin to hint at ways of cripping this cyborg legacy.

In a 1991 interview in the *Socialist Review*, Donna Haraway notes that her articulation of the cyborg stems from a commitment to ecofeminism, and theorists from Stacy Alaimo to Catriona Sandilands take Haraway at her word, incorporating the figure into their own ecofeminist theorizing. Following this cyborgian trail, I turn in chapter 6 to the role disability and able-bodiedness play in representations of nature and environmentalism. Ecofeminist visions of the future cannot be reduced to one coherent story: there are many different ecofeminist futures and perhaps even more different ways of imagining ecofeminist politics. Many of these visions, however, are rooted in contemporary ableist assumptions about how bodies look, move, sense, communicate, and think. Environmental conceptualizations of nature tend to assume that everyone accesses nature in the same way, and it is this presumption that colors environmental political visions. Nonnormative approaches to nature and the limitations of the body are erased; able-bodiedness becomes a prerequisite for imagining environmental futures. If disabled people are believed to lack the physical and mental capacities to access and experience nature in the present, then they can play no role in environmental understandings of nature in the future. Drawing on the work of crip artists and writers, I argue that the embodied experience of illness and disability presents alternative ways of understanding ourselves in relation to the environment, understandings which can then expand ecofeminist frameworks and current practices in environmental activism.

Each of these future visions—cyborg theory, environmentalism, and genetic utopianism—is characterized by a normalizing impulse, an impulse that is made apparent when viewed through the lens of disability. Adhering to ideologies of wholeness, cyborg theory attempts to normalize the disabled body through prosthetics and technological intervention, striving to make disabled bodies (appear) whole. Environmentalists often predicate their theories on the experiences of the nondisabled body, normalizing the body itself by marginalizing its limitations, buttressing ideals of hyper-ability and able-bodiedness, and erasing the experiences and insights of disabled people. Finally, genetic discourses frequently advocate genetic testing and selective abortion, normalizing the body/mind by testing disability out of existence.

It is possible, however, to theorize an "elsewhere," to provide a political framework for a more just world that does not rely on a normalizing impulse. Queer theorists are committed to forging a politics that does not marginalize, normalize, or criminalize queer bodies, practices, or desires; feminist theorists are engaged in imagining open-ended politics that do not attempt to normalize all women under a unified category of "woman." Building on these frameworks, disability theorists are actively imagining anti-ableist futures, theorizing what Robert McRuer and Abby Wilkerson call "desirably disabled" worlds that are not founded on the normalization of disabled people.[65] I position my text as part of this queer/feminist/disability project of imagining desirably queer/feminist/disabled worlds. By exposing the ableist assumptions embedded in future visions of genetic and biomedical intervention while simultaneously suggesting ways in which these ableist ideologies can be subverted, I reject the widespread depoliticization of disability.

It is this refusal that fuels, at least in part, my attempt to offer anti-ableist political visions of "elsewhere." Chapter 7, "Accessible Futures, Future Coalitions," represents my attempt to counter this erasure of disability from the political, this tendency to marginalize disabled people in political visions of the future. Building on the insights of feminist and queer theorists, queer disability activists, and disability studies scholars, I sketch the parameters of yet another idea of how to get "elsewhere," but one that welcomes, relishes, and desires disability, one that recognizes disability as political. This crip vision of elsewhere remains, by definition and by design, incomplete. In this final chapter, I explore three potential sites for coalition politics—trans and genderqueer bathroom access, environmental justice, and reproductive rights and justice—in order to develop a crip futurity that finds value in dissent and disagreement, that recognizes loss, that remains open. Using these three sites of possibility, I speculate on how we might extend and challenge the parameters of disability theory and politics, a theory and politics which too rarely engages in serious coalition work with other movements, communities, and inquiries. Reading narratives and movements as crip, even when they do not explicitly mention disability, might lead all of us to begin thinking disability, and disability futures, otherwise.

1 Time for Disability Studies and a Future for Crips

> Queerness should and could be about a desire for another way of being in both the
> world and time, a desire that resists mandates to accept that which is not enough.
>
> —José Esteban Muñoz, *Cruising Utopia*

WHAT WOULD IT mean to explore disability in time or to articulate "crip time"? Temporal categories are already commonly used in formulations of disability; one aspect of cripping time might simply be to map the extent to which we conceptualize disability in temporal terms. The medical field in particular has a long tradition of describing disability in reference to time. "Chronic" fatigue, "intermittent" symptoms, and "constant" pain are each ways of defining illness and disability in and through time; they describe disability in terms of duration. "Frequency," "incidence," "occurrence," "relapse," "remission": these, too, are the time frames of symptoms, illness, and disease. "Prognosis" and "diagnosis" project futures of illness, disability, and recovery. Or take terms such as "acquired," "congenital," and "developmental," each of which is used to demarcate the time or onset of impairment. "Developmental" does double duty, referring both to lifelong conditions, including those that develop or manifest in childhood and adolescence, but also implying a "delay" in development, a detour from the timeline of normative progress.[1]

Temporal frameworks are not limited to the medical field, however. Disability studies and disability movements also draw on discourses of temporality in their framings of disability, often using the same temporal terms mentioned above. Indeed, part of the work of these movements has been to reveal "nondisabled" and "able-bodied" as temporal, and temporary, categories; think here of the "TAB" tag (temporarily able-bodied), intended to remind nondisabled people that the abled/disabled distinction is neither permanent nor impermeable.[2] Disability studies' well-rehearsed mantra—whether by illness, age, or accident, all of us will live with disability at some point in our lives—encapsulates this notion, suggesting that becoming disabled is "only a matter of time." Sharon Snyder, Brenda Brueggemann, and Rosemarie Garland-Thomson call this temporality of inevitability "the fundamental aspect of human embodiment."[3] Of course, disability is more fundamental, more inevitable, for some than others: the work that one does and the places one lives have a huge impact on whether one becomes disabled sooner or later, as do one's race and class positions.[4] Yet these patterns can also be understood in terms of temporality: *frequency, incidence, occurrence.* Familiar categories of illness and disability—congenital and acquired, diagnosis and prognosis, remission and relapse, temporarily able-bodied and "illness, age, or accident"—are temporal; they are orientations in and to time, even though we rarely recognize or discuss them as such, and could be collected under the rubric of "crip time."

Exploring disability in time also includes speculation on temporalities of disability: how might disability affect one's orientation to time? Irv Zola and Carol Gill were perhaps the first disability studies scholars to mention the temporal orientation of "crip time," describing it as an essential component of disability culture and community. Tellingly, neither one of them defined the term but rather focused on its frequent appearance in disability communities; they wrote as if the concept would be already familiar to their readers. For Zola, discussing "the intricacies of crip time" was an important act of political reclamation for disabled people; Gill reports feeling pleasure and surprise at discovering "the common usage and understanding" of crip time among the diverse groups of disabled people she encountered.[5] By locating crip time in disabled people's in-group conversations, Gill and Zola center community-based temporalities, ones which they equate with disability culture and resistance.

Crip time emerges here as a wry reference to the disability-related events that always seem to start late or to the disabled people who never seem to arrive anywhere on time.[6] As one slang dictionary puts it, "crip time" means both "a flexible standard for punctuality" and "the extra time needed to arrive or accomplish something."[7] This need for "extra" time might result from a slower gait, a dependency on attendants (who might themselves be running late), malfunctioning equipment (from wheelchairs to hearing aids), a bus driver who refuses to stop for a disabled passenger, or an ableist encounter with a stranger that throws one off schedule. Operating on crip time, then, might be not only about a slower speed of movement but also about ableist barriers over which one has little to no control; in either case, crip time involves an awareness that disabled people might need more time to accomplish something or to arrive somewhere.[8]

Recognizing some people's need for "more" time is probably the manifestation of crip time most familiar to those of us in the academy. Disabled students (or at least those with approved paperwork) are permitted more time on exams, for example, or granted extended reading periods. But "crip time" means more than this kind of blanket extension; it is, rather, a reorientation to time. As Margaret Price explains, "[A]dhering to crip time . . . might mean recognizing that people will arrive at various intervals, and designing [events] accordingly; and it might also mean recognizing that [people] are processing language at various rates and adjusting the pace of a conversation. It is this notion of *flexibility* (not just 'extra' time)" that matters.[9] Crip time is flex time not just expanded but exploded; it requires reimagining our notions of what can and should happen in time, or recognizing how expectations of "how long things take" are based on very particular minds and bodies. We can then understand the flexibility of crip time as being not only an accommodation to those who need "more" time but also, and perhaps especially, a challenge to normative and normalizing expectations of pace and scheduling. Rather than bend disabled bodies and minds to meet the clock, crip time bends the clock to meet disabled bodies and minds.

How might thinking about time open new perspectives on and for disability studies? Or how might observations on "crip time" lead to more expansive notions of both time and futurity? Questions about time, temporality, and futurity continue to animate queer theory, but this work has yet to have much of an impact in disability studies, and disability studies scholars have rarely been participants in these discussions.[10] In articulating crip temporalities, then, I am calling for a mutual engagement in these discourses: What can disability studies take from queer work on critical futurity and, simultaneously, how might attention to disability expand existing approaches to queer temporality? How might our understandings of queer futurity shift when read through the experiences of disabled people, or when interpreted as part of a critique of compulsory able-bodiedness or able-mindedness? What does it do to queer time to place it alongside crip time, or queer futurity alongside crip futurity? Can we crip queer time?[11]

In offering these questions, my call is not only for disability studies to enter into theoretical discussions about time, temporality, and futurity, but also for us to wrestle with the ways in which "the future" has been deployed in the service of compulsory able-bodiedness and able-mindedness. Ideas about disability and disabled minds/bodies animate many of our collective evocations of the future; in these imaginings, disability too often serves as the agreed-upon limit of our projected futures. This book is about imagining futures and futurity otherwise.

My understanding of crip time and my desire for crip futurity exist in stark contrast to the temporal framing more commonly applied to disability and disabled people, what I call "curative time." I use "curative" rather than "cure" to make clear that I am concerned here with compulsory able-bodiedness/able-mindedness, not with individual sick and disabled people's relationships to particular medical interventions; a desire for a cure is not necessarily an anti-crip or anti-disability rights and justice position. I am speaking here about a *curative imaginary*, an understanding of disability that not only *expects* and *assumes* intervention but also cannot imagine or comprehend anything other than intervention.

Futurity has often been framed in curative terms, a time frame that casts disabled people (as) out of time, or as obstacles to the arc of progress. In our disabled state, we are not part of the dominant narratives of progress, but once rehabilitated, normalized, and hopefully cured, we play a starring role: the sign of progress, the proof of development, the triumph over the mind or body.[12] Within this frame of curative time, then, the only appropriate disabled mind/body is one cured or moving toward cure. Cure, in this context, most obviously signals the elimination of impairment but can also mean normalizing treatments that work to assimilate the disabled mind/body as much as possible. The questions animating a curative temporality include: Were you born that way? How much longer do you have to live this way? How long before they invent a cure? How long will a cure take? How soon before you recover?[13]

In this chapter, I engage in the process of articulating other temporalities, other approaches to futurity beyond curative ones. I do so by speculating on the possibilities of cripping queer time. First, I briefly summarize Lee Edelman's infamous queer polemic against the future. Although my larger project is concerned with how notions of the future have been used against disabled people, I argue that abandoning futurity altogether is not a viable option for crips or crip theory. Second, I read queer temporality through the lens of disability, exploring how illness, disability, and crip time are always already present in queer time. Third, I continue this reading of queer time through disability to pinpoint places where disability seems to exceed queer time. My interest is in how we might use these points of disconnection to expand both queer and crip time. Finally, I close with a few reflections on thinking disability in time. As critics of utopian thinking have long argued, the futures we imagine reveal the biases of the present; it seems entirely possible that imagining different futures and temporalities might help us see, and do, the present differently.

No Future for Crips

Lee Edelman has famously argued that queers and queer theory would be better off refusing the future altogether. ("Fuck the Future," as Carla Freccero puts it.)[14] Building on Lauren Berlant's work on the figure of the child in American politics, Edelman argues that futurity—an investment in and attention to the future or futures—is almost always figured in reproductive terms: we cannot "conceive of a future without the figure of the Child."[15] As a result, the Child serves as "the telos of the social order," the one for whom we all act, "the fantasmatic beneficiary of every political intervention."[16] He offers as an example abortion rhetoric, noting that both pro-choice and antiabortion activists frame their fight as on behalf of the children.[17] Patrick McCreery traces a similar parallel among both opponents and supporters of gay marriage: depending on one's stance, gay marriage either destroys children's well-being or enhances it, but both sides agree that the future of children is what is at stake in the debate and therefore what should guide our decisions.[18] For those in both fights, then, the struggle becomes no longer about rights or justice or desire or autonomy but about the future of "our" children. Both of these examples show the slipperiness of arguments based on the Child and reproductive futurity; one can mobilize the same rhetoric toward mutually opposing goals. What Edelman draws out is the coercive nature of such frames: it is not only that we *can* use the "future of our children" frame but that we *should* or *must* use it; politics itself is and can only be centered around the Child, foreclosing all other possibilities for action.

Reading from a queer crip perspective, I can easily see the ways in which "the future," especially as figured through the "Child," is used to buttress able-bodied/able-minded heteronormativity. First, the proliferation of prenatal testing, much of which presumes that all positive diagnoses will be "solved" through selective abortion, is a clear manifestation of compulsory able-bodiedness and able-mindedness. As we will see in the following chapters, pregnant women with disabilities and pregnant women whose fetuses have tested "positive" for various conditions are understood as threats to the future: they have failed to guarantee a better future by bringing the right kind of Child into the present.[19] Thus the idealization of the Child as the frontier of politics, the framing that troubles Edelman, should concern crip readers as well; discourses of reproduction, generation, and inheritance are shot through with anxiety about disability. These sites of reproductive futurity demand a Child that both resembles the parents and exceeds them; "we" all want "our" children to be more healthy, more active, stronger and smarter than we are, and we are supposed to do everything in our power to make that happen. The Child through whom legacies are passed down is, without doubt, able-bodied/able-minded.

Second, a politics based in futurity leads easily to an ethics of endless deferral. "We're held in thrall by a future continually deferred by time itself," Edelman notes, and this deferment serves to consolidate the status quo.[20] Focusing always on the better future, we divert our attention from the here and now; "We are rendered docile," in other words, "through our unwitting obedience to the future."[21] This phrasing is telling: "held in thrall," "rendered docile," "unwitting obedience"—each phrase signals stagnation and acquiescence, an inability to move in any direction because of a permanently forward-looking gaze. This deferral, this firm focus on the future, is often expressed in terms of cure and rehabilitation, and is thereby bound up in normalizing approaches to the mind/body. Disability activists have long railed against a politics of endless deferral that pours economic and cultural resources into "curing" future disabled people (by preventing them from ever coming into existence) while ignoring the needs and experiences of disabled people in the present.[22] This kind of focus on futurity does disabled people no favors, yet it is one of the most common ways of framing disability: we must cure Jerry's kids now so that there will be no more Jerry's kids in the future. Moreover, everything from sterilization to institutionalization, from bone-lengthening surgeries to growth attenuation, has been justified on the grounds that such acts will lead to better futures for the disabled person and/or for their communities. Within these discourses, disability cannot appear as anything other than failure.

Third, eugenic histories certainly bear the mark of reproductive futurity. Even keeping only to the United States, and only to the past one hundred years or so, examples abound of how concerns about the future of the "race" and the future of the nation (futures often depicted as intertwined) have been wrapped up in fears and anxieties about disability. Tens of thousands of people diagnosed with various "defects" were targeted by eugenic professionals and policies for the first half of the twentieth century, classified, and managed in order to contain the alleged risks they posed to public health. The category of "defectives" included not only people with disabilities but also people from "suspect" racial, ethnic, and religious groups as well as poor people, sexual "delinquents," and immigrants from the "wrong" countries. All were united under flexible concepts of degeneracy, defect, and disability, with "feeble-minded" serving as one of the most effective, and expansive, classifications of all. People placed into one or more of these categories might be tracked by family records offices, institutionalized and segregated from the public, sterilized against their will, barred from entering the country, or, in extreme cases, euthanized. Schools and universities included the study of eugenics in their curriculum, both disseminating and reifying these concepts of degeneration and defect. In many states, sterilization came to be seen as a necessary means of protecting the health of the race and the nation from further degeneration; as Oliver Wendell Holmes asserted in the infamous 1927 *Buck v. Bell* decision upholding Virginia's compulsory sterilization policies, "Three generations of imbeciles are enough."[23] While many overtly eugenic policies began to wane in the 1930s and 1940s, eugenic ideologies and practices did not fully disappear but rather flourished well into the Cold War and beyond.[24]

Virginia's sterilization law was not repealed until 1974, and coerced or forced sterilization of women of color, poor women, indigenous women, and disabled women persisted throughout most of the twentieth century; even today, under certain circumstances, disabled people can be sterilized without their consent, and poor women, immigrant women, and women of color continue to have their reproductive futures curtailed by the courts and the legislature.[25] Institutionalization remains a common response to disabled people, particularly those with "severe" disabilities; despite the Supreme Court's 1999 decision in *Olmstead*, which affirmed the right of disabled people to live in their home communities, many states continue to prioritize funding for institutions over funding community-based care.[26] State governments across the country are responding to budget crises with cuts to health care and disability services, especially in-home attendant care; given that many disabled people require such services in order to live independently, disability rights activists and health advocates note that even more disabled people, especially disabled people of color and low-income disabled people, are being forced into nursing homes or out onto the street. These trends do not bode well for the futures of disabled people, even as they are touted as necessary for preserving the future health of the state and the nation.

Indeed, at one time or another, each of these practices—sterilization, segregation, exclusion, institutionalization—has been justified by concerns about "the future" and particularly future children. For example, Mary Storer Kostir, an assistant at the Ohio Bureau of Juvenile Research, argued in a 1916 publication that *"physically rigorous but mentally feeble persons are a social menace.* . . . Their children threaten to *overwhelm the civilization of the future.* . . . [We] must also consider our children, and *not burden the future with an incubus of mental deficiency."*[27] In making her case for segregating those labeled "feeble-minded," Kostir weighs the futures of "our" children against those other children, the ones who are mentally deficient, threatening, and burdensome. A 1933 pamphlet by the Human Betterment Foundation similarly warns against the "burden" of "feeble-minded" children, noting that the failure to practice "eugenic sterilization" produces effects that are "disastrous . . . in future generations."[28] In these kinds of eugenic discourses, children serve as the sign of the future; the kind of future that awaits us will be determined by the kind of children we bear. Illness, "defect," "deviance," and disability are positioned as fundamentally damaging to the fabric of the community: polluting the gene pool, or weakening the nation, or destroying a family's quality of life, or draining public services (or, often, some combination of the four). To put it bluntly, disabled people were—and often are—figured as threats to futurity.

Whole books have been written about each of these practices, and this brief, sweeping history cannot begin to do justice to the material or, especially, to the bodies invoked by this material. Such broad summaries all too easily erase differences among people with disabilities, differences not only of race, class, sexuality, gender, and history but also of impairment; there are many bodies falling through the cracks of this overview. And yet, it is imperative to establish a pattern, to demonstrate that we have long felt and acted on the belief that disability destroys the future, or that a future with disability must be avoided at all costs. It is this pattern, these histories, that makes the question of the future so vexed. I can see clearly how futurity has been the cause of much violence against disabled people, such that "fuck the future" can seem the only viable crip response.

And yet, these very histories ultimately make such a refusal untenable, and it is here that I part ways with Edelman. I do not think the only response to no future—or, rather, to futures that depend upon no futures for crips—is a refusal of the future altogether. Indeed, "fucking the future," at least in Edelman's terms, takes on a different valence for those who are *not* supported in their desires to project themselves (and their children) into the future in the first place.[29] Edelman acknowledges that "the image of the Child [is] not to be confused with the lived experiences of any historical children," and his imperative to reject the future is therefore not so much about the futures of actual children as about "the whole network of Symbolic relations and the future that serves as its prop."[30] I am, then, writing in a different register, and somewhat simplifying Edelman's argument in the process. Yet, at the same time, Edelman's warnings of reproductive futurism, of idealizing the child, read quite differently when they *are* read alongside "the lived experiences of . . . historical children." As Heather Love urges, "What one wants more of . . . are things that *No Future* excludes from the start: an account of the relation between the idealization of children and their actual treatment in the world."[31] José Esteban Muñoz offers the kind of accounting we need here, noting that the futures of some children are neither protected nor fetishized: "Racialized kids, queer kids, are not the sovereign princes of futurity. Although Edelman does indicate that the future of the child as futurity is different from the future of actual children, his framing nonetheless accepts and reproduces this monolithic figure of the child that is indeed always already white."[32]

This always already whiteness is a whiteness framed by and understood through regimes of health and hygiene; health and hygiene have long served as "potent symbolic marker[s] of racial difference" in terms of both immigration policies and conceptualizations of disability and illness.[33] Anna Stubblefield details, for example, the ways in which the label of "feeble-mindedness" worked in the early twentieth century to signify a whiteness "tainted" by poverty and ethnicity; "[T]he racialized understanding of cognitive ability was used to signify not only the difference between white and nonwhite people but also the difference between pure and tainted whites." Whiteness, in other words, depended on the linkage of race, class, and disability for meaning.[34] Citizenship has been similarly policed; Sarah Horton and Judith C. Barker offer the example of oral health campaigns targeted toward Mexican immigrant families in the early 2000s, with the children's poor dental health cast as evidence of the parents' "'unfitness' for inclusion in the body politic."[35]

Queer kids, kids of color, street kids—all of the kids cast out of reproductive futurism—have been and continue to be framed as sick, as pathological, as contagious. The histories of eugenic segregation and sterilization I mention above offer multiple examples of this conflation of race, class, and disability; so, too, does Daniel Patrick Moynihan's infamous 1965 report *The Negro Family: The Case for National Action*. In it, he warns that "most Negro youth are in danger of being caught up in the tangle of pathology that affects their world, and probably a majority are so entrapped." They are "entrapped," explains Moynihan, because this "pathology" is endemic to black families; the black family is always already sick.[36] We can locate a more recent example of the linkages among race, class, and illness in the 2009 finding that doctors are four times more likely to prescribe antipsychotic drugs to children on Medicaid than children on private insurance; children on Medicaid are also far more likely to be prescribed such medications for "less severe conditions" than other children. As Dorothy Roberts notes, such differential treatment suggests the persistence of stereotypes about the mental health and behavioral stability of poor children and children of color.[37] I offer these examples not to make the case that racism and classism are really ableism, or that what Muñoz is *really* talking about is disability, as if everything collapses into disability; rather, I want to insist that these categories are constituted through and by each other. The always already white Child is also always already healthy and nondisabled; disabled children are not part of this privileged imaginary except as the abject other.

In highlighting this abjection, I am not simply arguing for an expansion of the privileged imaginary to include disabled children; as Robert McRuer makes clear, the crip call is not to become normate.[38] On the contrary, I want to interrupt this privileged imaginary by making apparent its assumptions; echoing Love's desire for a careful accounting of real children's lives, I call for critical maps of the practices and ideologies that effectively cast disabled people out of time and out of our futures. Let us return, then, to some of the terms with which I began this exploration of crip futures and temporalities: "frequency," "incidence," "occurrence." Jasbir Puar argues that the task at hand is not to repudiate reproductive futurities but to trace "how the biopolitics of regenerative capacity already demarcate racialized and sexualized statistical population aggregates as those in decay, destined for no future, based not on whether they can or cannot reproduce children but on what capacities they can and cannot regenerate."[39] She speaks, then, not only of disability futurity but of futures of disability: how are incidents of illness and disability inextricably bound, and differentially bound, to race/class/gender/nation?

Noam Ostrander's interviews with young black men in Chicago, each with violently acquired spinal cord injuries, are a useful illustration of these concerns. Several of these men describe being treated as if their current disablement were a foregone conclusion; people act as if they had always expected to find disability in these men's futures because of their gender, race, and class: of course you're in a wheelchair, what other futures could you possibly expect? As Isaac explains, "'[B]ecause I'm black, I'm supposed to get in trouble—stuff like this is supposed to happen . . . I'm supposed to be dead in jail or in a chair. Some people look at it like that and that kinda bothers me. Just because I'm an African-American that means what? . . . This is how our lives is?'"[40] The statistical likelihood that young, black men living in particular Chicago neighborhoods will be paralyzed (if not killed) by gunshot wounds serves to push them out of time, facing a future of no future, and a no future best embodied by a wheelchair. Disability, in other words, becomes the future of no future, with "dead in jail or in a chair" recognized as all the same, all signs of no future. In more mainstream, sentimental accounts of disability (i.e., those not featuring poor people of color living in "bad" neighborhoods), disability is what ends one's future; it is the familiar narrative of disability as tragedy and loss. But for the men Ostrander profiles, disability is the sign that one never had a future in the first place; loss is not the defining frame because there was nothing to "lose."

This assumption is laid bare in the results of a 2008 study of Medicare claims that describes the impact of race and region on health care. Researchers found, for example, that "blacks with diabetes or vascular disease are nearly five times more likely than whites to have a leg amputated"; an earlier study found similar racial disparities in medical responses to prostate cancer, with black men more likely than whites to have their testicles removed as part of treatment.[41] These differences are due in no small part to the larger disparities in our health care system; black people likely face more drastic treatments because their diagnoses come later and/or because they lack regular access to the high-quality care needed to manage chronic illnesses successfully. But whether we look at the end result—higher rates of amputation and thus of disability—or at the process—unequal access to care—it is hard to deny that some futures (and some bodies) are more protected than others.

The task, then, is not so much to refuse the future as to imagine disability and disability futures otherwise, as part of other, alternate temporalities that do not cast disabled people out of time, as the sign of the future of no future. It is to do the work Love, Muñoz, and Puar call for, and to do it with attention to how different populations are demarcated differently. The questions that then hang around us, that require sustained attention from queer disability scholars, would be the very ones raised by these queer theorists: How does the Child differ from historical children? How do some kids become the "sovereign princes of futurity" while others don't (or perhaps *because* others don't)?[42] Pursuing these kinds of questions makes clear that some populations are already marked as having no future, as destined for decay, as always already disabled.

Queer Time, Crip Time

One could argue that queer time *is* crip time, and that it has been all along. Queer time is often defined through or in reference to illness and disability, suggesting that it is illness and disability that render time "queer." Not only might they cause time to slow, or to be experienced in quick bursts, they can lead to feelings of asynchrony or temporal dissonance; depression and mania are often experienced through time shifts, and people with various impairments move or think at a slower (or faster) pace than culturally expected. These shifts in timing and pacing can of necessity and by design lead to departures from "straight" time, whether straight time means a firm delineation between past/present/future or an expectation of a linear development from dependent childhood to independent reproductive adulthood. Glimpses of these possibilities can be seen in recent queer theory. Elizabeth Freeman, for example, begins the "Queer Temporalities" issue of *GLQ* with a hint that illness and disability might be catalysts to thinking time differently, or *queerly*; riffing on Shakespeare's "the time is out of joint," she links this description of "skeletal dislocation" to a queer asynchrony, an experience of time in, on, and across the body. Imagining time as "out of joint" allows the possibility that time's "heterogeneity can be felt in the bones," that time "*is*" a body.[43] Just as quickly as she names this dislocation or disability, however, she moves away from it, focusing only on queer temporalities "beyond somatic changes like puberty, aging, or illness."[44] What happens, though, if we do not move "beyond somatic changes" but think about queer/crip temporalities *through* such changes, through these kinds of skeletal dislocations, or illness, or disease?

In an attempt to begin that kind of inquiry, I use this section to trace potential links and overlaps between queer temporalities and what we can call "crip time." I focus primarily but not exclusively on Judith Halberstam, not only because she has written extensively on the possibilities of queer temporalities but also because her work so clearly approaches the terrain of disability studies (even though she has yet to mark that closeness).[45] If queerness is, in Freeman's terms, "a set of possibilities produced out of temporal and historical difference," and thus a kind of temporality (or temporalities), then thinking through queer disability requires thinking about crip temporalities.[46] I am particularly interested in highlighting the work of illness and disability in articulations of queer time, drawing out the ways in which queer theorists deploy ideas of illness or disability to define queer time. Although I argue that disability categories are already at work in queer temporalities, I think there is more to be done in terms of tracing or creating connections, and I begin some of that work here, using queer temporalities to read disability experiences and reading crip temporalities as resembling queer time.

For Halberstam, queers are queer not only because of their objects of desire but also because they do too much of the wrong thing at the wrong time; attending to queer temporalities enables us to see queerness as "more about a way of life than a way of having sex."[47] She argues that time is foundational in the production of normalcy, such that engaging in particular behaviors at particular moments has become reified as the natural, common-sense course of human development. "Normative narratives of time," in other words, "form the base of nearly every definition of the human in almost all of our modes of understanding, from the professions of psychoanalysis and medicine, to socioeconomic and demographic studies on which every sort of state policy is based, to our understandings of the affective and aesthetic."[48] These normative narratives of time presume a linear development from a dependent childhood to an independent adulthood defined by marriage and reproduction.[49] Halberstam thus focuses most of her attention on how queer subcultures operate outside "the paradigmatic markers of life experience—namely, birth, marriage, reproduction, and death."[50] In articulating queerness through temporality, Halberstam highlights "strange temporalities, imaginative life schedules, and eccentric economic practices."[51] How might we read each of these categories of queer temporality in and through illness and disability?

Let's begin with "strange temporalities": Halberstam introduces her notion of queer time by talking about the early time of the AIDS epidemic, when "[s]ome gay men responded to the threat of AIDS . . . by . . . making community in relation to risk, disease, infection, and death."[52] Although Halberstam does not limit queer time to the time of illness and infection, she describes it as "emerg[ing] from the AIDS crisis," a context that forced gay communities to focus on "the here, the present, the now." That focus, argues Halberstam, pushed gay communities out of more mainstream temporal logics, ones in which the future was not continually diminishing with each death, or each diagnosis, or each symptom.[53] Instead, the queer time of the epidemic deflects attention away from the future altogether, attending only to this moment, finding urgency in the present. By Halberstam's reading, it was living, and dying, with AIDS that pushed (some) gay men out of a normative life course and into queer ruminations on urgency and emergence. Given that Halberstam's iteration of queer temporality stresses illness as much as sex, one could certainly make the argument that the time of the epidemic is both queer and crip time.[54]

Tom Boellstorff offers "the time of coincidence" as another queer temporality, one in which time "falls rather than passes"; he refers here to the coincidence of two cycles of time, as in "May 23rd 'falls' on a Tuesday," finding in this concept of synchrony a way to move beyond strict linear time. It allows for two cycles of time (such as days of the week and numbers of the month) to be running simultaneously yet not perfectly parallel, creating circular moments of coincidence rather than straight (in both senses of the word) lines of forward movement.[55] Is it possible, though, to read more into this notion of "falling" time, a phrasing that suggests a modality more akin to stumbling, tripping, and impaired bodies than walking ones? What is the time of falling, and how might we read disability into this focus on coincidence, on simultaneity? Or how might we read the distinction between falling and passing time as a distinction between falling and passing *in* time?

I am reminded here of Eliza Chandler's meditation on falling on the sidewalk, her exploration of how tripping up her feet leads to tripping up categories of identification and disidentification. Falling on the sidewalk, she explains, becomes a moment of falling into disability; it is the falling that identifies her to others as disabled, plunging her into categories and identifications that trip her up. Falling makes passing impossible, even as she moves from one to the other moment by moment, even as she inhabits one category in her mind at the same time as she inhabits another in the eyes of others. The experience of falling in time leads Chandler to recognize how shame and pride coincide in her body on the sidewalk, a queer awareness of how her body falls into, exceeds, and fails expectations all at the same time.[56] It is, at least in part, this link between falling and failure that renders crip temporalities queer. Notions of failure and excess, and acts of failing to adhere to some societal norms while or by exceeding others, run throughout discussions of queer temporality. Chandler knows that by falling she lives up to expectations about what *disability* does, even as she fails expectations about what the *body* does; failure and success thus coincide in the moment of falling.

We can move from "falling" to "falling ill" as another form of strange temporality. As Freeman herself suggests, living with illness can push time "out of joint," opening up alternative logics and orientations. Anthropologist Sarah Lochlann Jain explores how cancer diagnoses and prognoses interrupt "the idea of a time line and all the usual ways one orients oneself in time—one's age, generation, and stage in the assumed lifespan."[57] Living in "prognosis time" is thus a liminal temporality, a casting out of time; rather than a stable, steady progression through the stages of life, time is arrested, stopped. Paradoxically, even as the very notion of "prognosis" sets up the future as known and knowable, futurity itself becomes tenuous, precarious. But this very precariousness can, as Halberstam finds in AIDS narratives, become an impetus for erotic investment in the present, in one's diagnosed body.

Laura Hershey reports that inadvertently learning the nature of her diagnosis—and, as a result, her prognosis—changed her whole orientation to the world; she was familiar with living with disability, but discovering her prognosis fundamentally altered her relationship to futurity, even though her body remained unchanged. Sitting alone at school, she ran across the definition of muscular dystrophy in the dictionary: "A genetic disorder in which the body's muscles weaken and eventually waste away." At that moment, she writes, "All the futures I had imagined for myself were now replaced by this newly-revealed, short future: 'eventually waste away.'"[58] For Hershey, the time of prognosis is a single moment of telling but also an extended, if not indefinite, period of negotiation and identification. During that period, past/present/future become jumbled, inchoate. The present takes on more urgency as the future shrinks; the past becomes a mix of potential causes of one's present illness or a succession of wasted time; the future is marked in increments of treatment and survival even as "the future" becomes more tenuous.[59]

The strange temporality of diagnosis/prognosis seems all the more dislocating, all the more dis- and reorienting, for those falling out of or exceeding diagnostic categories. How might we understand the experiences of those with chronic fatigue and chronic pain, or those with multiple chemical sensitivities (MCS), struggling for years to find a medical professional or social services provider to recognize their impairments? Or the veteran trying again and again to get the government to acknowledge and address the effects of Agent Orange or Iraq War Syndrome or PTSD?[60] "What is the 'time,'" in Christopher Nealon's framing, "of the repeated attempt?"[61] Nealon pushes here for an understanding of queer time that includes the temporal experiences of marginalization and disavowal; how, he wonders, is the repeated experience of being denied recognition an orientation to time?[62] His question reminds me of the stories and images in Rhonda Zwillinger's powerful *The Dispossessed*, a profile of people with MCS who have lived through years of failed attempts to get their condition recognized, years that clearly took a toll; some of those Zwillinger profiled ran out of time, ultimately committing suicide out of frustration and isolation. As Roberta S. puts it, "For the past 16 years I have lived in my car, traveling from place to place looking for a 'safe' place so I can be indoors. I am so worn out I think I will die soon."[63] With these stories in mind, I supplement Jain's "prognosis time" with the time of undiagnosis: the shuttling between specialists, the repeated refusal of care and services, the constant denial of one's experiences, the slow exacerbation of one's symptoms, the years without recognition or diagnosis, the waiting.

Thinking about diagnosis and undiagnosis as strange temporalities opens the door to still other framings of crip time, of illness and disability in and through time. What would constitute a temporality of mania, or depression, or anxiety? If we think of queer time as involving archives of rage and shame, then why not also panic attacks or fatigue? How does depression slow down time, making moments drag for days, or how do panic attacks cause linear time to unravel, making time seem simultaneously to speed up and slam shut, leaving one behind?

"Strange temporalities" could then include the experiences of those with PTSD or MCS who live in a kind of anticipatory time, scanning their days for events or exposures that might trigger a response. Such scans include moving both forward and backward in time while remaining present in this moment: What has caused reactions before? What might cause reactions now? What reactions lie ahead? Writing about MCS, Mel Chen explains, "I now have a strategy of temporally placed imaginations; if my future includes places and people, I pattern-match them to past experiences with chemically similar places and chemically similar people."[64] Surviving with MCS requires an embodied awareness of one's location in space and time, "turning toward . . . or correspondingly away from" other bodies in the desire to survive from this moment into the next.[65] This time of anticipation is itself a kind of queer liminality, living always in anticipation of the moment that has not yet arrived: the rogue fragrance, the invisible gas, the passing smoke. Queer, too, in that it requires, and is born of, an erotic attachment to the surrounding environment. Chen writes poignantly about how this temporality of anticipation and response fosters queer orientations to objects and people; her sofa—familiar, safe—becomes more present, more of a home to her body than the bodies of others, while people—with their unexpected, undesired fragrances and smokes—become foreign, disorienting.[66] Encountering them in real time means being exposed to their chemical pasts (the shampoo they used that morning, the cigarette they smoked after class), which then impact one's immediate future (feeling fatigue, fog, nausea). MCS, then, leads to a strange temporality, one of coincidence and multiplicity. The constantly forward-looking stance, the stance of anticipation, is, of necessity, bound also to the constant glance back. Chen experiences her present body in relation to past exposures, with both determining how future not-yet exposures will play out. The strange temporalities of MCS thus include not only Chen but also those around her, offering glimpses of how our individual choices can affect the temporalities of others; I can unwittingly, unknowingly, cast someone else out of time by my chemical consumption.[67]

And what of Halberstam's "imaginative life schedules"? I think here of those crip families who juggle attendant care, receiving hours for one person but unofficially using them for another. For example, one adult might be "more" disabled in the eyes of the state and therefore qualify for more hours than her lover; once in the home, however, an attendant might do work that benefits the lover, or their children. Or what about the very scheduling of attendant care itself and the ways in which it requires a simultaneous inhabiting of present and future? Harriet McBryde Johnson explains that working with attendants requires scheduling "in advance each bathroom trip, each bath, each bedtime, each laying out of our food and . . . books, each getting in and out of our chairs."[68] The immediate future then mixes with the present, as Johnson uses this moment to plan the next and the next and the next. On one level, this kind of scheduling is more a difference in degree than in kind to the planning everyone does, regardless of attendant care. At another level, though, it requires a different orientation to one's body, a foregrounding of physical needs—eating and sleeping and shitting— and the ways in which they shape our days. It is a literal projecting of one's body *as a body* into the future even as one inhabits one's body in the present. What orientations to space and time might this embodied dualness allow?

Indeed, this kind of anticipatory scheduling is not limited to working with attendants, but often extends to working with and in one's own mind/body. For those who live with chronic fatigue or pain, for example, the present moment must often be measured against the moment to come: if I go to this talk now, I will be too tired for that class later; if I want to make that show tomorrow night, I need to stay home today.[69] This idea of conserving energy, of anticipating, can be read as queer in that it bucks American ideals of productivity at all costs, of sacrificing one's body for work. In other words, how might we begin to read these practices of self-care not as preserving one's body for productive work but as refusing such regimes in order to make room for pleasure?

"Eccentric economic practices," Halberstam's third category, can then include this kind of refusal of productivity; it might also include the many disabled people who operate on the barter system, trading services and products below the radar of the state. Attendant services, health care, and disability payments often come with strict requirements about how much one can earn and still receive services, an amount that keeps many disabled people hovering near the poverty line. Eccentric economic practices can ease some of the financial pressure while also enabling crips to write or create without putting their health care in jeopardy. We can think here, too, of disabled people who create their own cooperatives and collectives of attendant care, negotiating their own terms apart from the requirements of the state.

Imagining these kinds of practices brings me right back to Halberstam and her articulation of queers as those who

> will and do opt to live outside of reproductive and familial time as well as on the edges of logics of labor and production. By doing so, they also often live outside the logic of capital accumulation: here we could consider ravers, club kids, HIV-positive barebackers, rent boys, sex workers, homeless people, drug dealers, and the unemployed. Perhaps such people could productively be called "queer subjects" in terms of the ways they live (deliberately, accidentally, or of necessity) during the hours when others sleep and in the spaces (physical, metaphysical, and economic) that others have abandoned, and in terms of the ways they might work in the domains that other people assign to privacy and family.[70]

This definition, too, could easily be applied to disability, rendering disabled people "queer subjects." Most immediately we can recognize that disability likely inhabits the categories named here: many disabled people are homeless and unemployed/underemployed; HIV falls under the rubric of illness and disability, as does drug addiction; and disability does not preclude one from being a sex worker (and may, in fact, facilitate it or compel it). Moreover, as I noted above, the mechanisms of state services certainly push one out of the logic of capital accumulation and onto the edges of labor and production.

But we can think, too, of the blurring of boundaries between public and private. How does the use of attendants to assist with dressing and toileting disrupt the binary between private and public? Or what of the disabled people who use paid attendants to assist them with sex, either by positioning them in bed with their partners or by setting up and turning on sex toys? Or what of disabled people who engage in sex with their attendants? Each of these practices involve paid work "in the domains that other people assign to privacy and family," suggesting at the very least productive overlaps between queerness and disability.

Ellen Samuels explores this possibility of crip time as resistant orientation: "Crip time refuses to define itself in terms of either the ideal or the average: Schedules for work, parenting, and the social are thus shaped by individual needs, desires, and abilities, rather than by regimented economic and cultural imperatives."[71] By attending to the individual and the private, Samuels paradoxically indexes the social and the public; to refuse the regimentation of economic imperatives across the terrain of one's body, or one's time, is to reimagine what public time and social relations can look like. "Eccentric economic practices" challenge the normative modalities that define time, such as productivity, accomplishment, and efficiency, and they urge us toward something different.[72]

On Longevity, Lost History, and Futurity

Crip and queer temporalities clearly overlap, but reading them in relation to each other reveals areas of disconnect as well. In this third section, I highlight two ways that disability seems to exceed queer temporalities: first, the oppositional relationship between queer time and longevity; and second, the queer desire for reformulated histories. Early in Halberstam's definition of queer time, on one of the first pages of *In a Queer Time and Place*, she laments that "we create longevity as the most desirable future, applaud the pursuit of long life (under any circumstances), and pathologize modes of living that show little or no concern for longevity."[73] This critique appears again, almost verbatim, in the book's conclusion, thereby bookending Halberstam's depiction of queer time and alternative temporalities.[74] Although she never explicitly explores the notion of longevity in depth, its appearance at defining moments in the text suggests that her understanding of queer time draws its meaning, at least in part, from its opposition to longevity.

At first blush, this claim resonates; challenging the fetishization of longevity seems essential to both queer and crip politics, both queer and crip theory. Halberstam first issues this challenge in her discussion of HIV/AIDS and its effects on gay communities. As we saw earlier, she frames the time of the epidemic as a temporality that refuses futurity, one prompted by gay men who had been forced by death and disease to rethink the cultural focus on living long lives. No longer able to project their young selves far into the future, they were compelled to live for the moment, this moment, in all of its urgency, the future be damned.[75] I hear this call as an equally crip move: we can certainly read "longevity" as a code for both "health" and "stability," two terms disability studies is invested in troubling. I think, for example, of activists such as Hershey, who lived most of their lives knowing that a long life span was not in their future, but saw that fact as a call for love and justice rather than a sign of tragedy or shame. Or, as Robert McRuer argues in his queercrip reading of performance artist Bob Flanagan, "[S]urviving well can paradoxically mean surviving sick"; longevity is not the only rubric that matters.[76] A critique of longevity, then, can be easily articulated through disability studies; the devaluation of disabled bodies is due in no small part to those bodies' failure to adhere to norms of bodies as unchanging, impermeable, long-lasting, and stable.

This is not the only crip reading of this text, however; it bumps up against another possible reading of this passage, one that opposes queer time not only to longevity but to disability. Reading again, "[W]e create longevity as the most desirable future, applaud the pursuit of long life (under any circumstances), and pathologize modes of living that show little or no concern for longevity."[77] What is a crip to do with that troubling parenthetical? The insertion of "(under any circumstances)" seems to signal anxieties about illness, physical and mental degeneration, and disability; I read "under any circumstances" and hear "extraordinary measures," "breathing through a machine," "dependent on others." I read "under any circumstances" and hear "better off dead" and "life not worth living." Halberstam's lack of specificity about what she means by "long life (under any circumstances)" and "longevity" suggests an assumption of shared meaning or common understanding; apparently, we all know which circumstances would render life not-queer.

Halberstam undercuts her own arguments here, allowing culturally embedded fears of age, illness, and disability to dilute her critique. Thinking through disability suggests that at the very least we do *not* value longevity under any circumstances or by any means necessary; we do, indeed, "pathologize modes of living that show little or no concern for longevity," but one such mode of living *is* those bodies/minds who insist on living "under any circumstances." A critique of longevity can begin to feel misplaced in a culture that continually supports cutting services to disabled poor people, and that continues to warehouse disabled people in institutions and nursing homes, two practices that very well may ensure those disabled people do not live long lives.

Halberstam herself recognizes that the "hopeful reinvention of conventional understandings of time," as in her articulation of the time of the epidemic, is more possible for some bodies—and, we might add, some populations—than others.[78] Drawing on the work of Cathy Cohen, she notes, "[S]ome bodies are simply considered 'expendable,' both in mainstream and marginal communities, and the abbreviated life spans of black queers or poor drug users, say, does not inspire . . . metaphysical speculation on curtailed futures, intensified presents, or reformulated histories."[79] In focusing so closely on Halberstam's dismissal of a "concern for longevity" and "long life (under any circumstances)," I am insisting that we see disability—and more importantly, *living* with a disability, or living as disabled—as one of the positions that needs attention here. I argue for a disability studies that sees both "black queers" and "poor drug users" as within its purview, precisely because of their depiction as expendable, so I want to be clear that I am not suggesting a mere substitution of "disabled people" for "black queers or poor drug users" in Halberstam's quote. Rather, reading her queer critique of longevity through the lens of institutionalization—a lens which can encompass "disabled people" right alongside "poor drug users" and "black queers"—has a similar effect: "curtailed futures" sounds a lot less romantic, a lot less queer, when we think through the precise circumstances under which we do, and do not, fetishize longevity.

So, too, can the focus on "reformulated histories." The reimagining of lost pasts, or the conjuring of imagined pasts, animates much recent queer theory on time and futurity. Queer philosopher Shannon Winnubst, for example, urges an imagining of "lost pasts, where meanings and discourses are contested and practices and pleasures are forged."[80] As with critiques of longevity, her call to lost pasts can be deployed provocatively for crip ends. I think, for example, of Georgina Kleege and Brenda Brueggemann writing letters to the dead, not only contesting histories (of Helen Keller and Mabel Hubbard Bell, respectively) and the meanings attributed to them but refusing boundaries of place and time.[81] Writing open letters to the dead can surely be read as a queer crip interruption of the linear time of past/present/future as separate and distinct planes.[82] Kleege inserts herself into Keller's frame, arguing with her, disputing her accounts, imagining alternate endings; in so doing, she contests mainstream sentimental accounts of both Keller and of disabled people more generally, presenting the past (rather than the future) as a viable and necessary site for politics, for rage, and for pleasure. ·

And yet, this reimagining of lost pasts can bleed easily into a normalizing nostalgia; Muñoz warns of the difference between "queer utopian memory" (such as Winnubst's "lost pasts") and the desire for "a nostalgic past that perhaps never was."[83] Thinking through crip temporalities and futurities requires, then, a grappling with nostalgia, a recognition of the powerful role nostalgia plays in approaches to the body. Indeed, fears about longevity "under any circumstances"—fears of disability, in other words—are often bound up in a kind of *compulsory nostalgia* for the lost able mind/body, the nostalgic past mind/body that perhaps never was.

People with "acquired" impairments, for example, are described (and often describe themselves) as if they were multiple, as if there were two of them existing in different but parallel planes, the "before disability" self and the "after disability" self (as if the distinction were always so clear, always so binary). Compulsory nostalgia is at work here, with a cultural expectation that the relation between these two selves is always one of loss, and of loss that moves in only one direction. The "after" self longs for the time "before," but not the other way around; we cannot imagine someone regaining the ability to walk, for example, only to miss the sensation of pushing a wheelchair or moving with crutches. Contrast this nostalgia for the (imagined) nondisabled body with the before-and-after imagery in weight-loss advertisements. As Le'a Kent argues, "The before-and-after scenario both consigns the fat body to an eternal past and makes it bear the full horror of embodiment, situating it as that which must be cast aside for the self to truly come into being."[84] Elena Levy-Navarro extends Kent's argument, describing fat people as "history itself—that is, they are the past that must be dispensed with."[85] Fat bodies and disabled bodies appear in different temporal frames here, but neither is permitted to exist as part of a desired present or desirable future.

This assumption that disability cannot be a desirable location, and that it must always be accompanied by a nostalgia for the lost able mind/body, is what animates "the cure question" so familiar to disabled people: Wouldn't you rather be cured? Wouldn't you like to be as you were before? Wouldn't you prefer to be nondisabled?[86] The repetition of the question, the fact that disabled people are consistently expected to address it, is part of what gives the question its strength, its compulsory and coercive power. It has become inescapable, and the answer is assumed to be self-evident.

Yet, as Susan Wendell explains, such positionings are rarely so straightforward. In the same breath that she wishes for a cure to her chronic fatigue and pain, she notes that a complete return to her "before" state would lead to "dissonance": "I cannot wish that I had never contracted ME [myalgic encephalomyelitis], because it has made me a different person, a person I am glad to be, would not want to have missed being, and could not imagine relinquishing, even if I were 'cured.'"[87] Wendell works to inhabit both the before and the after at once, refusing the bifurcation of her identity into two distinct temporal planes.

But even those who have been disabled since birth are confronted with questions of temporal longing, expected to mourn what they never had. Eli Clare refuses this notion of the lost and longed-for body, this alleged desperation to return: "[F]or me having CP [cerebral palsy] is rather like having blue eyes, red hair, and two arms. I don't know my body any other way."[88] This presumption of loss, one that extends even to people who never "possessed" what they allegedly "lost," is a symptom of the compulsory able-bodiedness/able-mindedness challenged by disability studies scholars and activists. It illustrates the extent to which the nondisabled body/mind is the default position, as if all bodies/minds are purely abled until something happens to them, as if mind/body variation were not a common occurrence. We are expected to take up nostalgic positions toward our former selves, mourning what we have lost and what can now never be.

Thus the lost pasts I mention here—lost able-bodies, lost able-minds—are not queer but hypernormative; they rely on an assumption that all disabled people long for a lost whole, pre-illness, pre-disability body. In this framing, illness and disability can, and should, be left behind; these lost pasts are compulsorily hypernormative in that they are presented as futures disabled people would give anything to inhabit. Past, present, and future each become vexed, fraught: we lost what we had in the past, we exist in a present consumed by nostalgia for that loss, and we face futures far unlike the ones we had previously imagined. The futures we now face are then both unimagined and unimaginable, inconceivable. Compulsory nostalgia figures these futures as futures no one could possibly want; they have always already failed to achieve the ideal normalcy of our (imagined) able-bodied/able-minded pasts. The only culturally acceptable—culturally recognizable—future in this context is a curative one, one that positions a medicalized cure as just around the corner, as arriving any minute now. But this kind of cure-driven future positions people with disabilities in a temporality that cannot exist fully in the present, one where one's life is always on hold, in limbo, waiting for the cure to arrive. Catherine Scott traces a version of this limbo in Christopher Reeve's memoirs, describing them as a "struggle between the longed-for past, the pain-filled present, and the hoped-for future."[89]

Returning to Halberstam's caution that "the abbreviated life spans of black queers or poor drug users ... does not inspire ... metaphysical speculation on curtailed futures, intensified presents, or reformulated histories," how might we respond not by refusing such speculations altogether but by revising them, expanding them?[90] How might the life and times of "black queers or poor drug users" or disabled people lead to temporal understandings quite different from the ones sketched out in *No Future* or *In a Queer Time and Place* or *Feminist, Queer, Crip*, but still quite queer? What is the time of incarceration, an experience known as "doing time," or the time of institutionalization, fates familiar to the two populations Halberstam names here? Both institutionalization and incarceration are defined through overlapping temporal frames: *temporarily* committed, *permanently* placed, *consecutive life* sentences; both raise questions of chronology and development, such as the treatment of juveniles as adults (in prisons) and of young(er) adults as elderly ones (in nursing homes). How then do our/my notions of crip time shift if we/I think not only of institutionalization but also of incarceration as a sign of disability oppression?[91]

Or, returning to Nealon's notion of the "repeated attempt," how do our metaphysical speculations change if we see antiracist interruptions of monolithic whiteness as moments in and of queer time? Or what if I were to take seriously Chen's insistence that "the time of recovery" includes the time it takes to recover from a racist encounter on the street as much the time it takes to recover from a chemical exposure, with both temporalities constitutive of and important to crip time?

These questions are, for me, bound up in questions of analogy and experience, romanticism and metaphor. How can I articulate a queercrip time that does not oppose queerness to longevity yet maintains a critical stance toward hegemonic expectations of (re)productivity? Or, to put it differently, how do I respond to the fact that the theories we deploy, the speculations we engage, play out across different bodies differently?[92]

Future Desires, Present Despair

I have written this book because I desire crip futures: futures that embrace disabled people, futures that imagine disability differently, futures that support multiple ways of being. I use this language of desire deliberately. I know how my heart can catch when I see a body that moves oddly or bears strange scars. I know how my body shifts, leans forward, when I hear someone speak with atypical pauses or phrasing, or when talk turns to illness and disability. Part of what I am describing is a lust born of recognition, a lust to see bodies like my own or like the bodies of friends and lovers, as well as a hope that the other finds such recognition in me.[93] Perhaps most important to this examination of disability futures, it is a desire born largely of absence. We lack such futures in this present, and my desires are practically inconceivable in the public sphere. There is no recognition that one could desire disability, no move to imagine what such desire could look like.[94]

In 1989 Eve Kosofsky Sedgwick lamented the cultural pervasiveness and acceptance of "the wish that gay people *not exist.*" "There are many people in the worlds we inhabit," she explains, "who have a strong interest in the dignified treatment of any gay people who may already happen to exist. But the number of persons or institutions by whom the existence of gay people is treated as a precious desideratum, a needed condition of life, is small." The notion that someone could dispense "advice on how to help your kids turn out gay" is almost inconceivable, but, she warns, oppression will continue until we can both imagine and experience people and institutions doing exactly that.[95] What we desperately need is "a strong, explicit, *erotically invested* affirmation of some people's felt desire or need that there be gay people in the immediate world."[96]

I have avoided the temptation to substitute "disabled" for gay in the preceding quote, partly because I want to avoid any suggestion that Sedgwick's desire is now mere history. There are unfortunately far too many ways in which 2012 does not look that different from 1989. But I also worry about the other dangers of substitutive logics and practices, such as the rhetorical erasure of people inhabiting both locations, of queers with disabilities. More to the point, such easy paralleling fails to tease out the specificities of the queer/disability relationship. Facile parallels or quick substitutions make it more difficult to recognize how queerness continues to be read through the lens of disability, with both queers and crips rendered unnatural, sick, degenerate, and deviant. (This reading seems especially common for people on the trans spectrum or for intersex folks.) I use the quote here because it still feels all too true in 2012, and I, too, long for that kind of embodied investment in queer lives. I use it, too, because I think the inability to value queer lives is related to the inability to imagine disabled lives. Both are failures of the imagination supporting and supported by the drive toward normalcy and normalization. Not wanting to cultivate queerness, or to build institutions supporting that kind of cultivation, is intertwined with fears about cultivating disability. (I have a hard time even typing "cultivating disability" because it is almost impossible to imagine what a just version of that would look like. This book serves as my attempt.)

Thus my desire for crip futures is, as Heather Love puts it, "a hope inseparable from despair."[97] I feel this hope—and the hope has the fierce intensity that it does—because it is birthed out of and coexists with this despair about our impoverished imaginations. What I need is to follow some of these longings out, even if they put me in the realm of fantasy. Changing our imaginations, suggests Judith Butler, allows us to change our situations. Fantasy carries a "critical promise," she argues, "allow[ing] us to imagine ourselves and others otherwise."[98]

This intermingling of recognition and absence, of despair and hope, renders my desire quite queer. Queer in that my want, my longing, my pleasure intensifies with the queerness of these crip bodies, these crip futures. Queer, too, in that in imagining crip futures, I mean more than particular, identifiable bodies. I mean possibility, unpredictability, promise: the promise of recognizing crip where I did not expect to find it, the possibility of watching "crip" change meanings before my eyes. I name this desire "queer" in part because of its ambiguity. Becoming more "visible"—by increasing and publicizing the presence of disabled people in public, perhaps—does not guarantee acceptance or inclusion, especially for those not already privileged by race and class.[99] As feminists from Minnie Bruce Pratt to Bernice Johnson Reagon to Chandra Talpede Mohanty have cautioned, the desire for home, for familiarity, often leads to naïve evocations of community.[100] Thus, in naming and experiencing this desire, I am likely misreading and misrecognizing the bodies and practices of others. I am, in other words, finding both disability and desire where they don't necessarily belong—surely a potentially queer and crip move.

This desire, these imaginings, cannot be separated from the crip pasts behind us or the crip presents surrounding us; indeed, these very pasts and presents are what make articulating a critical crip futurity so essential. To put it bluntly, I, *we*, need to imagine crip futures because disabled people are continually being written out of the future, rendered as the sign of the future no one wants. This erasure is not mere metaphor. Disabled people—particularly those with developmental and psychiatric impairments, those who are poor, gender-deviant, and/or people of color, those who need atypical forms of assistance to survive—have faced sterilization, segregation, and institutionalization; denial of equitable education, health care and social services; violence and abuse; and the withholding of the rights of citizenship. Too many of these practices continue, and each of them has greatly limited, and often literally shortened, the futures of disabled people. It is my loss, our loss, not to take care of, embrace, and desire all of us. We must begin to anticipate presents and to imagine futures that include all of us. We must explore disability in time.

2 At the Same Time, Out of Time

Ashley X

The stories of women with disabilities must be told, not as stories of vulnerability, but as stories of injustice.

—Sherene Razack, "From Pity to Respect"

In thinking about crip futurity, I find myself haunted by Ashley X. Born in 1997, the girl known as Ashley X was diagnosed with "static encephalopathy" a few months after her birth. "In the ensuing years," doctors note, "her development never progressed beyond that of an infant," and her doctors held no hope that her cognitive or neurological baseline would improve.[1] "At the age of 6 years, she [could] not sit up, ambulate, or use language."[2] Concerned about their daughter's long-term future, Ashley's parents met with doctors in 2004 to discuss the potential effects of puberty and physical growth on their ability to care for her at home. Together they crafted a two-pronged plan: "attenuate" Ashley's growth by starting her on a high-dose estrogen regimen; and, prior to the estrogen treatment, remove Ashley's uterus and breast buds in order "to reduce the complications of puberty" and mitigate potential side effects of the estrogen treatment.[3] According to her parents and doctors, these interventions were necessary for Ashley's future quality of life: they would reduce her pain and discomfort (by removing the possibility of her menstruating or developing breasts) and would enable her parents to continue caring for her at home (by keeping her small enough to turn and lift easily). Her parents worried that, without the Treatment, Ashley would become too cumbersome for them to lift safely, and, as a result, her participation in social and recreational activities would decrease dramatically.[4] Ashley's doctors took this concern a step further, expressing fear that caring for her at home might eventually become "untenable" and that Ashley's parents would need to place her "in the hands of strangers."[5]

From the moment this case became public, in late 2006, it has garnered widespread attention. Both Ashley's doctors and Ashley's parents have written extensively about the case, carefully articulating their respective positions on the appropriateness of the Treatment. Bioethicists, disability rights activists, pediatric specialists, parents of disabled children, policy makers, disability studies scholars, legal experts, bloggers, and journalists have joined the fray, debating the ramifications of this case in particular and of growth attenuation/sterilization in general.[6] Critics of the Treatment have condemned the hospital for violating sterilization regulations, challenged the parents' presumption that they know what is best for their daughter, and debated the appropriateness of reshaping children's bodies without their consent. Supporters of the Treatment have stressed the difficulties of parenting severely disabled children, the noble intentions of the parents, and the alleged benefits of growth attenuation and sterilization. Rather than rehash that work here, parsing the legalities of the case or determining the proper decision-making authority or debating the moral permissibility of surgically shaping children, I want to take a different tack, rereading Ashley's case through the lens of time and futurity.

As becomes clear in both parental and medical justifications of the Treatment, the case of Ashley X offers a stark illustration of how disability is often understood as a kind of disruption in the temporal field.[7] Supporters of the Treatment frame Ashley's disability as a kind of temporal disjuncture; not only had she failed to grow and develop "normally," but her mind and body were developing at different speeds from each other. According to this logic, Ashley's body required intervention because her body was growing apart from her mind; physically, her body was developing rapidly, but mentally, her mind was failing to develop at all. As a result, she was embodied asynchrony; her mind and body were out of sync. By arresting the growth of Ashley's body, the Treatment could stop this gap between mind and body from growing any wider. In order to make this argument, Ashley's parents and doctors had to hold her future body—her *imagined* future body—against her, using it as a justification for the Treatment. Without intervention, the asynchrony between mind and body would only grow wider; Ashley's body would become more and more unbearable to her, to her parents, and to those encountering her in public. This future burden, brought on by the future Ashley, could only be avoided by arresting the present Ashley in time. Adding to the future framing of the case is the fact that both parents and doctors have offered the Treatment as a template for other children; they have expressed the hope that the Treatment will, in the future, become more widespread. The Ashley case, in other words, is shot through with temporal framings of the mind/body, especially the disabled mind/body, and with rhetoric about the future.

Before examining the temporal framing of the case, I will first present an overview of the Treatment and its legal aftermath, as well as a summary of how Ashley's parents and doctors explain and justify the Treatment. The bulk of the chapter reads the case through a temporal framing, focusing on the ways in which Ashley was cast, and cast

as, out of time; from the beginning of the case, she has been represented as temporally disjointed, as an eternal child, and as threatened by her future self. In addition,
I explore the gendered dimensions and assumptions of the Treatment, detailing how
Ashley's femaleness, or future femaleness, rendered her atemporality particularly grotesque. As this story makes painfully clear, not all disability futures are desirable; in
other words, the problem is not only the inclusion of disability in our futures but also
the nature of that inclusion. I conclude the chapter, then, with a brief reflection about
how to imagine desirably disabled futures.

A Case History of the Ashley Treatment

Ashley's surgery took place under the direction of Dr. Daniel Gunther in July of 2004,
at Seattle Children's Hospital; the procedure, which was "uneventful," included a hysterectomy, a bilateral mastectomy, and an appendectomy.[8] For the next two and a half
years, Ashley received high doses of estrogen in an attempt to stunt her growth. (Estrogen accelerates the "maturation of the epiphyseal growth plates," which means one's
bone plates fuse quickly, arresting growth).[9] At the conclusion of the estrogen regimen,
Ashley's size was about average for a nine-year-old girl: fifty-three inches tall and sixty-
three pounds. Three years later, in January 2010, her parents reported that her size had
remained virtually unchanged (fifty-three inches tall and sixty-five pounds). X-rays of
her hands revealed that the gaps between her finger bones had fused, indicating that
she had indeed reached her maximum height.[10] By her doctors' and her parents' measure, the Treatment was a success.[11]

For many disabled people and disability activists, however, the Treatment was
nothing to celebrate. As the case became public, disability rights organizations, disability activists, and disability studies scholars spoke out against the hospital's actions,
and the Washington Protection and Advocacy System (WPAS) launched an investigation in January 2007.[12] In May of that year, reviewers from WPAS issued their report
on the case, finding that "[t]he sterilization portion of the 'Ashley Treatment' was conducted in violation of Washington State law, resulting in violation of Ashley's constitu-
tional and common law rights."[13] According to WPAS, the hospital should have sought
a court order before moving forward with the sterilization; state regulations mandate
judicial review prior to the sterilization of patients who do not or cannot consent.

Although the hospital's own ethics committee had noted in regard to the hysterectomy that "there is need for a court review of this aspect of [the] proposal," no such
review took place.[14] Instead, after the ethics committee issued its report, Ashley's parents consulted with attorney Larry Jones about the sterilization. In a June 2004 letter
to Ashley's father, Jones asserts, "It is not necessary to have a court hearing on sterilization when the object of the medical procedure is not sterilization, but to obtain another
medically necessary benefit."[15] Rather, sterilization would be "merely a byproduct of
surgery performed for other compelling medical reasons," namely the prevention of
bleeding associated with estrogen therapy and the cessation of menstruation.[16] Since

sterilization was not the main goal of the Treatment, Jones argued, a court order was unnecessary. Moreover, he explained, the sterilization policies were intended to protect those patients who might develop or regain the capacity to raise children; Ashley would never have the ability to make child-bearing decisions, so there was no need to protect her from the permanence of sterilization.[17] Ashley's father sent the letter to Ashley's doctors, who later told WPAS that they had accepted the letter as a form of "court review" and acted accordingly.[18]

The Washington Protection and Advocacy System disagreed with this logic, arguing not only that the parents' consultation with Jones did not qualify as judicial review, but that his legal opinion "is not supported by a reasonable interpretation of pertinent law."[19] They explained that existing policy clearly required the hospital to safeguard Ashley's interests through a thorough judicial review. Seattle Children's Hospital accepted the findings in the WPAS report, agreeing that they had acted inappropriately in not following their own ethics committee's push for a court review. According to a joint statement signed by both parties in May 2007,

> [Seattle] Children's [Hospital] agrees with the finding in the report that Ashley's sterilization proceeded without a court order in violation of Washington State law, resulting in violation of Ashley's constitutional and common law rights. Children's deeply regrets its failure to assure court review and a court order prior to allowing performance of the sterilization and is dedicated to assuring full compliance with the law in any future case.[20]

Dr. David Fisher, the medical director of Seattle Children's Hospital, issued a statement supporting the WPAS findings, admitting "an internal miscommunication which resulted in a violation of the law" and taking "full responsibility."[21] In their joint statement with WPAS, Seattle Children's Hospital agreed to obtain a court order before permitting growth attenuation or sterilization procedures on other disabled children; they also pledged to develop stronger oversight and monitoring programs over their sterilization practices and policies. Finally, the hospital consented to the addition of a disability rights advocate to their ethics committee.

Although the case of Ashley X is "closed"—WPAS has released their findings; Seattle Children's Hospital has apologized and issued new guidelines per their agreement with WPAS—the Ashley Treatment remains an open question. Ashley's doctors and parents continue to write (separately) about the Treatment, presenting it as a viable course of action for other families. The University of Washington held symposia devoted to the case in 2007 and 2009; in late 2010, the Seattle Growth Attenuation and Ethics Working Group (SWG), an offshoot of the first symposium, published a position paper on growth attenuation.[22] In that report, they argue that "growth attenuation can be morally permissible under specific conditions and after thorough consideration"; one of those conditions is that the patient be neither ambulatory nor communicative.[23] Although most of the twenty-person group were able to agree to this compromise position, two participants wrote brief dissents, spelling out continued points of disagreement among some members.[24] These points of dissension, combined with the report's call for additional research, suggest that more debates and reports lie ahead.

Documenting the Ashley Treatment

The details of the Ashley Treatment became public almost two and a half years after her surgery. In October 2006, two doctors centrally involved in the case—Dr. Daniel Gunther, a pediatric endocrinologist, and Dr. Douglas Diekema, a pediatric bioethicist—published the results of the growth attenuation therapy in the *Archives of Pediatric and Adolescent Medicine*. Several months later, Ashley's parents launched a blog called *The "Ashley Treatment": Towards a Better Quality of Life for "Pillow Angels."* As these titles suggest, both texts took a future-oriented approach; they presented the Ashley Treatment as a new tool in the care of disabled children, one that other parents and doctors might choose to replicate. Before addressing this future-orientation, or analyzing the rhetoric deployed in each text, I first offer a brief summary of each document.

In their initial article, which focused primarily on the growth attenuation therapy, Gunther and Diekema argue that Ashley will benefit both physically and emotionally from her smaller size:

> A child who is easier to move will in all likelihood be moved more frequently. Being easier to move means more stimulation, fewer medical complications, and more social interaction. Personal contact between parent and child is likely to be more direct and personal without the need for hoisting apparatus or other devices. Being easier to move and transfer also makes it more likely that the child will be included in family activities and family outings.[25]

Gunther and Diekema frame the growth attenuation therapy as essential to Ashley's future quality of life; without it, they claim, her parents would eventually be unable to care for her at home or to include her in family events.

Gunther and Diekema's article is as interesting for what it excludes as for what it includes. While the WPAS report stressed the hysterectomy, discussing it at length, the two doctors limit discussion of the procedure and its ramifications to a single paragraph. "A word here about hysterectomy is probably appropriate," they concede, casting discussion about the hysterectomy—and, by extension, the hysterectomy itself—as a mere side issue to the more important topic of growth attenuation.[26] The hysterectomy is apparently so trivial, or so incidental, as not to merit extensive analysis on its own; they do not even use the word "sterilization" in regard to Ashley, thereby avoiding that conversation altogether. In downplaying the hysterectomy, Gunther and Diekema echo the stance of attorney Larry Jones: as Jones argued in his letter to the family, the hysterectomy and resultant sterilization were only byproducts of treatment done for other reasons. The hysterectomy was performed not in order to sterilize Ashley but to mitigate the risks of uterine bleeding (a side effect of the estrogen regimen) and the anxiety and discomfort of menstruation. Since Ashley would never develop the ability to raise children, preserving her reproductive health was not an issue; she had no need of her uterus, so there was no need to discuss it.

Effectively rendering Ashley's breasts as even more expendable than her uterus, Gunther and Diekema do not mention the bilateral mastectomy at all—nor does Diekema in an interview with CNN a few months later.[27] When eventually pressed about this silence, Gunther and Diekema argue that the mastectomy was irrelevant to growth attenuation and high-dose estrogen therapy; there was nothing to discuss.[28] Although Diekema has addressed the mastectomy in more recent articles, he seems to do so only in response to criticism, not because he sees the mastectomy as anything meriting attention in and of itself.[29]

Ashley's parents, however, understand the mastectomy differently, representing it on their blog as an essential component of "the Ashley Treatment"; for them, the hysterectomy, mastectomy, and estrogen regimen are all of a piece. The mastectomy, or, to use their language, "breast bud removal," was necessary for three reasons.[30] The primary reason for the "removal" was that any breast development was likely to cause Ashley pain and discomfort. Breasts would make lying down unpleasant for Ashley ("large breasts are uncomfortable lying down with a bra and even less comfortable without a bra") and would "impede securing Ashley in her wheelchair, stander, or bath chair, where straps across her chest are needed to support her body weight."[31] Those straps would then compress Ashley's breasts, causing further pain and confusion. Buttressing this rationale for the procedure were two "additional and incidental benefits": the bilateral mastectomy would eliminate the possibility of breast cancer or fibrocystic growth, two conditions present in the family; it would also prevent Ashley from being inappropriately "sexualized." According to Ashley's parents, the mastectomy "posed the biggest challenge to Ashley's doctors, and to the ethics committee," but the parents ultimately convinced them of the benefits of the procedure.[32]

Ashley's parents launched their blog on January 2, 2007, not long after Ashley completed her estrogen regimen, and it was this text that generated worldwide attention. Such attention seemed to be the parents' goal, as they started the blog "for two purposes: first, to help families who might bring similar benefits to their bedridden Pillow Angels; second, to address some misconceptions about the treatment and our motives for undertaking it."[33] The blog covers much of the same terrain as Gunther and Diekema's article, although more informally; it discusses Ashley's medical history and diagnosis, the details of the Treatment, and a point-by-point justification for the procedures. These pieces are supplemented by family photographs of Ashley (with her parents' and siblings' faces blurred for privacy), "testimonies" from other parents of "pillow angels," letters of support, and excerpts from sympathetic editorials and commentaries.[34] The blog also offers definitions for two key terms that did not appear in the original article by Gunther and Diekema: "the Ashley Treatment" and "Pillow Angel." "The Ashley Treatment" refers to the combination of growth-attenuating estrogen regimen, hysterectomy, and "breast bud removal," while "Pillow Angel" signifies people with a cognitive and mental developmental level that will never exceed that of a 6–month old child as well as associated extreme physical limitations, so they will never be able to walk or talk or in some cases even hold up their head or change position in bed. Pillow Angels are entirely dependent on their caregivers.[35]

Given the intent of the blog, it is not surprising that Ashley's parents see the Treatment as an unmitigated success. As they told CNN in 2008, "Ashley did not grow in height or weight in the last year, she will always be flat-chested, and she will never suffer any menstrual pain, cramps, or bleeding."[36]

Out of Line, Out of Time

Always flat-chested, never menstruating, finished growing: for Ashley's parents, the Treatment was undeniably about arresting Ashley's development so that they might continue to lift and carry her without difficulty. Mention of Ashley's flat chest and hysterectomy, however, suggests that more than weight was at stake in their decision. They were also concerned about the developmental disjuncture taking place as her body, which was developing more typically, grew further away from her mind, which "stopped growing . . . when she was a few months old." They understood Ashley's body as en route to "adulthood," even though her mind was permanently mired in "child-hood," and this disconnect required intervention. Doctors and bioethicists following the case echoed this concern; the Treatment was necessary to keep Ashley's cognitive self and physical self aligned. The Ashley Treatment thus enacted a circular temporal logic: Ashley's disabilities rendered her out of time, asynchronous, because of this developmental gap between mind and body; her development needed to be arrested to correct this mind/body misalignment; this arrested development then cast her further out of time, more befitting her permanent cognitive infancy.

From the beginning, the Treatment was described as a way to correct the disjuncture between Ashley's body and mind. "When you see Ashley," Dr. Diekema tells CNN, "it's like seeing a baby in a much larger body."[37] Without the Treatment, this disjuncture would only become more pronounced, as Ashley would eventually become not only a baby in a much larger body, but a baby in an *adult*'s body. What was needed, as her parents put it, was to bring Ashley's "physical self closer to [her] cognitive self."[38] As John Jordan argues, "Despite her otherwise healthy prognosis, Ashley's body had to be articulated as 'wrong' in such a way that the Treatment could be recognized as the best way to make her 'right.'"[39] This "wrongness" was framed in terms of a temporal and developmental misalignment between mind and body, "the brain of a 6–month-old" in the body of one much older; to the extent possible, the Treatment corrects that disjuncture.[40]

In this desire for mind and body to align, what we see is a temporal framing of disability dovetailing with a developmental model of childhood. In classical child development theory, children move through a defined sequence of stages toward adulthood, a one-way and linear march "upward." Children can be seen in this framework as "unfinished" adults, or as people who have yet to move through the necessary stages of growth and development.[41] What this understanding of childhood often means is that disabled people, particularly those with intellectual disabilities (or "developmental" disabilities, as they are often known), are also cast as "unfinished" adults. Diekema's description of Ashley as a "baby in a much larger body" reflects an extension of this logic: regardless of how old Ashley is chronologically, she will always be a "baby" developmentally. (Similar logics are at work when Jerry Lewis refers to adults with multiple dystrophy as "kids" or when Christopher Reeve describes paralysis as having "suddenly transformed [him] into a forty-two-year-old infant."[42] Reeve aligns physical dependence with infancy, and Lewis frames disability as inherently infantilizing.)

The linkage of intellectual disabilities with childhood has a long history. Licia Carlson, explaining that people classified as "idiots" in the late nineteenth and early twentieth centuries were seen as "remain[ing] at an early stage of development," notes that superintendents of state institutions often referred to their wards as "man-baby," "woman-baby," and "child-baby."[43] Within this framework, there is no room for the adult with intellectual disabilities; if adulthood is about independence, autonomy, and productivity, then adulthood becomes both unachievable and inconceivable in relation to profound intellectual impairment like Ashley's.

In their initial defense of the Treatment, Gunther and Diekema stress that Ashley faces a future of no future: she is "an individual who will never be capable of holding a job, establishing a romantic relationship, or interacting as an adult."[44] Within the logics of normative time, adults work, marry, and live independently; but according to Gunther and Diekema, disability renders too many of such practices impossible. As a result, the interventions can do no harm; she is already prohibited by her disabilities from having romantic relationships (or children), so her breasts and uterus are easily removed.

Notice, too, in their description the conflation of adulthood with productivity; interacting as an adult is paralleled with holding a job. Disability, then, is defined as a lack of productivity; in a move that brings the word closer to its roots, being disabled means being unable to work. Bioethicist Norman Fost makes plain this perspective in his summary of the case: "It [the Ashley case] reminds [me] of the scandal some years ago when it was discovered that some Cadillacs had Chevrolet engines."[45] In positioning Ashley as "a Cadillac with a Chevrolet engine," Fost not only references the "deceptive" nature of her imagined future appearance—a child in an adult's body—but reveals the degree to which we view normal adulthood as a time of, and as defined by, productivity. We are all to be smoothly running engines, and disability renders us defective products. Ashley does not merit the protections offered adults or other children because she will never be an adult.

The term "pillow angel" both reflects and perpetuates this linking of disability with infancy and childhood. Ashley's parents explain that they "call her our Pillow Angel since she is so sweet and stays right where we place her—usually on a pillow."[46]

This phrasing paints a picture of infant-like dependency and passivity; it makes it difficult to imagine Ashley as a teenager or a woman-to-be. Thus, much as the estrogen therapy and mastectomy make Ashley look like the permanent child she allegedly is, the "pillow angel" label names her as such. Within this schema, her body, mind, and identity all line up perfectly.

Such alignment is necessary not only to ensure that people treat Ashley "in ways that are more appropriate to [her] developmental age," but also to protect those around her from disruptions in their temporal fields.[47] Dr. Norman Fost, a bioethicist who has often written about the case, echoes Diekema's concerns about the problem of mind/body misalignment:

> [H]aving her size be more appropriate to her developmental level will make her less of a "freak." . . . I have long thought that part of the discomfort we feel in looking at profoundly retarded adults is the aesthetic disconnect between their developmental status and their bodies. There is nothing repulsive about a 2 month old infant, despite its limited cognitive, motor, and social skills. But when the 2 month baby is put into a 20 year old body, the disconnect is jarring.[48]

In invoking the image of an adult body with a baby's brain, and assuming such an image prompts repulsion, Fost enters the realm of the grotesque. He positions Ashley as the embodiment of category confusion, of "matter out of place"; the imagined Ashley blurs infancy and adulthood together, troubling cultural understandings of the normative life course.[49] We are to imagine an adult that looks like "us" but can never function or think like us, and this collision of sameness and difference makes us uncomfortable. George Dvorsky, another bioethicist commenting on the case, makes explicit this link to the grotesque. Writing in support of the Treatment, he too praises its ability to "endow her with a body that more closely matches her cognitive state—both in terms of her physical size and bodily functioning." He then goes on to argue that the "estrogen treatment is not what is grotesque here. Rather, it is the prospect of having a full-grown and fertile woman endowed with the mind of a baby."[50] The disjuncture between mind and body is apparently all the more jarring, all the more *grotesque*, because of Ashley's gender. Within this framework, Ashley's imagined future body is held against her present body and deemed excessive and inappropriate: too tall, too big-breasted, too fertile, too sexual, too *adult* for her true baby nature. The Treatment was thus necessary to prevent this imagined big and breasty body—this grotesque, fertile body—from coming into being. Dvorsky makes clear the unspoken reason why the growth attenuation had to be combined with a hysterectomy; without the latter, Ashley would remain grotesquely fertile.

The definitions that Ashley's parents provide on their blog reveal their own anxieties about the too-big, too-fertile body to come: they describe the hysterectomy as the "removal of *tiny* uterus" and the mastectomy as "breast bud removal: removal of *almond sized* glands."[51] Both procedures must be done quickly, they argue, before "rapid growth of breasts and uterus" begins.[52] Of course, any such "rapid growth" would be caused, at least in part, by the estrogen regimen itself, but the rhetoric has the effect of depicting Ashley's body as out-of-control; it is as if the imagined future Ashley, with her large breasts and uterus, is going to take over, to *consume*, the angelic pillow angel with her "almond sized breast buds." The Treatment is positioned as a cure for adult womanhood as much as adult disability.

Feminists have long challenged the reduction of women to their reproductive capacities, and the case of Ashley X reveals how disability both complicates and enables that reduction. On the one hand, despite the surgical focus on her reproductive organs, Ashley is understood to be completely removed from the realm of reproduction. What makes the bilateral mastectomy and hysterectomy permissible is the underlying conviction that Ashley will never need or use her breasts and uterus. Her parents explain that the only reason to forgo the "breast-bud removal" is if child-bearing and breastfeeding are in Ashley's future; since they are not, her breasts can be removed without any problem.[53] They present the hysterectomy in similar terms. In their diagram describing the treatment, the hysterectomy is placed next to the appendectomy, suggesting that for Ashley, her uterus is an appendix: useless, unnecessary, and expendable.[54] Thus, Ashley's disabilities prevent her from being reduced to her reproductive organs; unlike nondisabled women, she is not to be understood in those terms.

At the same time, however, the Treatment reveals the extent to which the female body is always and only framed as reproductive. Dvorsky's anxieties about Ashley's fertility suggest that disability only renders such fertility more threatening, more in need of containment and intervention. Furthermore, her parents' presentation of her breasts and uterus as irrelevant and unnecessary testifies to the persistence of a reproductive use-value understanding of female bodies. The only purpose of these body parts is reproductive; if reproduction is not in one's future, then these parts can be shed without ethical concern. The centrality of reproductive frameworks to our understanding of what constitutes a woman or a female is what made the mastectomy and hysterectomy possible or imaginable. Ashley's breasts and uterus were never going to serve their real purpose, so they could be dismissed.

Indeed, a dismissive attitude toward mastectomy and hysterectomy pervades Gunther and Diekema's original article. Their approach makes sense, in that to focus on the hysterectomy *qua* hysterectomy might prompt questions about state sterilization protections. But their discussion of the procedure makes clear that they had no real concerns about it; sterilizing someone like Ashley takes on the appearance of common sense. Indeed, they acknowledge concerns about forced sterilization only to brush them away:

> Hysterectomy in children, particularly in the disabled, is controversial and invariably associated with the negative connotations and history of forced "sterilization." But in these profoundly impaired children, with no realistic reproductive aspirations, prophylactic hysterectomy has several advantages as an adjunct to high-dose estrogen treatment.[55]

Placing "sterilization" in scare quotes suggests that Gunther and Diekema do not see it as a real concern, almost as if it were not an accurate description of a hysterectomy. The history of forced sterilization apparently has no bearing on cases of such profound impairment. Nor, apparently, do feminist critiques of sterilization, as the procedure is completely degendered in this passage. They describe hysterectomy in *children*, as if boys also have hysterectomies, as if there were no gendered dimension to such procedures.[56] Or, perhaps, the use of "children" is an indication that Diekema and Gunther do not recognize disabled children as gendered at all; they cannot be boys or girls because both categories presume an able-bodied/able-minded norm. The Treatment is thus a surgical manifestation of the conceptualization of Ashley as a permanent child. As a child, Ashley has no need of reproductive organs; as a disabled person, she has no sexuality. Maintaining her small size and keeping her flat-chested and infertile ensures that her physical appearance matches her cognitive functioning, and that both reflect the lack of sexuality befitting a disabled person/baby.

At first blush, it makes no sense to describe Ashley as cured or the Treatment as a kind of cure for her condition. The Treatment did not improve her cognitive or physical functioning nor was it intended to do so. Yet it is undoubtedly a curative response to disability. Ashley had to be cured of her asynchrony, at least to the fullest extent possible. She also had to be freed of the specter of her future body, the full-sized, large-breasted, menstruating and fertile body to come. Ashley had her imagined body held against her, and held against her in both senses of the phrase: it was this imagined body that justified the Treatment, and it was this imagined body that became grotesque when compared to her present body.

"Towards a Better Quality of Life for 'Pillow Angels'"

Ashley's parents and doctors are concerned not only about Ashley's future (and future body), both real and imagined, but also about the futures of other disabled children. The very fact of their writing proves as much, with each publication geared toward presenting the Treatment as effective, morally permissible, and ethically appropriate for others. Blogging enables Ashley's parents to communicate with other families worldwide and generates press coverage to further their message; publishing in medical journals is a way for Gunther and Diekema to gain peer validation, approval, and, ultimately, adoption of a new treatment beyond the featured case.

One need look no further than the title of Gunther and Diekema's article for proof that they see the growth-attenuating estrogen therapy as having an application beyond Ashley: "A New Approach to an Old Dilemma." The "old dilemma" is how best to care for children with severe disabilities, particularly how to keep them out of nursing homes and state institutions; the "new approach" to this problem is growth attenuation (and its accompanying surgeries).[57] Indeed, they frame their whole article in terms of the struggle against institutionalization. The first sentence of the article sets this tone, noting that the "American Academy of Pediatrics recently endorsed the goal of

Healthy People 2010 to reduce the number of children and youth with disabilities in congregate care facilities to zero by the year 2010."[58] For Gunther and Diekema, such an ambitious goal both requires and justifies bold new approaches such as growth attenuation; it also requires other doctors to take up the practice with their own patients.

Throughout the piece, Gunther and Diekema stress the efficacy of high-dose estrogen treatment in order to make the case for its use with other disabled children. Quite simply, their goal is to

> make an argument for the careful application of such a treatment strategy in nonambulatory, profoundly impaired children. We believe that foreshortening growth in these children could result in a positive benefit in the quality of life for both child and caregiver, and we propose that in situations in which parents request such an intervention, it is both medically feasible and ethically defensible.[59]

As this passage suggests, Gunther and Diekema see the Treatment as more appropriate for some children than others ("nonambulatory, profoundly impaired children"), but they refrain from setting out strict or definitive criteria, opening the door for even wider applicability. Aware that the Treatment might be controversial, they suggest the formation of a decision-making board to determine the appropriateness of the Treatment in particular cases; this recognition of the need for outside observers proves that they imagined the Treatment as having a life beyond Ashley.

Similarly, Ashley's parents imagine their blog as a resource for other parents seeking such treatments for their children; the subtitle of the blog makes this desire plain: "Towards a Better Quality of Life for 'Pillow Angels.'" The plural "angels" makes clear that they do not see Ashley as a unique case. "It is our hope," they explain, "that this treatment becomes well-accepted and available to such families, so they can bring its benefits to their special needs child if appropriate and at an optimal age in order to obtain the most benefits." They insist that the blog is not a defense or justification of the Treatment but rather a place to "share their learned lessons."[60] To that end, they offer a one-page summary of the Treatment—"The 'Ashley Treatment' for the wellbeing of 'Pillow Angels'"—that breaks down each component of the Treatment in terms of its primary and secondary benefits to Ashley. They urge other parents interested in the Treatment to contact them for advice and assistance, stressing that the Treatment is not limited to girls; in fact, they suggest, "it even makes more sense in [boys'] case, since boys tend to grow taller and bigger."[61]

Ashley's parents claim to have heard from "about a dozen" families who have successfully acquired the Treatment for their children (both boys and girls). Other families have apparently tried to do so, but without success; the blog mentions a family whose request was denied at the last minute, not by the ethics committee but because of "PR concerns."[62] More promisingly, from Ashley's parents' perspective, is the growing acceptance of growth attenuation by pediatric specialists. On their blog, they mention a packed session on growth attenuation at the 2008 Pediatric Academic Societies Meeting; according to a doctor present at the session, "half of the room said they had been approached by a family seeking growth attenuation, and about a dozen raised their hands when asked if they had offered it to a family."[63] Moreover, the recent report by the SWG proves that Ashley's parents and doctors have been successful in getting the medical and bioethics communities to take the Treatment seriously; the group's finding that growth attenuation is morally permissible under certain conditions and guidelines suggests that the practice may very well become more common.[64] Even when the Treatment first made news, and the voices of critics were more prominent, many observers saw the procedures as acceptable. A 2007 MSNBC poll, for example, found that 59 percent of respondents supported the decisions by Ashley's parents.[65]

Reading the "testimonials" and "letters of support" posted on the parents' blog drives home how persuasive Ashley's parents and doctors have been in making their case. Countless medical professionals, caregivers, and parents of disabled children have written to voice their support and, often, their wish that the Treatment had been available to the people in their care. Many of these responses illustrate the slippery expansiveness of categories like "pillow angel" and "severely disabled." While Ashley's parents, her doctors, and ethicists have all offered guidelines for the degree of impairment required for the Treatment to be appropriate (the most common criteria are "nonambulatory" and "noncommunicative"), those parameters are not universally accepted.[66] One parent writes, for example,

> I am the father of a child (now 16) born with Spina Bifida. Whitley is paralyzed [sic] from the waist down. We were talking about your daughter and the treatment that you were giving Ashley. . . . Whitley agrees with me that if she was much smaller the effort she would need to "get around" would be much easier. She weighs about 120 lbs and is 4'11" tall. She is a handful to lift. God bless you and Ashley and keep up the good work for her, God is guiding you in a good direction.[67]

Whitley and her father would perhaps not get their wish for the Treatment; not only is she likely too old to benefit, an ethics committee might not approve its use with someone of her level of impairment. She is able not merely to communicate, but to evaluate her situation and express her own desires; she may not be able to walk, but she is able to "get around." She is not impaired enough, in other words, to qualify for the Treatment, at least according to the criteria recommended by the SWG. But, according to her father, she *is* sufficiently impaired. His comments reveal that the attempt to draw bright lines between classes of disability is rarely successful; one person's "severe" may be another's "moderate" or "mild." Supporters of the Treatment insist that it is to be used only in rare cases, cases of "profoundly impaired" children, and that concerns of its being expanded to cover ever-broader categories of disability are overblown. They may be right; yet, as Whitley's father makes clear, defining "profound" impairment constitutes contested, and slippery, terrain.

The Future Will Be Privatized: The Ashley Case in Context

Discourses surrounding the Ashley Treatment serve as a template not only for future medical interventions or standards of care but also for how to view the place of disability and caregiving in the early twenty-first century. The future invoked by the Ashley treatment is a wholly privatized one: disability and disabled people belong in the private sphere, cared for by and within the nuclear family; and the nuclear family should be the sole arbiter of what happens within it. This is not to say that such cases have no bearing on the public sphere, but rather that the public sphere is to have little bearing on such cases. Even as the case is debated in public, it is repeatedly cast by supporters of the Treatment as a private matter. We can see traces of this position in the family's insistence that there was no need for judicial review in this case. In their response to the WPAS investigation, they go so far as to suggest that judicial oversight should never play a role in private, familial deliberations involving children like Ashley:

> While we support laws protecting vulnerable people against involuntary sterilization, the law appears to be too broadly based to distinguish between people who are or can become capable of decision making and those who have a grave and unchanging medical condition such as Ashley, who will never become remotely capable of decision making. Requiring a court order for all hysterectomies performed on all disabled persons regardless of medical condition, complexity, severity, or prognosis puts an onerous burden on already over-burdened families of children with medical conditions as serious as Ashley's.[68]

This rejection of judicial oversight dovetails with long-standing cultural presumptions about the objectivity and authority of Western medicine. Within this framework, doctors and scientists are objective observers of the truth of the body, uniquely able to read, interpret, and understand the mind and body. Logically, then, medical experts are better able to evaluate and adjudicate questions of medical ethics because they can bracket their own political or emotional investments and focus only on the case at hand. They are able, as Donna Haraway puts it, to perform the "god trick of seeing everything from nowhere," making decisions free from bias or subjective opinion.[69] Dr. Diekema's response to the WPAS recommendations serves as a case in point. Challenging the WPAS demand for the addition of disability advocates to hospital ethics committees, Diekema asserts that "ethics committees are not for people with political agendas."[70] With this claim, Diekema positions people living with disability—family members, disability advocates, and disabled people, i.e., those constituting community members within the framework of the WPAS report—as political actors in ways that doctors and bioethicists are not. Such professionals apparently have no such "political agendas" and therefore are the only proper members of ethics committees. Families—such as Ashley's parents—play an integral role in medical decisions, but only in terms of their own families' cases; their agendas turn political if directed outward, beyond their individual situations. Noteworthy is Diekema's depoliticization not only of doctors and bioethicists but of the whole decision-making process. Both disability and decisions about disability are private concerns rather than political ones.

Thus, parents, with guidance from doctors, are the only ones with standing in such cases. As Ashley's parents explain on their blog, "In our opinion, only parents with special-needs children are in a position to fully relate to this topic. Unless you are living the experience, you are speculating and you have no clue what it is like to be the bedridden child or their caregivers."[71] Leaving aside for the moment their assumption that parents are always the best—indeed the only—spokespeople for disabled children, I want to focus on how their rhetoric excludes all other voices from this debate. Parents are not only the ultimate arbiters but also the only ones with any right to speak or reflect on the case; both decision making and debate belong only within the realm of the family. As a result, outside observers are invited to participate only within the terms of the parent-child relationship. Many editorials, commentaries, and blogs personalized and thereby privatized the debate by phrasing it exclusively in terms of familial questions: What would you do if this were your child? Who would you want caring for your child? How would you feel if the state/the medical establishment/disability activists took away your right to determine your child's care? What would you do if an ethics committee refused you access to a treatment you knew was in your family's best interest? The very phrasing of the questions reveals how pervasive this private framing is.

One of the main themes running throughout critiques of the Ashley Treatment is the need for more social support for parents of disabled children. Supporters of the Treatment counter that such services are currently unavailable and that to "abandon" Ashley's parents to "these harsh social and economic realities" would be cruel; "Ashley does not live in a utopian world," Sarah Shannon notes in *Pediatric Nursing*, and to focus on the need for accessible houses or in-home attendant care is a "utopian view of care."[72] Shannon's read of current realities is unfortunately accurate, but calling any and all talk of social supports as utopian and therefore unreasonable denies the possibility of different futures and different presents. As Adrienne Asch and Anna Stubblefield explain, there are already-existing practices and technologies that make home care easier, such as mechanized lifts that can assist with transfers. Moreover, many "full-size" adults live successfully in independent settings and receive care outside of institutions, even without the kind of growth-stunting interventions that the Treatment involves.[73] Completely brushing aside frank talk of social supports renders these kinds of options invisible, such that the Treatment appears as the only real choice parents can make for their children.

Thus the dilemma described by Ashley's doctors is a choice between the Treatment and institutionalization: if we let her imagined grotesque body come into being, then the only possible future that can await her is the one of the institution, or what

Harriet McBryde Johnson calls the "disability gulag."[74] Ashley must be protected, then, from that future location and the future body that would put her there; the Treatment is her only hope for a future away from the institution. That this is a false choice—for surely these are not the only two options, and the Treatment by no means guarantees that she will never be institutionalized—does not take away from the rhetorical power of this justification for the Treatment.

Supporters of the Treatment make a compelling case, and its power is one of the reasons why this story is essential to an analysis of crip futures. The doctors involved in the case, Ashley's parents, their supporters: all draw on rhetoric and ideas nourished and developed from within disability rights movements, but to far different effects. In their initial article, for example, Gunther and Diekema stress the importance of moving as many disabled children as possible out of institutions and other long-term care facilities, keeping them with their families and in their communities. Ashley's parents and their supporters similarly tout the importance of keeping Ashley at home, allowing her to grow up with her siblings and surrounded by people who love her rather than isolated in an institution. (Indeed, they assert that they would never place Ashley in an institution, Treatment or not.) These are undoubtedly goals shared by, and long advocated by, disability rights and independent living movements.

The use of these arguments to justify growth attenuation, sterilization, and mastectomy—as if such practices were necessary to stave off institutionalization—requires those of us concerned and invested in these movements to challenge this appropriation of language and ideology. We need to be much more vigilant and aware of the risks inherent in touting the importance of family involvement and family care. Too easily, those calls can be reinterpreted to mean that the only care worth supporting is that provided by relatives, inadvertently demonizing and pathologizing the use of paid attendants. This is not to say that family members who provide attendant care for their disabled relatives should not themselves be compensated for their work; indeed, I support consumer-directed attendant services that allow disabled people to hire their own attendants, including family members. But, as Laura Hershey explains, seeing attendant care as something best provided by a family member too easily perpetuates the idea that disability is a private problem concerning the family that has no place in the public sphere. This attitude, in turn, leads to the continued devaluation of caregiving; abysmal wages and working conditions are justified on the basis that family members—almost always women—would be doing this work anyway and therefore any compensation, no matter how meager, is sufficient.[75] Moreover, casting disability as a private, familial problem, one properly confined to the home, makes it possible to remove caregiving—regardless of whether it is provided by a relative, regardless of whether it is compensated—from the political realm of public policy. This attitude suggests that the only thing that matters is having a loving relative by one's side, rather than attending to the resources, support, and training that a loved one might need to make such caregiving sustainable over the long term.[76]

Unknown Futures, Narrowed Futures: Measuring "Quality of Life"

The Ashley Treatment has been presented as necessary to Ashley's quality of life. Ashley will be "better off" as the result of these interventions, the story goes; her parents and doctors had to intervene in order to protect her from future harms. "Quality of life" is a familiar refrain in discussions of disability, as the term has often been used as a measure of the worth of disabled people's lives. "Measure" is perhaps too precise a term, as the meaning or criteria of "quality" of life are often taken to be common sense. Many people, regardless of dis/ability, may use the term to examine their own experiences, but disabled people often find their own quality of life described by others as if it were self-evident in their appearance or diagnosis; such discussions almost always include descriptions of the disabled person's (assumed) level of function and pain.[77] Yet accurately evaluating function is not as easy as it might seem. If a disabled person has never been given any kind of adaptive therapy or training, or if someone has no access to adaptive equipment (or only to substandard equipment), then one's function might be much lower than one's ability. Quality of life, then, is affected by one's access to resources and bodies of knowledge rather than a necessary fact of the body/mind. Indeed, descriptions of another's pain and suffering often rely more on assumption than fact, as do presumptions about what level of function is required for a good quality of life.[78]

As a result, analyses of other people's lives, ones intended to demonstrate a certain quality of life (or lack thereof), are often ambiguous and contradictory. Descriptions of Ashley are no different, rife with inconsistencies about the nature of her life. Ashley's doctors and parents describe her as having the cognitive functioning of an infant, but her parents also talk about her experiencing confusion, feeling boredom, and having musical preferences (she reportedly waves her arms along with music that she likes). Reading each of these reactions in relation to each other suggests that Ashley's cognitive abilities might be more advanced than justifications for the Treatment assert; or, perhaps, her family is reading more into her behaviors than others can see. In either case, the combination of observations suggests that function and quality of life are not as straightforward as some analyses might claim. Given someone like Ashley, who "cannot communicate," these questions of quality of life become all the more complicated; she cannot tell us what she thinks about her life.

The issue of communication is itself complicated. According to her parents and doctors, Ashley is unable to communicate and will always remain so. This lack of communication was one of the factors used to justify the Treatment (and one the SWG extended, casting "noncommunicative" as one of the criteria used to evaluate the appropriateness of growth attenuation). But, again, as I note above, if Ashley's parents are able to track boredom, confusion, and musical preferences in Ashley's reactions, then she does not sound completely noncommunicative. Perhaps she could eventually develop a means of communicating with others; in their analysis of the Ashley case, Adrienne Asch and Anna Stubblefield remind us that "there is a long history of experts underestimating the cognitive abilities of people who appear to be profoundly intellectually impaired."[79] Some parents of children with "severe" or "profound" disabilities have reported seeing changes in behavior or capacity over time, despite the fact that their children were given static, unchanging prognoses. They report that their children changed in their ability to interact with the world even if the world remained unable to recognize their interactions as communication or intent.[80] Ashley may never develop the ability to speak or interact in a normative fashion, but perhaps her "reactions" could be extended or enhanced through technologies such as assisted communication. Assisted communication—which often involves an aide helping a disabled person point toward letters, words, symbols, or pictures on a communication board (or, increasingly, electronic device)—remains controversial, but it does at least raise the question of whether Ashley's noncommunicative status is permanent or complete. There certainly are examples of people who claim to have received similar diagnoses and yet eventually learned ways to communicate with others.[81] Given that possibility, why engage in such an extensive medical intervention based in part on the fact of her noncommunication? Is there not a possibility that new technologies could enable some form of communication in the not-too-distant future?

I cannot know the answer to that question, and asking it seems only to raise a whole other set of problems and complexities. Stressing that Ashley might "get better" either through technological interventions or therapy (or both) suggests that it is the "getting better" that renders the Treatment offensive or inappropriate. And if that is the case, then the Treatment is appropriate as long as we make sure we are getting the "right" children, the ones who do not have a chance of improving their function. But drawing lines between levels of impairment is notoriously difficult and, as Eva Kittay points out, suggests that some people are more deserving of ethical concern and consideration than others.[82]

Rather the key seems to be to focus on the unknowability inherent in the case.[83] There is no way to know for certain whether the Treatment improved Ashley's quality of life. We have no baseline of "quality" by which to measure, for Ashley or for any of us. Supporters of the Treatment claim medical evidence for their assertion that the Treatment had a positive effect, but they are extrapolating from other cases or other situations. Ashley's parents' long-term quality of life likely improved, given that Ashley will remain easier to lift, and Ashley's quality of life is bound up in her parents'; if they are doing well, the odds are higher that she is doing well. But, again, we cannot know, not for certain, whether the Treatment benefited Ashley's quality of life.

Were the interventions a success in terms of reducing Ashley's pain? I don't know; I can't know. The surgery itself likely resulted in pain both physical and psychological, but perhaps that pain has faded from Ashley's memory. Perhaps that pain, now passed, is less significant than the constant pain of compressed breasts or the recurring pain of menstrual cramps. Or perhaps not. We cannot know the answers to these questions, but they are presented in Treatment-supportive discourses as self-evident. The claim that the Treatment reduced Ashley's pain is taken as fact.

Missing from this discussion of Ashley's quality of life is the possibility of pleasure; how might the Treatment have foreclosed upon a range of potential sites and sources of pleasure? It is possible that Ashley would have developed the large breasts that reportedly run in her family, and it is possible that she would have experienced discomfort from them. It seems equally possible, however, that she would have experienced pleasure from those imagined large breasts: the sensation of her shirt moving against her skin, or of her skin moving against her sheets, or of her own arms brushing against her breasts. Even the tight chest straps holding her in her chair could have been sources of pleasure: perhaps she would enjoy the sensation of support, or take pleasure in the alternation between binding and release as she was moved in and out of her wheelchair. The inability or unwillingness to imagine these pleasures is a manifestation of cultural approaches to female sexuality and disability. It is seemingly inconceivable to imagine Ashley's body—her disabled female body—as the source of any sensation other than pain. We have few tools for recognizing female sexuality, particularly disabled female sexuality, as positive; nor can we recognize the potential for a self-generated and self-directed sexuality.

Ashley's parents see the mastectomy as offering an "additional benefit to Ashley" beyond its elimination of imagined future pain; according to them, the mastectomy will also prevent "sexualization towards [her] caregiver."[84] Their syntax is odd here. To what does the "towards" refer? Is it meant to imply the possibility of a caregiver taking sexual liberties with Ashley, so that the mastectomy prevents caregivers from sexualizing her? Or does it refer to the possibility that Ashley might feel sexual when touched by her caregiver? In either case, it is a troubling rationale for the surgical removal of her breast buds. A lack of breasts does not render one safe from sexual assault or abuse, and many would argue that such assault is more the result of a desire for power and control than of sexualization.[85] Or, if their concern is more about Ashley feeling sexual (and it is profoundly unclear what they would imagine that to mean, given their positioning of her as a noncommunicative infant), then the surgery has been justified, in part, on the need to diminish Ashley's access to pleasurable sensations. Maybe Ashley experiences pleasure from being held or hugged, from being bathed in warm water or toweled off, from nestling into a fresh bed or feeling the sun on her face. And if we can recognize those physical sensations as human pleasures to which even the disabled are entitled, then why deny her the future possibility of feeling the sensations of her breasts?[86] The Treatment foreclosed on some of the ways Ashley might experience, or understand, or interact with her own body. Her inability to describe such interactions or even to understand them intellectually does not necessarily translate into an inability to feel them.

At the Same Time, Out of Time;
or, Looking for Ashley among Crips and Queers

"Out of time": I choose this phrase for its multiple meanings. First, Ashley's being "frozen in time" is a casting out of time; the development of her female body has been arrested, removing her from expected patterns of female development and aging. Second, the use of Ashley as a "case study" only exacerbates this frozen-ness, as scholars and activists—including myself—continue to focus on what happened to Ashley in the past, as if the intervening years never happened, as if she weren't continuing to live beyond the dates of our analyses. Third, the Treatment itself was justified on the basis of Ashley's being always already out of time: her mind and body were so asynchronous that medical intervention was necessary to prevent her from falling further out of time. Finally, Ashley has run out of time. We are too late to stop the Treatment, too late to interrupt this representation of her as endangered by her future self or as embodied asynchrony.

To return then to where I started: In thinking about crip futurity, I find myself haunted by Ashley X. Of course, Ashley is not the only one doing the haunting. Ashley's parents suggest that there have been other pillow angels who have undergone the Treatment, and, if so, their stories remain unknown; I am haunted by that unknown. I think also of those disabled children who were altered in more traditional but no less invasive ways, children whose stories have not been seen as worth remembering, let alone preserving or disseminating.[87] Perhaps the interventions in their bodies were considered a matter of course, a part of the standard of care, and therefore not prompting judicial review or public response; or maybe they were children who were seen not as figures in a sentimental narrative but as the inevitable and unremarkable casualties of poverty, violence, and inequality. Perhaps the details of their lives were unable to capture the public imagination in the same way a white pillow angel could. Sentimentality has historically and culturally been linked with white middle-class femininity, and Ashley's representation as a "pillow angel" calls to mind these racialized discourses of domesticity and passivity. As Patricia Williams points out, the "pillow angel" label held sway in public discussions of the case in no small part because of Ashley's race and class. Williams doubts, and with good reason, that "a poor black child would have been so easily romanticized as a 'pillow angel.'"[88] Williams uses the case as a reminder that we are more concerned with the quality of some lives than others (even as the steps ostensibly taken to "ensure" that quality reveal profound ableist and misogynist anxiety).

I draw on this language of haunting to mark the difficulty of this case, to recognize the power with which it hit. In the years since this story first broke, conversations about the Ashley case have repeated and repeated themselves, a citational frequency that reveals the emotional toll the case took—and continues to take—on disabled people. I know that I continue to feel a mixture of anger, shame, and betrayal about the Ashley case: betrayal that mainstream feminists largely kept silent about the case, perhaps seeing it as only a "disability" issue; anger that these medical and surgical interventions were allowed to happen and will likely happen again; and shame that we could not save her, that we cannot reach her.

Yet supporters of the Treatment argue that disability activists have no bearing on this case because Ashley is too severely disabled to be considered a disabled person.[89] Ashley's parents, for example, refer to her as "permanently unabled" in order to distinguish her from other disabled people; "unabled" is a "new category" that includes "less than 1% of children with disability."[90] Although she does not argue for this kind of new terminology, Anita J. Tarzian agrees that it might be a "misnomer" to call Ashley disabled. Both disability rights and people-first or self-advocacy movements are concerned with individuals who "have some level of cognitive capacity," she explains, which means that these movements do not have the tools or the rhetoric to address those with "severe neurological impairments."[91]

Predominant models of disability studies and activism too often *do* skim over such people, and Ashley's situation is not, and never has been, similar to most of us working in disability studies. How, then, are we to understand the differences between our experiences even as we name us all as disabled? Or, to move in the other direction, how might such an identification—we are all Ashley X—work to trouble the binaries of functional/nonfunctional, physical/developmental, or moderate/severe disability? What work are we enabled to do by placing Ashley in the center of disability scholarship and activism, or by positioning her as part of disability communities and movements? If crip theory and critical disability studies remind us to attend not only to the experiences of disabled people but also, and especially, to the ways in which disability and ability work in the world, then we need to contest this representation of some minds and bodies as beyond the reach of disability analysis and activism.

I want to caution, then, against viewing Ashley as exceptional or her case as a spectacular anomaly. After all, there remains a very real possibility that growth attenuation (and its attendant surgeries) will be performed on other disabled kids, which means that we cannot dismiss the case as a one-time event. More to the point, Ashley herself is *not* wholly unlike the other disabled people inhabiting the pages of this book or the movements and scholarship discussed here. To see her differently, to accept the representation of her as "unabled" rather than "disabled," is to accept an ableist logic that positions impairment—if "severe" enough—as inherently depoliticizing; "unability" becomes the category that allows "disability" to separate itself from those bodies/minds that remain in the margins.

We will remain haunted by the Ashley case, in other words, if we refuse to look for her among crips and queers, if we refuse to recognize her as part of our work. How might we imagine futures that hold space and possibility for those who communicate in ways we do not yet recognize as communication, let alone understand? Or futures that make room for diverse, unpredictable, and fundamentally unknowable experiences of pleasure? If, as I discussed in the previous chapter, queerness entails nonheteronormative approaches to temporality, then how might we learn to approach asynchronous bodies and minds as something other than grotesque or pathological? Reading Ashley through the lens of temporality is likely going to require changes to both our theories of disability and our approaches to queer/crip futurity. As we intervene in the representation of Ashley as abnormally asynchronous or grotesquely fertile, as we interrupt the depiction of her as developmentally and temporally other, we must take care, as feminist disability scholars and crip theorists, not to write Ashley out of our own desirably disabled futures.

3 Debating Feminist Futures

*Slippery Slopes, Cultural Anxiety,
and the Case of the Deaf Lesbians*

> The fear that lesbians and gay men will start to fabricate human beings, exaggerating the biotechnology of reproduction, suggests that these "unnatural" practices will eventuate in a wholesale social engineering of the human. . . . But it seems a displacement, if not a hallucination, to identify the source of this social threat, if it is a threat, with lesbians who excavate sperm from dry ice on a cold winter day in Iowa when one of them is ovulating.
>
> —Judith Butler, *Undoing Gender*

THE PERVASIVENESS OF prenatal testing, and especially its acceptance as part of the standard of care for pregnant women, casts women as responsible for their future children's able-bodiedness/able-mindedness; prospective parents are urged to take advantage of these services so as to avoid burdening their future children with any disabilities.[1] This notion of "burdening" children finds an echo in the debate over same-sex marriage, with LGBT couples cast as selfish parents, placing their own desires over the physical and mental health of their children (and, by extension, of all children). Moreover, according to Timothy Dailey of the Family Research Council, homosexual parents often "'recruit' children into the homosexual lifestyle" by modeling "abnormal sexuality."[2] The possibility that same-sex parents might produce queer children is one of the most common reasons given for opposing such families, a reasoning that takes for granted the homophobic worldview that queerness must be avoided at all costs.

It is in the literature of reproductive technologies and their "proper" use that heterocentrism and homophobia intersect powerfully with ableism and stereotypes about disability. These stories reveal profound anxieties about reproducing the family as a normative unit, with all of its members able-bodied/able-minded and heterosexual. At sites where disability, queerness, and reproductive technologies converge, parents and prospective parents are often criticized and condemned for their alleged misuse of technology. Assistive reproductive technologies are to be used only to deselect or prevent disability; doing otherwise—such as selecting for disability—means failing to properly reproduce the family.

In this chapter, I explore one such story in which ableism and heterocentrism combine, a situation in which parents were widely condemned for failing to protect their children from both disability and queerness. Sharon Duchesneau and Candace McCullough, a deaf lesbian couple in Maryland, attracted publicity and controversy for their 2001 decision to use a deaf sperm donor in conceiving their son. What most interests me about their story, and what I focus on here, is the consistency with which cultural critics and commentators took for granted the idea that a better future is one without disability and deafness. In order to illustrate this dimension of the story, I frame their account with an analysis of Marge Piercy's influential utopia, *Woman on the Edge of Time*.[3] In that novel, as in the responses to McCullough and Duchesneau, "common sense" dictates that disabled minds/bodies have no place in the future, and that such decisions merit neither discussion nor dissent. Both stories, in other words, center around the proper use of assistive reproductive technology and the future of children.

This is What the Future Looks Like: Reproduction and Debate in *Woman on the Edge of Time*

In 2001, I served as a teaching assistant in an introduction to women's studies course at a liberal arts college in Southern California. One of the assigned texts was Marge Piercy's novel *Woman on the Edge of Time* (1976), chosen by the professor in order to spark discussion about feminist futures. Published over three decades ago, the novel continues to be popular among feminists for its representation of an egalitarian society. Students responded enthusiastically to Piercy's book, finding its imagined utopia hopeful, enviable, and desirable. As a disability studies scholar, however, I found the novel troubling for its erasure of disability and disabled bodies, an erasure that is never debated or discussed in the novel. With the marked exception of mental illness, an exception to which I will return, *Woman on the Edge of Time* simply assumes that a feminist future is, by definition, one without disability and disabled bodies.

Woman on the Edge of Time is a feminist utopia/dystopia that chronicles the experiences of Connie Ramos, a poor Chicana woman who has been involuntarily institutionalized in a New York mental ward. The novel moves back and forth among three settings: mental institutions and Connie's neighborhoods in 1970s New York; Mattapoisett, a utopian village in 2137; and a future, dystopic New York City inhabited by cyborgs and machines in which all humans have been genetically engineered to fulfill certain social roles.[4] While incarcerated in the violent ward of a mental institution in 1976, Connie develops the ability to travel mentally into the future, interacting with a woman named Luciente who lives in the utopian Mattapoisett community. During one attempt at mental travel, Connie's attention is diverted and she finds herself in the dystopic future Manhattan, but the rest of her time travels involve Mattapoisett.

Piercy lovingly describes Mattapoisett. She has clearly thought a great deal about difference in constructing this world, trying to envision a thoroughly feminist, antiracist, socially just, and multicultural community. All sexual orientations and identities are present and respected in her vision of Mattapoisett, everyone possesses equal wealth and resources, and all have access to education according to their interests. People in Mattapoisett have developed harvesting and consumption patterns intended to redress the global imbalance of wealth, resources, and consumption wrought during Connie's era. The world is viewed holistically, with Mattapoisett's inhabitants aware of how their actions affect others both within the borders of their community and beyond.

Luciente explains to Connie that Mattapoisett's communal harmony has been achieved through radical changes in the system of reproduction. All babies are born in the "brooder," a machine that mixes the genes from all the population's members, so that children are not genetically bound to any two people. Three adults co-mother each child, a task that is undertaken equally by men and women. Through hormone treatments, both men and women are able to breast-feed, exemplifying the community's belief that equality between the sexes can be engineered through technological intervention and innovation. By breaking the traditional gendered nature of reproduction, explains Luciente, the brooder has eliminated fixed gender roles and sexism within the community. It has also eradicated racism by mixing the genes from all "races," thereby rendering everyone mixed-race and making notions of "racial purity" impossible to maintain. Cultural histories and traditions have been preserved, but have been separated from the concept of "race." Luciente's friend Bee tells Connie that the community has recently decided to create more "darker-skinned" babies in order to counteract the historical devaluation of people of color, resulting in a village inhabited by people of all skin tones: "[W]e don't want the melting pot where everybody ends up with thin gruel. We want diversity, for strangeness breeds richness."[5]

All decisions concerning the community are publicly debated during open meetings. Decisions are made on the basis of consensus, and every community member is allowed and expected to participate. People volunteer to serve as representatives to intercommunity meetings at which decisions affecting a larger population are debated. No decisions are made for other people by other people. Every person has the right to speak out on issues that affect him or her.

To illustrate the way this participatory democracy works, Piercy gradually introduces Connie, and the reader, to a conflict currently being played out in Mattapoisett. The "Mixers" and the "Shapers" are involved in a heated disagreement about the next direction the brooder should take, with the Shapers advocating a more aggressive stance. The Mixers would prefer to maintain the status quo: the brooder currently screens out genes linked to birth defects and disease susceptibility, thereby preventing "negative" characteristics from being passed down to children. The Shapers, however, want to program the brooder to select for "positive" traits as well, ensuring that children will have the traits most desired by the community. Luciente and her friends are on the side of the Mixers, arguing that it is impossible to know which traits will be necessary or valued in the future. Piercy makes it clear that Luciente's perspective mirrors her own; the genetically engineered inhabitants of her dystopian New York suggest the logical, and undesirable, result of a Shaper victory. Piercy refuses, however, to simply impose a Mixer victory on Mattapoisett; she depicts a continuing process of respectful dialogue and public debate between the two groups, creating a vision of a feminist community in which all people participate equally in the decisions that affect them. The Mixers-Shapers debate is never resolved in the novel, illustrating Piercy's notion of the importance of open-ended dialogue and group process.

It is this description of democratic decision making, of a community debating publicly how it wants technology to develop in the future, that has made *Woman on the Edge* such an attractive text to feminist scholars of science studies and political theory. Decades after its initial publication, the novel continues to inspire feminist thinkers with its image of an egalitarian future in which all people's voices are heard, respected, and addressed. A quick glance at the women's studies syllabi collected on Internet databases reveals the continued popularity of the book in conversations about "feminist futures," "feminist utopias," and "ecofeminisms"; *Woman on the Edge of Time* is often taught in introductory women's studies classes to initiate discussion about feminist worldviews.[6]

Similarly, several feminist political theorists and science studies scholars cast the book as a vital exploration of political and technological processes influenced by feminist principles. José van Dijck, for example, praises Piercy for depicting science as "a political and democratic process in which all participants participate," a depiction that recognizes genetics "as a political, rather than a purely scientific," practice. Political theorist Josephine Carubia Glorie shares van Dijck's assessment, noting that Piercy's novel features a society in which all community members are able to engage in social critique. Even those who disagree with Piercy's pro-genetic engineering and pro-assisted reproduction stance, such as ecofeminists Cathleen McGuire and Colleen McGuire, find *Woman on the Edge of Time* to be a compelling vision of a world without social inequalities.[7] As these comments suggest, over thirty years after its initial publication, *Woman on the Edge of Time* remains a powerful, productive text for feminist theorists concerned with the role of technology in the lives of women and committed to envisioning an egalitarian, just world. Piercy's articulation of the "Mixers vs. Shapers" debate—should we breed children for desired traits?—seems prescient in the early twenty-first century as bioethicists and geneticists debate the morality and feasibility of allowing prospective parents to create or select embryos on the basis of such traits as sex, hair color, or height.[8]

What has gone unnoticed in these praises of Piercy's novel, however, is the place of disability, and specifically disabled bodies, in her imagined utopia. In a world very carefully constructed to contain people of every skin tone and sexual orientation, where people of all genders and ages are equally valued, disabled people are absent.

This absence cannot simply be attributed to oversight or neglect; it is not that Piercy forgot to include disability and disabled people among her cast of characters and life experiences. On the contrary, the place, or rather the absence, of disability in Piercy's utopia is at the heart of the Mixers-Shapers debate: both the Shapers and the Mixers agree on the necessity of screening the gene pool for "defective genes" and "predispositions" for illness and "suffering." It is taken for granted by both sides—and by Piercy and (presumably) her audience—that everyone knows and agrees which genes and characteristics are negative and therefore which ones should be eliminated; questions about so-called negative traits are apparently not worth discussing. Thus, disabled people are not accidentally missing from Piercy's utopia; they have intentionally and explicitly been written out of it. Mattapoisett, an influential feminist fictional utopia, has wiped out congenital disability. The apparent lack of any physically or cognitively disabled inhabitants of Mattapoisett, coupled with the genetic screening of all congenital disabilities, suggests that even disabilities acquired through age, illness, or accident are lacking in this utopia; presumably medicine has advanced to such a degree that all impairments can be cured or prevented.

At first glance, mental disability seems to be an exception to this absence. Not only is the novel highly critical of the institutionalization of people with mental disability, it also casts "crazy" as a diagnosis more likely to be attached to poor women of color and to those who refuse to adhere to cultural norms. Unlike the stigma and forced institutionalization Connie faced in 1970s New York, the inhabitants of Mattapoisett recognize mental disability as part of a normal course of life, with people "dropping out" of their communities as needed to tend to their mental and emotional needs. But this requirement to drop out, to separate oneself from the community until one's functioning returns to "normal," enacts another version of this erasure of disability. People with disabilities have no place in this feminist future. Indeed, it is their very absence, whether permanent or temporary, that signals the utopian nature of this future.

Neither Piercy, writing in the mid-1970s, nor theorists such as van Dijck and Glorie, writing in the late 1990s, seem to have noticed that the entire Mixers-Shapers debate rests on profound assumptions about whose bodies matter. Van Dijck and Glorie praise Piercy for articulating a vision of science as a democratic process in which all voices are heard, yet the assumptions underlying the Mixers-Shapers debate ignore the perspectives of an entire class of people, those with congenital disabilities. Never once do the nondisabled members of Mattapoisett debate the decision to eliminate ostensibly defective genes, never do they question how one determines which genes are labeled "defective" or what "defective" means. Van Dijck highlights Piercy's recognition that genetics is political—contested and contestable, subject to debate and disagreement—but fails to realize that screening the gene pool for allegedly negative traits is also political. In both the novel and interpretation of the novel, it is assumed that disability has no place in feminist visions of the future, and that such an assumption is so natural, so given, that it does not merit public debate.

What does it mean that disability appears in Piercy's utopia only as an unwanted characteristic in a debate over genetic engineering, a debate itself used to illustrate her ideas about democratic science? What does it mean that feminists writing and teaching about the United States in the 1990s and 2000s use this novel, and specifically the Mixers-Shapers debate, as an example of ideal democratic decision making and public critique, of a political community grounded in feminist principles of egalitarianism and democracy? What can be inferred about disability from the fact that contemporary feminists highlight a debate in which both parties assume from the beginning that "negative" traits are self-evident, natural, and therefore outside the scope of discussion? What can a feminist disability studies reader learn from the fact that feminist theorists have offered no critique of a debate in which disabled people do not participate because they have already been removed from this supposedly diverse, multicultural, egalitarian landscape?

I suggest that Piercy's depiction and, more importantly, feminist theorists' praise of it mean that disability in the United States is often viewed as an unredeemable difference. Disability and the disabled body are problems that must be solved technologically, and there is allegedly so much cultural agreement on this point that it need not be discussed or debated. Disability, then, plays a huge, but seemingly uncontested, role in how contemporary Americans envision the future. Utopian visions are founded on the elimination of disability, while dystopic, negative visions of the future are based on its proliferation; as we will see below, both depictions are deeply tied to cultural understandings and anxieties about the proper use of technology.

I turn now to one particular case of the alleged misuse of technology, moving from Piercy's fiction to the stories we tell ourselves about others' reproduction. The story of Sharon Duchesneau and Candace McCullough, a deaf lesbian couple who selected a deaf sperm donor for their pregnancies, has been presented to the public almost exclusively in terms of what the future can, should, and will include. Whether warning of a slippery slope, of other disabled people "manufacturing" disabled children, or of "unnatural" lifestyles, commentators see the couple's selection of a deaf sperm donor as a sign of a dangerous future. I am less interested in arguing for or against these women's decision than in detailing how critics of the couple utilize dystopic rhetoric in their condemnations, presenting deafness and disability as traits that obviously should be avoided. As with *Woman on the Edge of Time*, a world free of impairment is portrayed as a goal shared by all, a goal that is beyond question or analysis, a goal that is natural rather than political.

Deaf/Disabled: A Terminological Interlude

For most hearing people, to describe deafness as a disability is to state the obvious: deaf people lack the ability to hear, and therefore they are disabled. For some people, however, deaf and hearing alike, it is neither obvious nor accurate to characterize deafness as a disability and deaf people as disabled. Rather, Deaf people are more appropriately described as members of a distinct linguistic and cultural minority, more akin to Spanish speakers in a predominantly English-language country than to people in wheelchairs or people who are blind.[9] Spanish speakers are not considered disabled simply because they cannot communicate in English without the aid of an interpreter, and, according to this model, neither should Deaf people, who rely on interpreters in order to communicate with those who cannot sign, be considered disabled. Drawing parallels between Deaf people and members of other cultural groups, supporters of the linguistic-cultural model of deafness note the existence of a vibrant Deaf culture, one that includes its own language (in the United States, American Sign Language [ASL]), cultural productions (e.g., ASL poetry and performance), residential schools, and social networks, as well as high rates of intermarriage.[10] As Deaf studies scholar Harlan Lane explains, "[T]he preconditions for Deaf participation [in society] are more like those of other language minorities: culturally Deaf people campaign for acceptance of their language and its broader use in the schools, the workplace, and in public events."[11] This linguistic-cultural model of deafness shares a key assumption of the social model of disability—namely, that it is society's interpretations of and responses to bodily and sensory variations that are the problem, not the variations themselves.

Everyone Here Spoke Sign Language, Nora Groce's study of hereditary deafness on Martha's Vineyard from the early eighteenth century to the mid-twentieth century, provides an example of this perspective. Groce argues that genetic deafness and deaf people were so interwoven into the population that almost every person on the island had a deaf relative or neighbor.[12] As a result, "everyone [there] spoke sign language," a situation that proves it is possible for hearing people to share the responsibility of communication rather than simply expecting deaf people to lip-read and speak orally or alleviate their hearing loss with surgeries and hearing aids.[13] Groce's study challenges the idea that deafness precludes full participation in society, suggesting that the barriers deaf people face are due more to societal attitudes and practices than to one's audiological conditions. For those who subscribe to this worldview, deafness is best understood as a distinct culture in which one should feel pride, rather than as a disability.

Although some Deaf people are averse to the label "disabled," either because of their immersion in Deaf culture or because of an internalized ableist impulse to distance themselves from disabled people, others are more willing to explore the label politically. This kind of exploration is based on making a distinction between being labeled as "disabled" by others, especially medical or audiological professionals and the hearing world in general, and choosing to self-identify as disabled. Many Deaf people who choose to take up the label of disability do so for strategic reasons. For some, the decision stems from a desire to ally themselves with other disabled people. They recognize that people with disabilities and Deaf people share a history of oppression, discrimination, and stigmatization because of their differences from a perceived "normal" body. As a group, Deaf and disabled people can work together to fight discrimination, and they have done so since the birth of the modern disability rights movement in the late 1960s. Thus, while some Deaf people may be opposed to (or at the very least ambivalent about) seeing deafness as a disability, they may simultaneously be willing to identify themselves as disabled or to ally themselves with disabled people in order to work toward social changes and legal protections that would benefit both populations.[14]

Recognizing this affinity between disability and deafness is particularly important in an analysis of cure narratives and utopian discourse, because it is precisely the image of deafness as disability that animates these narratives. What makes the actions of parents who express a preference for a deaf baby—the case under consideration here—so abhorrent to the larger culture is the refusal to eradicate disability from the lives of their children.

Reproducing Cultural Anxiety: The Case of the Deaf Lesbians

In November 2001, the same year that I taught Piercy's novel, Sharon Duchesneau and Candace (Candy) McCullough, a white lesbian couple living in Maryland, had a baby boy named Gauvin, who was conceived by assisted insemination. Both Duchesneau, the birth mother, and McCullough, the adoptive mother, are deaf, as is their first child, Jehanne. Jehanne and her new brother Gauvin were conceived with sperm donated by a family friend, a friend who also is deaf. Duchesneau and McCullough had originally intended to use a sperm bank for the pregnancies, but their desire for a deaf donor eliminated that option: men with congenital deafness are precluded from becoming sperm donors; reminiscent of the eugenic concern with the "fitness" of potential parents, deafness is one of the conditions that sperm banks and fertility clinics routinely screen out of the donor pool.[15] Several months after he was born, Gauvin underwent an extensive audiology test to determine if he shared his parents' deafness.[16] To the delight of Duchesneau and McCullough, the diagnosis was clear: Gauvin had "a profound hearing loss" in one ear, and "at least a severe hearing loss" in the other.[17] Duchesneau noted that they would have accepted and loved a hearing child, but a deaf child was clearly their preference. "A hearing baby would be a blessing," Duchesneau explained, "a Deaf baby would be a special blessing."[18]

Liza Mundy covered Duchesneau and McCullough's story for the *Washington Post Magazine* in March of 2002, and her essay provided a detailed explanation of these women's reproductive choices. Although the piece acknowledged the criticisms lodged against Duchesneau and McCullough, it was largely sympathetic; Mundy took care to explain the women's understanding of Deaf identity and to situate them within a larger understanding of Deaf culture and community. She also, of necessity, mentioned the women's lesbian relationship, but it was not a central component of the piece. For Mundy, it was the women's deafness, and their decision to have deaf children within a larger Deaf community, that made their story newsworthy.[19]

The piece made quite a splash, and the story of the Deaf lesbian couple was picked up by other newspapers and wire services. Papers across the United States and England ran versions of and responses to the story, and cultural critics from across the ideological spectrum began to weigh in. The Family Research Council, a Washington-based organization that "champions marriage and family as the foundation of civilization," issued a press release with comments from Ken Connor, the group's president at the time. Describing Duchesneau and McCullough as "incredibly selfish," Connor berated the pair for imposing on their children not only the "disadvantages that come as a result of being raised in a homosexual household" but also the "burden" of disability. Connor linked disability and homosexuality, casting both as hardships that these two women "intentionally" handed their children. The Family Research Council's press release closed with a quote from Connor that not only continued to link homosexuality with disability but also depicted both as leading toward a dystopic future: "One can only hope that this practice of intentionally manufacturing disabled children in order to fit the lifestyles of the parents will not progress any further. The places this slippery slope could lead to are frightening."[20] The use of the term "lifestyles"—a word frequently used to refer derisively to queers and our sexual/relational practices—effectively blurs deafness and queerness, suggesting that both characteristics are allegedly leading "us" down the road to ruin.[21]

Indeed, the queerness of this future had everything to do with its portrayal as negative and imperfect. Although Ken Connor and the Family Research Council probably would not celebrate the use of a Deaf sperm donor by a heterosexual couple, it is highly unlikely that they would have condemned it as aggressively or as publicly as they did here, casting such a move as the first step on a slippery slope into the unknown. (They have not gone on record, for example, condemning Deaf heterosexuals who have children.) The case of the Deaf lesbians acquired the mileage that it did because of its evocation of a queer disabled future; heterosexism and ableism intertwine, each feeding off and supporting the other.

The Family Research Council was not alone in discussing these women's desire for a Deaf baby in the context of their sexuality. Indeed, even some queer commentators found something troubling, and ultimately dystopic, about the idea. Queer novelist Jeanette Winterson seemed to suggest that it was precisely these women's queerness that made their decision so anathema:

> If either of the Deaf Lesbians in the United States had been in a relationship with a man, Deaf or hearing, and if they had decided to have a baby, there is absolutely no certainty that the baby would have been Deaf. You take a chance with love; you take a chance with nature, but it is those chances and the unexpected possibilities they bring, that give life its beauty.[22]

It is worth noting that Winterson appears concerned only about the loss of some possibilities, namely the possibility of having a hearing child. Screening out deaf donors from sperm banks *also* removes the chance of "unexpected possibilities," at least in terms of genetic deafness, but apparently the denial of that chance does not trouble her.

Winterson condemned Duchesneau and McCullough for removing the element of "chance" from their pregnancy and guaranteeing themselves a deaf baby, a guarantee that could not happen "with nature."[23] However, her remarks obscure the fact that the women's use of a deaf donor provided no such guarantee, a fact made clear in Mundy's article.[24] Duchesneau, McCullough, and their deaf donor; Winterson's hypothetical deaf heterosexual couple: both groups would have exactly the same odds of having a deaf child, yet Winterson found no fault with the imagined heterosexual conception. She appears to believe that it is acceptable, if perhaps regrettable, for heterosexual deaf couples to have deaf children because such an act is "natural"; bearing deaf children becomes "unnatural" and thereby dangerous when it is done outside the bounds of a "normal, natural" relationship—an odd position for a queer writer to take and one that has certainly been influenced by dominant ableist culture.

Winterson clearly took for granted that "everyone" views these women's behavior as reprehensible; for her, it was a "simple fact" that life as a deaf person is inferior to life as a hearing person. Duchesneau and McCullough's refusal to accept this "simple fact," and their insistence that deafness is desirable, has made them the targets of criticism from across the political spectrum. Winterson echoed Connor's "slippery slope" rhetoric when she suggested that these women's actions will lead to other, allegedly even more troubling futures. "How would any of us feel," she asked, "if the women had both been blind and claimed the right to a blind baby?" The tone and content of Winterson's essay answers this question for her readers, making clear that "we" would feel justifiably outraged.[25] It is perhaps no accident that Winterson referred to "blind women" rather than "blind people," again implying that it might be "natural" for a heterosexual blind couple to reproduce, but not a lesbian one. She even drew on this image for the title of her essay, "How Would We Feel If Blind Women Claimed the Right to a Blind Baby?"[26]

This rhetorical move—shifting from an actual case involving deafness to a hypothetical situation involving a different disability—is a popular strategy to convince a disabled person that her decision to choose for disability, either by having a disabled child or by refusing technological fixes, is misguided, illogical, and extreme. By decontextualizing the situation, removing it from a Deaf person's own sphere of reference, it is assumed that the Deaf person will be able to recognize her error in judgment. This practice suggests that some disabilities are worse than others, that eventually one can substitute a particular disability that is so "obviously" undesirable that the disabled person will change her mind. Cross-disability alliances are presumed to be nonexistent; it is assumed that all Deaf people believe it would be best to eliminate the birth of "blind babies" or people with X disability.

This story is complicated by the fact that Winterson's stance is not without basis. In the *Washington Post* story, McCullough does express a preference for a sighted child. According to Mundy,

> If they themselves—valuing sight—were to have a blind child, well then, Candy acknowledges, they would probably try to have it fixed, if they could, like hearing

parents who attempt to restore their child's hearing with cochlear implants. "I want to be the same as my child," says Candy. "I want the baby to enjoy what we enjoy."[27]

McCullough and Duchesneau's position that Deaf babies are "special blessings" does not mean that they are not also simultaneously implicated in the ableism of the larger culture; their desire for deafness does not necessarily extend to a desire for any and all disabilities. Deaf and disabled people are not immune to the ableist—or homophobic—ideologies of the larger culture. (It is worth noting in this context, however, that McCullough does not express a desire for genetic testing and selective abortion).

Indeed, even some disabled queers mirrored the blend of heterocentrism and ableism circulating through mainstream responses to Duchesneau and McCullough's reproductive choices. A participant on the QueerDisability listserv, for example, found the couple's decision to choose a Deaf donor troubling, partly because of the hardships and social barriers their children would face, partly because of the alleged financial burden their children would place on the state. Echoing Winterson, the listserv member drew a distinction between the "naturally" Deaf children who result from heterosexual relationships and the "unnaturally," and therefore inappropriately, Deaf children who result from queer relationships. We are left to wonder how this community member would view the choice by an infertile heterosexual Deaf couple to use a Deaf sperm donor, whether that choice would be deemed more natural and therefore acceptable.[28] Her comments lead me to believe that she would, like Winterson, find less fault with the imagined heterosexual couple than with the real homosexual one: either deafness or homosexuality in isolation would be permissible, but the combination is too abnormal, too disruptive, too queer, even for some gays and lesbians and people with disabilities.

These kinds of responses to the use of assisted insemination by Deaf queers support Sarah Franklin's argument that, while reproductive technology "might have been (or is to a limited extent) a disruption of the so-called 'natural' basis for the nuclear family and heterosexual marriage, [it] *has instead provided the occasion for reconsolidating them.*"[29] With few exceptions, Franklin explains, the state has taken little action to guarantee queers and/or single parents equal access to assisted reproductive technologies, and prominent people in the field of reproductive medicine have been outspoken in their belief that these technologies should not be available to same-sex couples or single parents.[30] As sociologist Laura Mamo points out, "[A]ccess to reproductive technologies in the United States is from the outset a class-based and sexuality-based phenomenon, and the institutional organization of these services enacts the reproduction of class and sexuality hierarchies by assuring the survival and ongoing proportionality of middle-class (usually white) heterosexual families."[31]

Mamo details the ways in which lesbians and (single heterosexual women) are disadvantaged within the medical system. Insurance policies, for example, require a diagnosis of infertility before they agree to cover assistive technologies, yet such a diagnosis is difficult to make in the absence of heterosexual sex. Many lesbians want to use sperm donated by a friend or family member, yet some clinics forbid the use of sperm from a known donor unless the woman is married to the donor.[32] Dorothy Roberts and Elizabeth Weil note that many fertility clinics require proof of a "stable" marriage before initiating treatment, an open-ended requirement that has been used to block the treatment of queers, women of color, and poor people. California prohibits discriminating against queers in fertility treatments, but, as Elizabeth Weil argues, such discrimination can hide under other names. Guadalupe Benitez lost her case against the North Coast Women's Care Medical Group when they argued that they had refused to treat her not because she was a lesbian but because she was unmarried; in an earlier case, which the clinic lost, Benitez was able to prove that treatment had stopped because of her status as a lesbian.[33] Assisted insemination may make it easier for queers to bear children, thereby "unsettling the conflation of reproduction with heterosexuality," but heterocentric/homophobic attitudes may prevent, or at least hinder, their use of this technology.[34]

Dorothy Roberts notes that racism also plays a role in access to assisted reproductive technologies, as doctors are far less likely to recommend fertility treatments for black women than for whites.[35] Although clinics cannot legally discriminate against potential patients on the basis of race, they can neglect to inform people of color about all possible treatments.[36] Ableist attitudes pose similar barriers to disabled people's use of assisted reproductive technologies. Many disabled women report being discouraged by their doctors and families from having children, a fact that suggests that they might not receive all the fertility assistance they need.[37] The policing of these technologies serves to reinforce the dominant vision of a world without impairment and to perpetuate the stigmatization of the queer, disabled, nonwhite body.

The case of Kijuana Chambers deserves attention here, as her experience with a Colorado fertility clinic illustrates the kind of policing reconsolidation to which Franklin refers. In 1999, Chambers went to the Rocky Mountain Women's Health Care Center (RMWHCC) for assisted insemination. After three cycles of treatment, the clinic informed Chambers that they could no longer work with her because they had "concern[s] about her ability to safely care for a child." Chambers is blind, and the clinic believed that her blindness posed a direct threat to the welfare of any future child.[38] Until she could provide an assessment from an occupational therapist attesting to her ability to raise a child, the clinic would no longer treat her. Chambers sued the RMWHCC under the Americans with Disabilities Act and Section 504 of the Rehabilitation Act, claiming that the clinic illegally discriminated against her on the basis of her disability. Sighted women, her supporters noted, were not required to provide documentation of their ability to childproof their homes or raise their children. In November 2003, a US District Court jury in Denver found in favor of the defendants, deciding that the clinic behaved appropriately in questioning Chambers's fitness. The US Tenth Circuit Court of Appeals decided in the summer of 2005 not to rehear her case, letting the lower court's decision stand.

Chambers's race (African American) and her sexual orientation (lesbian) may well have factored into the clinic's decision, but the clinic's spokespeople and legal staff, and the media, have focused primarily on Chambers's status as a single disabled woman. An article in the *Denver Post*, for example, makes no mention of Chambers's race or sexual orientation, and other news reports on the case followed suit. Given the long history of disability being seen as more medical than political in this country, the exclusive focus on Chambers's blindness guaranteed that this case would be understood by the public as a matter of common sense and child protection rather than discrimination. This is not to suggest that race played no role in Chambers's treatment; during the hearing, she was portrayed in almost animalistic terms, with witnesses testifying to her dirty underwear, disheveled appearance, and emotional outbursts, claims that at least implicitly drew on histories of racist claims about Africans' and African Americans' allegedly primitive and uncivilized nature. (Contrast this portrayal with the depiction of Duchesneau and McCullough, white, middle-class, professional women, as "selfish." The condemnation of these women varied dramatically by their racialized positions.[39]) Rather, I want to suggest that discrimination on the basis of disability, in this case blindness, is often not seen as discrimination at all, and therefore not considered as having a place in the political arena. It is assumed to be self-evident that blind women cannot parent safely or appropriately, and there is nothing discriminatory or political about asking them to prove otherwise to a medical expert (as Chambers was required to do).

In her analysis of the case, disability rights activist Laura Hershey argues that the clinic drew on

> contradictory notions about disability and help. . . . On the one hand, Chambers felt confident she could raise a child largely by herself, yet because of her stubborn refusal to prove this to anybody, she was denied treatment. On the other hand, if Chambers sometimes did ask for assistance—perhaps with finding her clothes in an unfamiliar environment, for example [as happened during an appointment at the clinic]—this was viewed as reason enough to doubt her competence.[40]

Chambers challenged the clinic's assertion that medical professionals were the best judges of her ability to raise a child, and she disputed their suggestion that an occupational therapist could provide a more accurate assessment of her assistance needs than she herself could. The jury agreed with the clinic's position, however, that clinic staff were justified in requiring "expert" documentation of Chambers's parenting abilities. Unfortunately, explains Carrie Lucas of the Colorado Cross-Disability Coalition, presumptions of incompetence are common for parents and potential parents with disabilities: "[T]he public believes we [people with disabilities] must prove ourselves before we are allowed to do the things nondisabled people consider their right."[41] The Chambers case provides a powerful example of how the use of reproductive technologies by certain people—such as disabled people, queers, single parents, people of color, or, as in this case, a disabled queer single parent of color—is patrolled and restricted, with "nontraditional" users brought under strict surveillance. This surveillance is cast, then, not as a political decision, or a potentially discriminatory one, but as an obviously necessary step toward a better life.

None of the articles tracing the reproductive choices of Sharon Duchesneau and Colleen McCullough questioned the assumption that a future without disability and deafness is superior to one with them. As in Piercy's fictional debate between the Mixers and the Shapers, no one recognized the screening out of deaf sperm donors as a political decision; indeed, it was not recognized as a decision at all because no other possibility was even conceivable. The vast majority of public reactions to these women's choices tell a story about the appropriate place of disability/deafness in the future; it is assumed that everyone, both hearing and Deaf, disabled and nondisabled, will and should prefer a nondisabled, hearing child. Thus the future allegedly invoked by the couple's actions is dangerous because it advocates an improper use of technology; technology can and should be used only to *eliminate* disability, not to *proliferate* it. Such a goal is *natural*, not *political*, and therefore neither requires nor deserves public debate.

Open to Debate? Disability and Difference in a Feminist Future

This idea that disability is best conceptualized as a problem to be eradicated brings us back to how Marge Piercy addresses disability and other differences in *Woman on the Edge of Time*. In her utopian vision of a future Mattapoisett, diversity is highly valued, with the village's inhabitants rejecting the idea of a "thin gruel" in which everyone is the same. I want to suggest, however, that the community is actually founded on an *erasure* of difference. Sexism is rooted out not through the passing of antidiscrimination laws or a changing of attitudes but by erasing reproductive differences, rendering both sexes able to breast-feed and neither able to give birth. Similarly with racism: Mattapoisett uses the brooder to mix races together; different skin tones may result, but the practice is founded on the idea that racism can never be eliminated until everyone is, essentially, the same. Piercy removes the stigma of mental disability but only on the grounds that those who are unwell voluntarily remove themselves from the community, dropping out of society until they are back to "normal." Other disabilities she eliminates entirely from her vision of the future. In Piercy's utopia the problem is not ableism, the problem is disability itself, and it can best be solved by segregating people with mental illnesses and eradicating "defective" genes from the brooder. Moreover, this elimination of disability can take place without debate or discussion; the whole community apparently supports it. In Mattapoisett the problem of disability is best solved through its eradication, segregation, and erasure.

As illustrated by *Woman on the Edge of Time*, and as manifested in the furor surrounding McCullough and Duchesneau's reproductive choices, disability is often seen as a difference that has no place in the future. Disability is a problem that must be eliminated, a hindrance to one's future opportunities, a drag on one's quality of life. Speaking directly about the Duchesneau and McCullough case, bioethicist Alta Charo argues, "The question is whether the parents have violated the sacred duty of parent-hood, which is to maximize to some reasonable degree the advantages available to their children. I'm loath to say it, but I think it's a shame to set limits on a child's potential."[42] Similar claims are made in opposition to same-sex parenting; critics argue that children raised in queer households will have a lower quality of life than children raised in heterosexual ones.[43] However, in both of these situations, it is assumed not only that disability and queerness inherently and irreversibly lower one's quality of life but also that there is only one possible understanding of "quality of life" and that everyone knows what "it" is without discussion or elaboration.

In *The Trouble with Normal*, Michael Warner condemns the use of "quality of life" rhetoric, arguing that this terminology masks dissent by taking for granted the kinds of experiences the term includes. Although he is challenging the use of "quality of life" arguments in public debates about pornography and public sex, Warner's argument resonates with cultural constructions of disability, as becomes clear when we substitute "disability" for "porn":

> The rhetoric of "quality of life" tries to isolate [disability] from political culture by pretending that there are no differences of value or opinion in it, that it therefore does not belong in the public sphere of critical exchange and opinion formation. When [people] speak of quality of life, [they] never acknowledge that different people might want different qualities in their lives, let alone that [disability] might be one of them.[44]

Susan Wendell suggests that living with disability or illness "creates valuable *ways of being* that give valuable perspectives on life and the world," ways of being that would be lost through the elimination of illness and disability.[45] She notes, for example, that adults who require assistance in the activities of daily life, such as eating, bathing, toileting, and dressing, have opportunities to think through cultural ideals of inde-pendence and self-sufficiency; these experiences can potentially lead to productive insights about intimacy, relationship, and interdependence. "If one looks at disabilities as forms of difference and takes seriously the possibility that they may be valuable," argues Wendell,

> it becomes obvious that people with disabilities have experiences, by virtue of their disabilities, which non-disabled people do not have, and which are [or can be] sources of knowledge that is not directly accessible to non-disabled people. Some of this knowledge, for example, how to live with a suffering body, would be of enor-mous practical help to most people. . . . Much of it would enrich and expand our culture, and some of it has the potential to change our thinking and our ways of life profoundly.[46]

To eliminate disability is to eliminate the possibility of discovering alternative ways of being in the world, to foreclose the possibility of recognizing and valuing our interdependence.

To be clear, no policy decisions have been made as to which "defects" should be eliminated or about what constitutes a "defective" gene; with few exceptions, assisted reproductive technology remains largely unregulated in the United States. But the proliferation of prenatal testing and the increasing availability of pre-implantation genetic diagnosis certainly send a message about the proper and expected approach to disability. Public discussions of these technologies have lagged far behind their use and development, and they rarely include the perspectives of disabled people. As H-Dirksen L. Bauman argues, "Presumptions about the horrors of deafness are usually made by those not living Deaf lives."[47] The Prenatally and Postnatally Diagnosed Conditions Awareness Act (2008) is a step in the right direction, mandating that women receive comprehensive information about disability prior to making decisions about their pregnancies, but it remains unclear how well this policy will be funded or enforced. Moreover, as the debate surrounding Duchesneau and McCullough's reproductive choices makes clear, selecting for disability remains a highly controversial position, and hypothetical disabled children continue to be used to justify genetic research and selective abortion. "Curing" and eliminating disability—whether through stem cell research or selective abortion—is almost always presented as a universally valued goal about which there can, and should, be no disagreement.

I want to suggest that stories of Deaf lesbians intentionally striving for Deaf babies be read as counternarratives to mainstream stories about the necessity of a cure for deafness and disability, about the dangers of nonnormative queer parents having children. Their stories challenge the feasibility of technological promises of an "amazing future" in which impairment is cured through genetic and medical intervention, thereby resisting a compulsory able-bodied/able-minded heterosexuality that insists upon normal minds/bodies. It is precisely this challenge that has animated the hostile responses these families have received. Their choice to choose deafness suggests that reproductive technology can be used as more than a means to screen out alleged defects, that disability cannot ever fully disappear, that not everyone craves an able-bodied/able-minded future, that there might be a place for bodies with limited, odd, or queer movements and orientations, and that disability and queerness can indeed be desirable both in the future as well as now.

The story of the Deaf lesbians, Candace McCullough and Sharon Duchesneau, is only one among many. An ever-increasing number of memoirs, essays, and poems about life with a disability, as well as theoretical analyses of disability and able-bodiedness, tell other stories about disability, providing alternatives to the narratives of eradication and cure offered by Marge Piercy in *Woman on the Edge of Time*. There are stories of people embracing their bodies, proudly proclaiming disability as sexy, powerful, and worthy; tales of disabled parents and parents with disabled children refusing to accept that a bright future for our children precludes disability and asserting the right to bear and keep children with disabilities; and narratives of families refusing to accept the normalization of their bodies through surgical interventions and the normalization of their desires through heterocentric laws and homophobic condemnations. These stories deserve telling, and the issues they raise demand debate and dissent.

It is not that these tales are any less partial or contested than the others in public circulation; they, too, can be used to serve multiple and contradictory positions. Indeed, Lennard Davis argues that we need to question whether these kinds of reproductive decisions—choosing deafness and disability—are "radical ways of fighting against oppression" or "technological fixes in the service of a conservative, essentialist agenda."[48] I would only add that the two are not mutually exclusive; the same choice can serve both agendas. Just as selecting for girls can be as problematic as selecting for boys, with both choices potentially reliant on narrow gender norms and expectations, selecting for disability has the potential to reify categories of able-bodiedness as much as deselecting disability does.[49] What is needed then are examinations of how particular choices function in particular contexts; what does it mean for lesbian parents to choose deafness in this context, or a single mother to refuse to terminate a pregnancy after receiving a Down diagnosis in that context? Such explorations are impossible as long as selecting for disability remains largely inconceivable, as long as we all assume—or are assumed to assume—that disability cannot belong in feminist visions of the future and that its absence merits no debate.

4 A Future for Whom?

Passing on Billboard Liberation

[Advertising] is a world that works by *abstraction*, a potential place or state of being situated not in the present but in an imagined future with the promise to the consumer of things "you" will have, a lifestyle you can take part in.

—Marita Sturken and Lisa Cartwright, "Consumer Culture
and the Manufacturing of Desire"

"Super man," the billboard exclaims, the unfamiliar gap between the two words emphasizing both the noun and its adjective. Below this phrase is the word "STRENGTH," followed by the imperative "*Pass It On.*" At the bottom, in small print, runs the name and web address of the organization behind this public relations campaign: Values.com/Foundation for a Better Life. The "super man" referenced in the caption is, of course, the late Christopher Reeve, the white actor who starred in a series of *Superman* films in the 1980s before becoming a quadriplegic in a riding accident in 1995. A black-and-white photograph of Reeve's head and shoulders consumes the left half of the billboard; the only marker of Reeve's disability is the ventilator tube that is just visible at the bottom of the frame. Reeve smiles slightly, looking thoughtfully into the camera and the eyes of passersby.

Quadriplegics are not often presented as the embodiment of strength, but this sign suggests that, in Reeve's case, such a designation is accurate. According to the billboard, although Reeve was no longer able to run or jump or climb, he remained a strong man; his strength simply lay more in his character than in his body. Prior to his injuries, Reeve was "Superman," a fictional hero capable of leaping buildings and bending steel. Later, as a disabled person, Reeve was not Superman but a *super* man. The billboard informs its audience that Reeve's masculinity not only remained intact postinjury but increased, an improvement due primarily to his strong character and integrity. Indeed, his masculinity, disability, and strength are presented in the billboard as intricately related, each supporting the other: it was his disability that provided him the opportunity to prove his strength, and his strength testified to his masculinity. Reeve's ability to triumph over his disabilities, to continue living and working even after a life-changing injury, marked him as strong, and this strength in turn marked him as a super man. The billboard urges viewers to preach this message of self-improvement, to spread the word about the importance of developing and maintaining strength of character, even in, or especially in, the face of adversity.

According to the organization's website, "The Foundation for a Better Life is not affiliated with any political groups or religious organizations" but is rather an apolitical organization interested in fostering individual and collective betterment through values education and engagement.[1] It is this positioning that I want to examine here: this attempt to depoliticize notions of community, this assumption of shared values, and this articulation of what a better life entails. By presenting these concepts as apolitical, the Foundation for a Better Life (FBL) renders them natural, accepted, commonsense, and therefore beyond the scope of debate or discussion. The FBL operates on the assumption that we all know and agree what a better life entails, and what values are necessary to achieve it; there is no need for argument or critique. Representations of disability and illness play a large role in this campaign, with a significant number of billboards praising individuals with disabilities for having the strength of character to "overcome" their disabilities. The depoliticization mandated by these billboards and the FBL itself is made possible through reference to the disabled body; in other words, it is not just that the FBL depoliticizes disability, but that it does so in order to depoliticize all the values featured in its campaign. Indeed, the presence of the disabled body is used to render this campaign not as ideology but as common sense.

In order to show that the depoliticization mandated by these billboards is made possible through reference to the disabled body, I first examine the parameters of this "better life" sketched out by the FBL, highlighting the exclusions inherent in such articulations. Not all bodies, practices, or identities are welcome in this better life, especially those figures deemed too queer, or too political, or too dependent to be of value. Next, I uncover the ways in which these billboards strategically deploy this depoliticized view of disability to present their entire ideology as beyond reproach. Finally, I want to explore the possibility of queering and cripping these billboards, of offering alternative, and multiple, conceptions of what constitutes a better life. How might we turn this iconography back on itself, making apparent its political assumptions about "community values" by challenging its deployment of disability and disabled bodies?

Super Man's Values and the Quest for a Better Life

Persuading passersby of the importance of self-improvement, and encouraging them to engage in values-oriented conversations, is the raison d'être of the Foundation for a Better Life, the sponsor of the Reeve billboard and others like it. A privately funded nonprofit organization based in Colorado, the FBL uses its website and a series of billboards, bus shelter posters, and television public service announcements to advocate personal responsibility and character development.[2] According to the website, the FBL's mission is to remind people of the importance of "quality values." In order to promote these values, each of the organization's print pieces celebrates a different value, from ambition to self-respect, by highlighting a person or event that embodies that trait. The celebrities and private citizens featured in the campaign donated their images to the FBL in support of its efforts to foster values-based communities and individuals. In addition to the Reeve piece on strength, there are billboards of a New York City firefighter on 9/11 (who modeled *courage*), Benjamin Franklin (displaying *ingenuity*), and even the animated figure Shrek (who encourages you to *believe in yourself*), among others. All three of the "courage" signs are illustrated with an adult male figure (a 9/11 firefighter, a protestor at Tiananmen Square, and Muhammad Ali), suggesting that the values of the FBL's community adhere, at least partly, to traditional gender roles.[3] The values "helping others," "volunteering," "compassion," and "love," for example, are represented by women.

There are fifty-eight different billboards in the group's portfolio, almost a third of which feature disabled people[4] who, as the captions make clear, have overcome the limitations of their minds and bodies through the development of individual values: Muhammad Ali, whose face is shown in a black-and-white photograph edged by darkness, embodies *courage* in recognizing that, as someone with Parkinson's disease, "His biggest fight yet isn't in the ring"; Adam Bender, who lost a leg to cancer, stands one-legged in his baseball uniform as a symbol of *overcoming* ("Threw cancer a curve ball"); Brooke Ellison, smiling as she poses in her wheelchair and wearing her graduation gown, was able to graduate from Harvard ("Quadriplegic. A-. Harvard") because of her *determination*; Michael J. Fox, depicted in black-and-white with his face partly in shadow, models *optimism* ("Determined to outfox Parkinson's"); Whoopi Goldberg, pictured with lowered head, furrowed brow, and her eyes looking up at the camera through her dreadlocks, "Overcaem [sic] dyslexia" through *hard work*; Bethany Hamilton, a young surfer who lost an arm during a shark attack, demonstrates *rising above* adversity ("Me, quit? Never") as she poses on the beach next to her bitten surfboard; Dick Hoyt models *devotion* by pushing his adult son Rick in a modified racing wheelchair along a wooded path ("Dad's been behind him for 65 marathons"); Helen Keller, depicted as a young girl reading Braille and wearing an abundantly frilly dress, is praised for her *foresight* because she "could only see possibilities"; Christopher Reeve, as noted above, is a "Super man" because of his *strength*; Alexandra Scott, a young girl pictured sitting behind her homemade lemonade stand, is a figure of *inspiration* for raising millions of dollars for pediatric cancer research ("Raised $1M to fight cancer. Including hers"); Marlon Shirley, poised to begin a race with his sleek prosthetic leg, epitomizes *overcoming* ("Lost Leg. Not heart"); and Eric Weihenmayer, a blind hiker photographed in profile on a snowy mountaintop, succeeded ("Climbed Everest. Blind") thanks to his *vision*.[5]

In keeping with the foundation's focus on personal accountability, most of the people featured in these billboards are pictured alone, several of them depicted against an empty dark background. The accompanying text makes clear that whatever suc-cesses these people have achieved, whether graduating from college or reaching Ever-est, were achieved solely through an individual adherence to "community-accepted values." Within this individualist framework, disability is presented as something to be overcome through personal achievement and dedication. Although the Hoyt father-son team seemingly departs from this iconography of individualism, disability in this image remains firmly within a private familial framework; not only is a family member the only community imagined for Rick Hoyt, "devotion"—a virtue laden with notions of private faith and individual rather than social action—is presented as the operative value here. Moreover, despite their label "Team Hoyt," the father is positioned as the virtuous one; he is the agent of devotion and his disabled son its passive recipient.

In case the message of the billboards is too ambiguous, the FBL's website clearly delineates the group's perspective: by encouraging "adherence to a set of quality val-ues through personal accountability and by raising the level of expectations of perfor-mance of all individuals regardless of religion or race," the FBL places a high premium on individual responsibility. The billboards are intended "to remind individuals they are accountable and empowered with the ability to take responsibility for their lives and to promote a set of values that sees them through their failures and capitalizes on their successes."[6]

This narrative of overcoming is made explicit in the texts featuring Adam Bender, Whoopi Goldberg, Bethany Hamilton, and Marlon Shirley, but it underlies the other signs as well: Eric Weihenmayer, for example, overcomes the limitations of his eyesight by relying on his metaphoric *vision*, an intangible virtue that permits him to achieve a difficult feat, while Brooke Ellison and Christopher Reeve overcome quadriplegia through their respective *determination* and *strength*.[7] Disability appears as an indi-vidual physical problem that can best be overcome (and should be overcome) through strength of character and adherence to an established set of community values.

This focus on personal responsibility precludes any discussion of social, political, or collective responsibility. There are no billboards touting solidarity, or social change, or community development; none of the images celebrate disparate groups coming together to engage in coalition work. There is no recognition of ableism or discrimina-tion or oppression in these materials, only an insistence that individuals take respon-sibility for their own successes and failures. As a result, disability is depoliticized, pre-sented as a fact of life requiring determination and courage, not as a system marking some bodies, ways of thinking, and patterns of movement as deviant and unworthy.

This depoliticization is exacerbated by the campaign's erasure of the work of dis-ability rights activists. In the FBL worldview, disabled people thrive not because of civil rights laws and protection from discrimination, but because of their personal integrity, courage, and ability to overcome obstacles. Thus, Ellison's ability to go to Harvard is attributed solely to her individual determination, which, although a fac-tor in her success (and certainly a factor in her A- average), was surely facilitated by accessible buildings, antidiscrimination policies, and laws mandating equitable and inclusive education for disabled people. Her education was, in key ways, made possible by the disability rights activists who struggled before, and after, her.

Disability rights activists, however, aren't the only ones erased in this particular billboard, and it is worth sitting with the Ellison image a little longer in order to highlight the gendered assumptions of this campaign. Brooke Ellison's mother, Jean, was surely as determined as her daughter when it came to Brooke's education. Jean Ellison lived with Brooke during her tenure at Harvard, attending classes with her, helping with her personal care, and serving as her scribe during exams: doing whatever it took, in other words, to help Brooke survive and flourish at Harvard. Ellison's profile on the FBL website does acknowledge that she excelled at Harvard "[w]ith the tireless help of her mother," but this help is made invisible by the billboard image and text. Unlike Dick Hoyt, who is publicly celebrated for the (alleged) sacrifices he has made to assist his son, and lifted up as the embodiment of devotion, Jean Ellison is nowhere to be found in the image of her daughter. Comparing the representations of these two parent-child teams, one could easily argue that gender plays a role here: we expect women, as mothers, to devote their lives to their children, an expectation that then renders their devotion banal and uninteresting; but male, fatherly, devotion continues to be treated as an anomaly and therefore deserving of surprised celebration.

The FBL's attention to individual virtue obscures the ableist attitudes inherent in these billboards. Reeve appears strong and "super" to many Americans, and Ali "courageous," simply by virtue of their living with a disability. In the logic of ableism, anyone who can handle such an (allegedly) horrible life must be strong; a lesser man would have given up in despair years ago. Indeed, Reeve's refusal to "give up" is precisely why the FBL selected Reeve for their model of strength; in the "billboard backstories" section of their website, they praise Reeve for trying to "beat paralysis and the spinal cord injuries" rather than "giv[ing] up." Asserting that Goldberg is successful because of her hard work suggests that other people with dyslexia and learning disabilities who have not met with similar success have simply failed to engage in hard work; unlike Whoopi Goldberg, they are apparently unwilling to devote themselves to success. Similarly, by positioning Weihenmayer's ascent of Everest as a matter of vision, the FBL implies that most blind people, who have not ascended Everest or accomplished equivalently astounding feats, are lacking not only eyesight but vision. The disabled people populating these billboards epitomize the paradoxical figure of the supercrip: supercrips are those disabled figures favored in the media, products of either extremely low expectations (disability by definition means incompetence, so anything a disabled person does, no matter how mundane or banal, merits exaggerated praise) or extremely high expectations (disabled people must accomplish incredibly difficult, and therefore inspiring, tasks to be worthy of nondisabled attention).

The individuals featured in these billboards have been decontextualized and their lives have been depoliticized. They have been removed from the realm of health-care inequalities, inaccessible buildings, and discriminatory hiring practices. Those who have succeeded do not need legislative assistance because they have strong values; those who have failed simply lack those values and are in need not of a more equitable society but of character education. According to the FBL and its billboards, disability is not a political issue but a character issue, and should be addressed as such. There is no mention of the ways in which these individuals differ by race, gender, or class, presenting everyone as equally capable of succeeding, as possessing equal opportunities and resources. Reeve's many accomplishments, for example, are presented as solely the result of his immense inner strength of character; his reliance on a huge staff of attendants, therapists, and doctors—all made possible because of his personal wealth and quality insurance coverage—go unmentioned. All it takes is strength to survive, and thrive.

In this focus on individual virtue and personal responsibility, every other aspect of these individuals' lives is stripped away, making disability, and the overcoming of that disability, the only salient characteristic of their lives. Muhammad Ali's well-known battles with racism and his public protests against US imperialism in Vietnam—surely instances in which he embodied courage by speaking his conscience and challenging injustice—are erased in the presentation of Parkinson's disease as his biggest fight yet, or as his only fight outside of the ring.[8] To address those fights, the FBL would have to expand its vision of a better life to include not simply individual virtues but collective action. It would necessitate a contextualizing of disability as only a part of the fabric of people's lives, one always already inflected by categories of race, class, and gender. Such a portrayal would then require a reckoning with the politics of disability, thereby challenging the FBL's positioning of disability as mere fact of the mind/body, a presentation that enables their depiction of the entire Pass It On campaign as apolitical, noncontroversial, and commonsense. In other words, the campaign relies heavily on a depoliticized vision of disability in order to depoliticize the entire campaign.

A Better Life for Whom? Foundational Foreclosures

According to the FBL's website, the group is concerned about the current state of American culture and the direction in which the country is moving. It offers these billboards as part of its vision for what a better America would look like and what values it would embody. The very name of the organization—the Foundation for a Better Life—establishes the group's concern with the future and testifies to its belief that the principles it celebrates are integral to achieving this "better life." In an early version of the FAQ section of its website, the organization argues that the future depends on individual Americans dedicating themselves to "community values" and values-based education:

> The Foundation encourages others to step up to a higher level and then to pass on those positive values they have learned. These seemingly small examples of

individuals living values-based lives may not change the world, but collectively they will make a difference. And in the process help make the world a better place for everyone. After all, developing values and passing them on to others is the Foundation for a Better Life.[9]

The FBL mission statement claims that the organization's sole purpose is to remind people of the importance of the "quality values" that "make a difference in our communities." In recent years, the website has become increasingly interactive, and there is now a section where visitors can suggest people and values for future billboards. At first glance, this shift seems to signal a new openness on the part of the organization, a willingness to see the values we live by as subject to debate and disagreement, but the FBL continues to define the terms of the debate. Commentators must choose from a select list of values in making their recommendations: "perseverance" is an acceptable virtue, for example, while "resistance" is not; values-based communities apparently have room for "volunteering" but not "activism." Moreover, every posting on the site is subject to the organization's terms and conditions, and there is not a single negative or critical post on the FBL site. A values-based life may be key to the health of the community, but it is the FBL, not local communities, that determines what those values are. Nor, for that matter, is there any discussion of what "community" means in this context and whom the term was intended to include. Nonetheless, the Pass It On campaign has been running on billboards, on television stations, and in movie theaters nationwide for over a decade, suggesting that the FBL envisions a coherent national community with a single set of shared values. But what are these community values? Who constitutes the community imagined here, and based on what criteria? Whose better life is this?

Wholly absent from the website are details about the FBL itself: there is no address given for the organization, nor is there a description of its history or a directory of its members. According to Gary Dixon, identified in press releases as the president of the FBL, the family who created and funded the FBL wants to remain anonymous, but media reports and tax returns link the organization to billionaire developer Philip Anschutz and the Anschutz Family Foundation.[10] Since its inception in 1982, the Anschutz Foundation has supported a range of conservative organizations. In the early 1990s, it supported the antigay organization Colorado for Family Values, which was one of the driving forces behind Colorado's Amendment 2; declared unconstitutional by the US Supreme Court in 1996, this amendment to the state constitution would have prohibited local antidiscrimination laws on behalf of gays, lesbians, and bisexuals. More recently, the Anschutz Foundation has provided financial support to the Institute for American Values, which runs antipornography campaigns, warns of the dangers of single-mother households, supports reforms to make divorces more difficult to acquire, and favors marriage incentives for low-income people. If these affiliations provide a hint of what the "better life" promised by the FBL entails, then the future they envision is certainly a heteronormative one.

Although individuals with disabilities play a starring role in the Pass It On campaign, they are not the primary or intended audience for these billboards. They appear in these billboards to inspire—and contain—the nondisabled, who are the target audience for these spots. "If even severely disabled people like Christopher Reeve and Brooke Ellison can develop these values and improve themselves," the signs imply, "then so can you. Unlike them, you have no excuse. Stop complaining, buck up, work hard and overcome."

Visitors to the FBL website can post comments on each billboard, and even a cursory reading of the posts makes clear that (nondisabled) viewers respond in exactly this way to these images. As one respondent wrote regarding the Bethany Hamilton sign, "[She] is a inspiration. For all those who blame others or circumstances, I will say—'look at Bethany Hamilton.'" R. H. in Utah internalizes this message, writing in response to the Reeve billboard: "I printed this out/cut it out and thumbtacked it to my pod wall at work. I see it everyday and I am reminded that I am not paralyzed and I can do this! . . . My life isn't so hard—just somedays it feels like it is." Many of the comments regarding the disability billboards echo this notion that (nondisabled) viewers should be grateful for what they have because things could be much worse, a "much worse" best illustrated by the disabled body.[11]

The billboard format exacerbates this contrast. Each of these images is located far above ground level, so that passersby literally have to look up at the pictures of the virtuous people towering over them. This difference in scale mimics the difference in scale nondisabled viewers trace between themselves and the disabled people in the billboards: "Their problems are huge—paralysis, blindness, amputation—and mine are small because I'm not disabled."

Through these messages of individualism and compliance, the disabled bodies in these billboards are used to push other disabled bodies aside, beyond the margins of these texts. Populating the margins of the FBL billboards are those other disabled people, the ones who haven't managed to graduate from Harvard, or climb Mount Everest, or sport high-tech prosthetic limbs. The ones who demand and require access to quality elementary education, or who protest the institutionalization of mostly low-income disabled people, or who refuse to accept quietly the cultural narratives of cure and assimilation. The ones who aren't interested in easy celebrations of community values but rather in the right to live within one's community, on one's own terms. The ones who recognize that the marginalization of disabled people is due not to a lack of determination or hard work or courage but to pervasive and persistent economic, political, and social exclusions. These disabled bodies are relegated to the margins of the better futures promised by the FBL: we're admitted only insofar as we promise not to complain but only to inspire.

This articulation of a better life, illustrated through the strategic use of disabled bodies, conjures not only an able-bodied future, but a heteronormative one. Joining the failed disabled bodies on the margins of these billboards are the failed bodies of queers and other deviants. If the possession of already-agreed-upon and extrapolitical values are necessary for inclusion in the FBL dreamscape, then queers will be excluded by default. If, as David Halperin argues, queerness entails "a social space for the construction of different identities, for the elaboration of various types of relationships, for the development of new cultural forms," then queerness cannot—and would not—coexist with the FBL.[12] Rather than simply accepting such values as self-evident, queer theory would insist upon an interrogation of such values. Whose values are these, and whose experiences do they take for granted?

Although the FBL presents itself as committed to and concerned about diversity and tolerance of difference—two values highlighted on the organization's website—it is a diversity that is used to consolidate a white able-bodied heteronormativity. Images on the FBL website are carefully composed of people of all ages, religious affiliations, and racial/ethnic groups, but the insistence on shared community values constrains and contains that diversity. There is no recognition that different communities might value different characteristics at different historical moments and in different contexts. On the contrary, the FBL argues that its values, and its entire campaign, "transcend any particular religion or nationality," evoking a unified global community coming together to lead values-based lives. The FBL's "better life" and "positive values" rhetoric takes for granted the notion that "we" all agree what constitutes a better life, what values we hold dear, and, for that matter, who "we" are.

This taken-for-grantedness is made possible, at least in part, through strategic recourse to the disabled body. While the few FBL billboards that draw explicitly on 9/11 or make direct calls to patriotism have met with some criticism, the remainder of the billboards, and particularly those in what I call the disability series, serve to shield the entire FBL campaign from scrutiny. Images of inspirational cripples, from Reeve to Ellison, are used to testify to a shared set of values with which we can all easily agree. Who would publicly dispute the description of Mohammad Ali as courageous, or Alexandra Scott as inspirational, or Brooke Ellison as the embodiment of determination? Who would deny the value of perseverance, or inner strength, or foresight, particularly when embodied by people from a marginalized group? As one of my students said when I mentioned this campaign to her, "What kind of person says bad things about a billboard praising a little girl with cancer?"

Indeed, I can find little public criticism of the billboards, the "Pass It On" campaign, or the FBL itself.[13] A LexisNexis search turns up a few exposés on Philip Anschutz (his business deals, particularly his ownership of Qwest Communications, have sparked a handful of lawsuits), but nothing critical about the billboards themselves. Even in the context of an extended profile of Anschutz, the *New York Times*, for example, argues that these billboards are "largely noncontroversial, apolitical, and multifaith," ending the discussion there.[14] Anschutz, in other words, merits critical attention by the press, but the billboards apparently do not. There is no need for a critical look at these billboards because there is nothing there, no agenda, no politics, no exclusions. In the words of the FBL, "In this day and age, it can be hard to believe that an organization's only goal is to encourage others to do good—but that really is why we exist."

If this lack of critical attention is any indication, the FBL is being taken at their word, understood as existing only to foster good works and character development. But the predominance of disabled bodies in these billboards demands greater attention. What work does disability do in this campaign, and what are the assumptions on which these signs rely?

In order to address these questions, I want to deconstruct two more billboards, one that clearly belongs in the disability series of images, and one that, at least on the surface, seems not to be about disability at all. I first saw the Marlon Shirley billboard in 2006, three years into the US occupation of Iraq.[15] Shirley's amputation is not war-related; as his FBL backstory makes clear, his left foot was amputated in 1984 as the result of a childhood accident. The billboard itself, however, doesn't give any details of Shirley's injury, and it seems likely that at least some viewers will imagine this young black male amputee as one of the 45,329 US service members injured in Iraq and Afghanistan.[16] Shirley's age, gender, and race, together with his athleticism, feed into this misperception of him as an injured veteran; young men continue to be the image of the US military, news profiles of disabled athletes tend to focus on disabled veterans, and Shirley's youthful muscularity suggest his amputation was the result of accident rather than illness. Moreover, the nature of Shirley's impairment increases the likelihood that he will be read as an injured veteran. Although an astonishing number of veterans are returning from Iraq and Afghanistan with traumatic brain injuries and/or PTSD, the figure of the amputee remains the predominant image of the disabled veteran in the media.[17]

What are we to make of the fact that this image surfaced in this particular moment, as many wounded soldiers were returning home and attempting to claim disability assistance and health care? Or at a time when soldiers with PTSD were being denied treatment and discharged because they allegedly had preexisting conditions? What might "overcoming" mean in such a context? Or a focus on personal responsibility and individual character development? To be clear: I'm not suggesting that the Pentagon is behind the FBL, determining which images appear when; nor do I mean to suggest that the FBL is opposed to granting any medical care or social services to disabled veterans. But I do want to draw attention to the ideological frameworks and effects of these billboards. Given the other billboards in this campaign, and the responses viewers have had to such billboards, it seems reasonable to assume that many viewers will read Shirley's body and the accompanying text (Lost leg, not heart / OVERCOMING / Pass It On) as a reminder that all people, including wounded veterans, need to pull themselves up by their own bootstraps. The sign's imperative to overcome, and then to pass on such overcoming to others, makes clear that such personal achievement is the only acceptable response to tragedy; only then will we have the foundation for a better life.

To make clear how much the effectiveness of this message relies on the disabled body, I turn now to a billboard that doesn't appear to have anything to do with disability. In this billboard, Liz Murray, a young white woman, is seated in a classroom, holding a psychology textbook and smiling slightly at the camera. "From homeless to Harvard," the billboard proclaims, "AMBITION." I first saw this billboard in Austin, Texas, in the northern part of the city. The sign was directly over a clothes donation box and a bus shelter—two sites marked by poverty and homelessness—at an intersection with panhandlers on each corner. Looking up at the sign and down at the donation box, the insidiousness of this campaign hit me hard. How might the sight of this billboard affect drivers' responses to the panhandlers at the stoplight? Or how might it affect their responses to the city of Austin's changes to its panhandling laws, changes intended to push the homeless away from city streets and neighborhoods? More broadly, how might it influence their stance toward the public sector itself, and moves to further shrink public services? Does a values-based life mean that we should preach ambition to the homeless? Is ambition all that the homeless lack? Surely Murray's journey to Harvard was more complicated than that, but the juxtaposition of her smiling face and the donation box suggests otherwise.

Although this particular billboard does not seem at first to fit in my disability series, I want to position it as such. Not only are many homeless people disabled, homelessness is a threat all-too-real for many disabled people; homelessness *is* a disability issue. But even Murray's own "billboard backstory" draws a link with disability. Her parents were both drug addicts when she was a child, and it was their addiction that caused them to lose their housing. Her mother eventually died of AIDS, and Murray nursed her father through a long illness. These details emerge in reading her story on the FBL website, as do examples of the many kinds of assistance she received in her childhood. The sound-bite format of the billboard eclipses these details, however, completely removing her story from any social or political context.

Responses to the billboard suggest that this removal of context has been effective. Rafael, in Salinas, California, writes on the FBL website: "Thank you for this wonderful billboard and its prime location. I saw this billboard driving along highway 99 in California's Central Valley where unemployment and poverty is at double digits. Ambition lets us all know that everything is possible if you go after it." But can ambition really solve the problem of unemployment? How is Murray's story being used to push other bodies—disabled and nondisabled—out of the margins of the billboards, those who haven't managed to ride the wave of personal responsibility to success? Personal responsibility becomes the only factor that matters, the only thing standing between the homeless and a Harvard education.

What I want to suggest is that the predominance of disability billboards in the FBL campaign makes it easier for most people to read this kind of decontextualized paean to personal responsibility as apolitical and benign. Queer theorists Lauren Berlant and Lee Edelman suggest that the figure of the child is used to render certain positions as extrapolitical, as beyond the realm of politics, and I suggest that the disabled body performs a similar function within the logic of the FBL. To quote Edelman,

> Such "self-evident" one-sidedness—the affirmation of a value so unquestioned, because so obviously unquestionable, as that of the Child whose innocence solicits our defense—is precisely, of course, what distinguishes public service announcements from the partisan discourse of political argumentation. But it is also, I suggest, what makes such announcements so oppressively political . . . shap[ing] the logic within which the political can be thought.[18]

In the case of the FBL, the "unquestioned because so obviously unquestionable" position is that of praising disabled people for overcoming their disabilities. What could possibly be wrong with highlighting the character of people who have worked hard and succeeded?

This question runs throughout online discussions of the billboard campaign. Anytime someone challenges the neoliberal demands of the billboards, there are readers who respond with calls for more trust and less cynicism. As one commentator puts it, "Take the message you are given and stop trying to decipher hidden intentions. [I]t'll do you a lot of good."[19] Even some of those who are suspicious of Philip Anschutz's involvement with the FBL (and who therefore worry that there might be "hidden intentions") make distinctions between Anschutz's politics and the values he promotes. Maria Niles of *BlogHer*, for example, is wary of Anschutz's involvement, casting her politics as far different from his, but admits to liking and appreciating the uplifting messages of the billboards.[20] Justin Berrier, writing on the *MediaMatters* blog, stresses that he has "no problem with the Foundation for a Better Life's values messages" even as he condemns the secrecy surrounding Anschutz's involvement with the organization.[21] Respondents to a critical story on Portland's Indymedia site react similarly, with one explaining that his "concerns are hardly the message, but clearly the messenger"; another notes that, "while the info on Anschutz is disturbing to me, and I don't like the Unity/Spirit of America stuff, I thought the other messages passed along were good."[22]

There are bloggers challenging the FBL billboards, and some of them challenge the campaign for its exclusionary notions of community, much as I do here. But their critiques are almost always leveled at the explicitly, or recognizably, political billboards, those that make explicit reference to patriotism and nationalism. The disability billboards are given a pass, either not discussed at all or critiqued only for their "saccharine" or "cheesy" tone. Yet, as I detail here, the disability series is also political, and those images play a significant role in creating the exclusionary, and coercive, notions of community that pervade the campaign as a whole. We need to recognize and challenge this strategic deployment of disability, acknowledging that rhetorics of disability acceptance and inclusion can be used to decidedly un-crip ends.[23]

Advertising, including public service announcements, works by "reflect[ing] preexisting ideological narratives," and the FBL billboards are successful because they draw on commonsense, familiar understandings of disability.[24] The use of real-istic photographs facilitates the reception of these billboards as truth. As Rosemarie Garland-Thomson explains, "Photography's immediacy and claim to truth inten-sify what it tells viewers about disability, at once shaping and registering the public perception of disability."[25] Seeing disability as the site of and for personal struggle, overcoming, and triumph—one of the dominant frames for understanding disability in this culture—makes it easier to overlook the ideological underpinnings of this campaign.

As these responses suggest, most of the FBL billboards—and by extension, the entire Pass It On campaign—are seen to be not about politics but about hope and community and goodness. And it is the presence of disabled minds/bodies that makes this message possible, not because disabled minds/bodies are recognized as embodying hope, community, or goodness, but because we assume that anyone who finds Christopher Reeve inspiring or wants to say kind things about Marlon Shirley must embody these characteristics. These ads are effectively cast as beyond reproach because what oppositional stance could one possibly take to these texts? There is no need to explore whose values are celebrated in this campaign, whose bodies are seen as belonging to the community, whose practices are valued. As a result, those failed disabled bodies inhabiting the margins of the billboards remain on the margins, as do the bodies of others unable to meet the FBL's standard of virtue, unwelcome in the FBL community.

But "community" rests on the notion that people can come together in consensus and unity, putting aside their differences in order to create a unified whole grounded in common experiences and common values. This presumption of unity, however, excludes differences and dissent, thereby creating a self-perpetuating homogeneity.[26] Attempts to determine in advance how to adjudicate community values run the risk of solidifying existing understandings of community, thereby making it much more difficult to shift or expand definitions of "community" in the future. Current under-standings of such concepts then become the standard against which to measure future articulations, potentially keeping in place barriers to access that are not as yet rec-ognized as such, thereby prohibiting or marginalizing other bodies, identities, and practices. Instead, following Judith Butler, I propose "open[ing] up the field of possibil-ity . . . without dictating which kinds of possibilities ought to be realized."[27]

Queercrip Futures

There is another billboard in the Foundation for a Better Life's disability series that I have yet to address. Their final disability-related sign features a young baseball player dressed in his team uniform and holding a baseball bat. He sits proudly in his wheel-chair, and his fellow wheelchair-baseball teammates arc in a semicircle behind him, with a few nondisabled spectators standing in the borders of the photo. The word OPPORTUNITY appears on the right side of the billboard, over the phrase "A league of their own." According to the text, these young baseball players are flourishing thanks to their being given the opportunity to play in a "league of their own."

Drawing on the tools of feminist, queer, and disability studies scholars, I want to read this billboard differently, to crip and queer its representations. My oppositional reading begins by contrasting the picture in this billboard with the others in the disability series. This piece touting "opportunity" is the only one in which a disabled person is situated in a community, surrounded by other disabled people and their friends and family. Unlike Ali, Scott, Reeve, Keller, Goldberg, Ellison, Hamilton, Shirley, Fox, Bender, and Weihenmayer, all of whom are depicted alone, or Hoyt, who is featured with his "devoted" father, the baseball player is presented as part of a much larger community, one in which he is an active participant. He has gained recognition not for an individual achievement but for teamwork and collective action. Such a depiction seems appropriate, as this billboard is the only one to tout a value that hints at a larger social and political context. Unlike courage, determination, and hard work, each of which typically describes the character of an individual person, opportunity positions someone within a larger field of social relations. This sign, then, can be interpreted as a recognition that disabled people (like nondisabled people) need opportunities and resources in order to thrive. Rather than preaching a message of charity or individual accountability, this sign can be interpreted as a call for increased social responsibility, for working to ensure that all people have access to opportunity.

But this kind of reading requires working hard against the grain, and, as feminist and queer scholars have long noted, such readings can be far from satisfying.[28] For, even as I describe my imagined interpretation, I know that most viewers read this image through a heavily sentimental lens. Rosemarie Garland-Thomson argues that images of disabled children epitomize the sentimentalization of disability, a process by which disability appears as "a problem to solve, an obstacle to eliminate, a challenge to meet," thereby motivating the viewer to act on behalf of the "sympathetic, helpless child."[29] Within such a framework, it makes sense that the billboard backstory for this image includes quotes only from the parents of these children, not from the children themselves. We learn that the boy in the center of the frame is Justin, and that he has cerebral palsy, but we learn these facts only through the words of Justin's (unidentified) parent. Justin's visible presence in the billboard but verbal absence in the backstory suggests yet again that it is the nondisabled whom the FBL most wants to reach. Rather than read this billboard as a story about increased social responsibility, or about the vibrant communities that exist among and with disabled people, viewers are to discover yet another paean to personal virtues such as charity and tolerance. "Opportunity" reads not as part of a collective responsibility, as something tightly woven in structures of privilege and oppression, but as a personal obligation to those imagined as less fortunate than oneself, a private gift completely divorced from ableism, discrimination, or inequality.

Instead of resigning myself to the existing images, then, I want to imagine another disability series, another set of billboards that trumpet "a better life." My disability series imagines "community values" not in the FBL understanding, in which discrete individuals manifest a set of already-agreed-upon values in their own private lives, but in a feminist/queer/crip understanding of community and *coalition* values, in which both the parameters of the community and the values praised within it are open to debate. What does "courage," "determination," or "opportunity" mean? What kinds of practices and attitudes do they include, and which do they exclude? Who is involved in determining the characteristics valued in a particular community? Who is included in—or excluded from—the community itself? How can different communities come together to form coalitions? Rather than accepting the FBL proclamation that *unity* is "what makes us great," I envision a media campaign that favors *dissent* at least as much as unity, that recognizes political protest and activism as signs of courage, that is as concerned with collective responsibility and accountability as personal.

I am not the first to suggest alternate billboards to the ones created by the FBL. Billboard activists across the country have "liberated" some of these signs, with the "What makes us great/UNITY" billboard attracting the most attention. In the FBL version of this billboard, a young white girl waves an American flag while sitting on the shoulders of an adult male, perhaps her father. There are other people and flags in the background, suggesting a patriotic rally of some kind; the "billboard backstory" confirms this characterization, describing it as a rally in Arizona on September 12, 2001. In the reimagined versions, posted on Indymedia, one has been changed to read "What makes us great/IMPUNITY," while another states that "what makes us great" is "PROFIT$ AT ANY COST."[30] Such efforts literally and metaphorically disrupt the borders of the billboard, making the billboard itself into a contested and contestable site, positioning the message contained therein as part of a larger debate. The "us" invoked in the billboard is apparently not so unified after all.

As far as I know, however, these activists have yet to liberate the billboards in the disability series, and this fact supports my contention that the presence of disability positions these billboards—and, effectively, the overall Pass It On campaign—as beyond reproach. Unlike the UNITY billboard, which has consistently been claimed as a political space and statement, the disability billboards are assumed to be devoid of any political content, and therefore not in need of debate or dialogue. The combination of words such as "determination," "inspiration," and "courage" with the images of disabled people creates an appeal seen as impossible to refuse.[31] And this lack of debate is precisely my point: through the use of the disabled body, and the long history of representations of disability as natural, individual, and apolitical, the FBL casts its entire campaign as impossible to refuse.

In the face of this denial of politics, my extended disability series features Leroy Moore, a disabled African American poet and activist whose *courage* is evident in his writings condemning racism, ableism, and their interrelationships; Corbett O'Toole, a white lesbian polio survivor who models *coalition building* as she bridges queer, lesbian, and disability communities and concerns in her activism; disability rights activists from ADAPT crawling up the steps of the Supreme Court building who illustrate the vital importance of *dissent*; the coalition of genderqueer and disability activists involved in PISSAR—People In Search of Safe and Accessible Restrooms— who embody *direct action* when they map gender-neutral and disability-accessible restrooms on college campuses; and Mia Mingus, a disabled queer woman of color practicing *solidarity* in her work on reproductive justice. And, in order to challenge the realm of "positive thinking" mandated by the FBL billboards—itself a kind of able-mindedness—I also imagine billboards acknowledging *anger* over discriminatory policies and billboards *mourning* the loss of community activists.[32] Disability in these images is not something to be overcome through adherence to "community values" but an identity to be claimed and reinterpreted through collective action and coalition work. In this worldview, disabled people do not lack strength of character but legal protections, access to public spaces, adequate and affordable health care, and social and political recognition.

I call for a queer/crip team of billboard liberators, scrawling the word "pity" or "tokenism" underneath the word "overcoming" on the Marlon Shirley billboard. I want to pair "inspiration"—a word that has long been the bane of disabled people's existence—with Nomy Lamm's description of a prosthetic leg as an effective, and certainly inspired, sex toy.[33] I want to see Tee Corinne's famous photograph of two naked dykes getting it on in a wheelchair plastered over the picture of Bethany Hamilton: "Me, quit? Never." Or let's replace Helen Keller as the model of "only see[ing] possibilities" with Loree Erickson, a young activist pioneering the development of radical crip porn through her film *Want*. Not only would these text/image combinations trouble the staid, assimilationist images of disabled people favored by the FBL, they would also insist upon queer sexuality as valued.

After delivering an earlier version of this chapter at a talk in Berkeley, I joined two local crips in a small guerrilla campaign to kickstart these dialogues. We departed from the more established practice of billboard liberation and decided to liberate a bus shelter sign. With two of us in wheelchairs, and the third disabled by chronic fatigue syndrome and environmental illness (EI), the ground-level sign was easier to reach from our particular embodiments than a billboard would be. Moreover, the bus shelter seemed closer to crip communities and histories of crip activism than the billboard; public transit systems have long been targets of civil disobedience, with activists engaging in continuing struggles for accessible buses, bus and train stops, and stations.[34] We found a bus shelter in southwest Berkeley that featured the Marlon Shirley image, and, armed with spray paint and stencils, we began the liberation. Although we had not discussed it in advance, we each took on the task best suited to our impairments: Ellen Samuels served as lookout, because her EI required her to stay at a distance from the paint; my limited hand control made wielding the spray paint impossible, so I held the stencils in place, blocking the sign from public view with my body; and Anne Finger transformed the original caption "Lost Leg, Not Heart: Overcoming" into "Lost Leg,

Not Rights: Overcoming Pity." Ellen snapped a quick picture of the liberated sign with her phone, and we hurried away.

In hindsight, our careful surreptitiousness was probably unnecessary. The depoliticization of disability that I trace in this chapter likely made our political acts unintelligible; no one would suspect three white women, two of them in wheelchairs, of vandalism or destruction of property. Indeed, as we moved away from the sign, we noticed two women waiting on the other side of the shelter, neither one of whom seemed to even notice what we were doing, despite our immediate proximity and excited conversation about our intent and action. Unfortunately, our liberating text was removed within days, and not long after that the FBL poster was replaced with an advertisement for *America's Next Top Model*, a different manifestation of heteronormative able-bodiedness.

I want to close with one more tweaked billboard to drive home the point that simply substituting the FBL billboards with my own, tempting though that may be, is not a permanent solution, as the *America's Top Model* ad suggests, nor is it an unambiguous one. In this final billboard, courtesy of the Billboard Liberation Front, we have the familiar image of the young white girl waving an American flag, but the text has been radically altered. NATIONALISM, the reworked ad now exclaims, "What Makes Us Blind." The billboard liberators have managed to highlight and challenge the nationalism inherent in the original advertisements, but only by relying on the same kind of normalizing logic found within the campaign as a whole. By figuring "blindness" as the sign of ignorance and exclusion, the alleged liberators of this billboard remained trapped in the ableist logic of the FBL. This time, rather than using disability to foreclose debate, the text's creators have used disability as a sign of such foreclosure. Either way, the better life heralded by the billboard isn't welcoming of disabled people.

Taking my cue from the work of queer cultural critics who remind us that "queer" is not always transgressive, I want us to reckon with the inevitability that in dealing with notions of a better life, of a better future, it is not enough to simply insert new billboards in the place of old ones; that, too, would signal a foreclosure of other potentialities and possibilities.[35] I am not merely arguing for a progress narrative of images, moving from "bad" images of disability to "good" ones.[36] I offer these cripped, queered billboards not as the real tools of a better life, not as the real future, but as a catalyst to get us thinking about what might equal a more livable life, and for whom, under what conditions and at what costs.

5 The Cyborg and the Crip

Critical Encounters

> Who cyborgs will be is a radical question; the answers are a matter of survival.
> —Donna Haraway, *Simians, Cyborgs, and Women*

CONTROVERSY CAME QUICKLY to the cyborg. In 1983, *Socialist Review* invited several feminist theorists, among them Donna Haraway, "to write about the future of socialist feminism in the context of the early Reagan era."[1] Haraway responded with "A Manifesto for Cyborgs," framing the cyborg as a figure of feminist critique.[2] Her cyborg was a radical border-crosser, blurring the boundaries between human and animal, machine and organism, physical and non-physical.[3] Such a cyborg, she argued, could "guide us to a more livable place," an "elsewhere," in which "people are not afraid of their joint kinship with animals and machines, not afraid of permanently partial identities and contradictory standpoints."[4] This potential arose from the cyborg's hybridity, its transgression of boundaries and categories; because it does not, or cannot, privilege unity or sameness, it offers "a way out of the maze of dualisms" that characterize Western thought.[5]

Haraway positioned her cyborg as an intervention not only in Western dualism but especially in Western feminism, and her critique was focused along two fronts: first, feminist dismissals of science and technology, and second, feminist reliance on "universal, totalizing theory."[6] She argued that the cyborg's non-innocence—its origins in a militarized and colonizing technoscience—was precisely what made it a potentially productive tool for feminist analysis. It could lead to "the final imposition of a grid of control on the planet" or to a feminist politics in which we take pleasure and responsibility in technology; the key is to recognize this risky dual capacity as opening new possibilities for resistance.[7] The fragmented cyborg pushes us to see from multiple perspectives at the same time, stressing that every perspective "reveals both dominations and possibilities unimaginable from the other vantage point."[8] Capable of "holding incompatible things together because both or all are necessary and true," the cyborg rejects binary logic and embraces contradiction.[9]

Nowhere is its contradictory stance more apparent than in terms of science and technology. As Haraway describes it in an interview, the manifesto is "neither technophobic, nor technophilic, but about trying to inquire critically" into the assumptions, uses, and implications of technoscience; it urges feminists to engage in and take responsibility for "the social relations of science and technology."[10] Thus, she warns against feminist approaches that serve only to heighten the dualism between science and nature by rejecting technology outright. Her manifesto is an alternative to those feminisms that "have insisted on the necessary domination of technics and recalled us to an imagined organic body."[11] The feminist task, then, is not to plot some escape from technology, or to map our return to a preindustrial Eden, but rather to contest for other meanings of, or other relations with, technoscience. The cyborg serves as a theoretical framework for such contestations.

Haraway describes her project as a challenge to "versions of Euro-American feminist humanism" that assume "master narratives deeply indebted to racism and colonialism."[12] The valorization of nature and the desire on the part of some feminists to cast all technology as phallocentric is one such master narrative; another is the development of a universalizing feminist theory dependent on monolithic ideas of "woman," articulations that prioritize gender over race and class. Haraway's second intervention, then, was in "some streams of the white women's movement in the United States" that naturalize "woman."[13] For Haraway, the boundary-crossing cyborg could be a productive intervention in such debates, shifting the terrain of feminist thought and practice from monolithic identities to shifting affinities. Drawing on Chela Sandoval's work on women of color and "oppositional consciousness," Haraway pushes for a feminism not "on the basis of natural identification, but . . . on the basis of conscious coalition, of affinity, of political kinship."[14] Through her cyborg figure, she suggests that "the future of socialist feminism" requires a politics open to the possibility that "[g]ender might not be a global identity after all, even if it has profound historical breadth and depth."[15]

Although Haraway explicitly positioned both the cyborg and its manifesto as feminist, not all readers shared that interpretation. Reflecting on the history of the manifesto, Haraway recalls that the *Socialist Review*'s East Coast Collective found the essay politically unsuitable, antifeminist, and devoid of critique; like many readers since then, they found the piece a naïve embrace of technology and urged that it not be published. The Berkeley Collective disagreed, ushering the piece into publication.[16] But the questions raged: Was the cyborg figure emancipatory or reactionary? Was the manifesto based in critique or was it an undertheorized celebration of technology? Could the cyborg figure point to a socialist feminist future? Were we all cyborgs, as Haraway claimed?[17]

These questions linger over twenty-five years later. Ecofeminists, queer theorists, and historians of new reproductive technologies, among others, continue to debate whether the cyborg figure provides a potentially emancipatory vision for the future.[18] Even theorists who dismiss the cyborg as passé engage in versions of this question; their challenge to the cyborg's continued relevance is only the latest iteration of the questions that have faced the figure from the beginning.[19] It is this question of the cyborg's efficacy in imagining different futures that leads me to take up the figure: Can the cyborg offer an effective model for disability theory and politics? Is it a useful figure for analysis? Is its usefulness tied to its status as metaphor, or should we approach it more literally? In other words, are disabled people cyborgs, and, if so, what can be gained through such an identification? What, finally, is the relationship between disability and the cyborg?

Haraway herself initiated a focus on disability. In the manifesto, she suggested that "[p]erhaps paraplegics and other severely handicapped people can (and sometimes do) have the most intense experiences of complex hybridization" because of their reliance on machines and prosthetics.[20] Other theorists quickly followed Haraway's lead, using disability and disabled bodies as illustrations or examples of cyborgism in their own articulations of cyborg theory.[21] Disability studies scholars joined the conversation as well, exploring the possibility that the cyborg as boundary-blurring hybrid could be a useful model for conceptualizing disabled bodies and theorizing disability.[22]

Even with all this attention given to the cyborg, however, there are few disability studies pieces that focus exclusively on the figure; the cyborg appears in passing as part of a larger exploration of disability and postmodern body theory, contemporary performance, or technological advances. The article-length analyses that do exist tend to focus on a specific cyborg technology, such as cochlear implants, or on a specific cultural representation, such as the Bionic Woman, rather than on the manifesto itself or on the cyborg as a political figure.[23] As a result, the cyborg's feminist histories are downplayed or ignored; the cyborg as a critical intervention in feminist theory is often not the cyborg that appears in disability studies.[24] Yet it is this cyborg we most need. Consider this chapter, then, an intervention in disability studies, one that recognizes key texts and terms in feminist theory, such as feminist commentary on the cyborg, as part of the archive of disability studies.

Of course, cyborg theory requires an intervention as well, for, far too often, disability functions in cyborg theory—including Haraway's manifesto—solely as an illustration of the cyborg condition. Markedly absent is any kind of critical engagement with disability, any analysis of the material realities of disabled people's interactions with technology. Disabled bodies are simply presented as exemplary, and self-evident, cyborgs, requiring neither analysis nor critique. If, as Haraway insists, cyborg bodies are not innocent, but are "maps of power and identity," then a close crip reading of the cyborg is long overdue.[25]

The cyborg figure certainly holds much promise for a disability politics; from its suspicion of essentialist identities to its insistence on coalition work to its interrogation of ideologies of wholeness, the cyborg offers productive insights for developing a feminist disability vision of the future. Its disinterest in and refusal of temporalities ruled by "salvation history," "oedipal calendar[s]," and "rebirth without flaw" suggest the possibility of crip futurities, futurities grounded in something other than the compulsory reproduction of able-bodiedness/able-mindedness.[26] Moreover, Haraway's desire for a politics based on political affinity rather than biological identity can be a useful resource for disability studies scholars and activists crafting a movement among people with different impairments. A cyborg politics would not require an amputee, a blind person, and a psychiatric survivor to present their identities and experiences as the same, or even all amputees' experiences as the same, but rather would encourage the formation of flexible coalitions to achieve shared goals. Finally, Haraway's manifesto marks one of the first moments that disability and disabled people appear in feminist critical theory, and although that appearance leaves much to be desired, it serves as a vital opening into feminist and queer thought.

Rather than abandon the cyborg because of its ableist rhetoric and manifestations, I argue for a continued struggle with the figure, using it to stage our own blasphemous interventions in feminist theory. This struggle entails not only reimagining the cyborg from a critical crip position but also engaging seriously with existing critiques of the figure. In other words, what might disability studies learn from criticisms of the cyborg by women of color, by antiracist scholars, or by activists working to contest globalization? How can we use the figure of the cyborg not only to imagine disability differently but to imagine a cripped coalition politics? Thus, this chapter has two goals: first, to trace in detail the ways in which cyborg discourses universalize the experience of disability, removing it from the realm of the political; and second, to explore the possibility of a cripped cyborg politics, one that draws on the practices of feminist and queer disability activists and theorists. To twist Haraway's iconic, ironic prose: "Crip the Cyborg for Earthly Survival!"[27]

"Rise of the Cyborgs"

The cyborgs of popular culture bear little resemblance to the cyborgs of Haraway's manifesto. Robocops and Terminators, they are more likely to engage in spectacular acts of violent hypermasculinity than in feminist theory and practice; their enhanced bodies seem to reify gender differences rather than critique them. Indeed, feminist critics from Anne Balsamo to Claudia Springer warn that such cyborgs will do little to transform existing gender relations, and their exaggerated able-bodiedness suggests that they offer few resources to disability theory or politics.[28] My focus, then, is not on these cyborgs, but on the cyborgs of critical theory; I leave the disability critique of science fiction to others.[29] Jennifer Gonzalez argues, however, that cyborgs "function as evidence" of "differences, histories, stories, bodies, [and] places,"[30] making it important to mark the multiple articulations of the cyborg/disability relation. Before turning to Haraway and other cyborg theorists, then, I want to briefly engage the disabled cyborg as it figures in the mainstream news media. Articles in the popular press frequently draw on the image of the cyborg in their coverage of disability and technology, suggesting a seamless link between "cyborg" and "disabled person" thanks to adaptive technology. This assumption of identification is one that runs throughout academic approaches to the cyborg.

"The immediate future is filled with hope for the disabled," exclaims Sherry Baker in her article "Rise of the Cyborgs" in *Discover*. Thanks to new developments in medical technology, we are "soon" going to be living in an era when "brainpower will let the paralyzed walk, [and] allow the mute to speak." Enabling "the paralyzed" to walk is one of the most common expectations for these technologies. A similar article in *Forbes*—also, and not coincidentally, called "Rise of the Cyborg"—showcases a hybrid assisted limb that "one day . . . may even let recovering stroke victims and paraplegics walk again." That story was followed a year later by "Cyborg Waiting List," which described disabled consumers' enthusiasm for the still-under-development device.[31]

The term "cyborg" in these stories, associated with the forward-looking "rise," operates as evocative shorthand for adaptive technology, associating such technology with a promising future for "the disabled." It quickly becomes clear, even after only a cursory reading of these kinds of cyborg stories, that "cyborg" and "physically disabled person" are seen as synonymous. Or, rather, that "person with physical disabilities" is a self-evident, commonsense category of cyborgism. The reporters do not explain what they mean by "cyborg" or what leads them to describe disabled people in cyborgian terms. They assume that their readers will easily and uncritically understand disabled people as cyborgs and link their future to one of medical technology; no explanation or definition is apparently required.

Representing the cyborg/disabled person relationship as both seamless and self-evident obscures the facts of these very technologies. In a context in which most disabled people in the United States are un- or underemployed, and in which almost a third of disabled people live below the poverty line, many of these cyborg technologies remain out of reach of the people for whom they are imagined.[32] The "cyborg-style iLimb Hand" heralded in the UK *Register*, for example, costs eighteen thousand dollars, and the price tag leaps higher if we include not only the device itself but the training and maintenance it likely requires.[33] The ability to become cyborg is too often economically determined.[34]

Presenting the cyborg/disability connection in a purely positive light also ignores the fact that, for many people, adaptive technologies can be painful; the same brace that makes it easier to walk may cause skin breakdown or other difficulties. Yet these news stories tend to focus only on the advantages brought by these technologies, describing the latest inventions in the language of healing and restoration. Tobin Siebers explains that such accounts presume that "[p]rostheses always increase the cyborg's abilities; they are a source only of new powers, never of problems."[35] As a result, these celebratory news stories present high-tech technology as solving the "problem" of disability;

pity and discrimination are rendered irrelevant here. So, too, are issues of adaptation and negotiation: as Siebers suggests, these cyborgian tales assume an easy melding of body and machine. The relationship between disability and technology is discussed only in terms of the devices' ability to normalize the body and/or to restore its previous function; there is nothing else to discuss, apparently, and the devices' value is assumed.

Many of these articles position cyborg technology as affecting only disabled people; nondisabled people may eventually use these devices, but they are not currently cyborgs in the same way as disabled folks. Baker predicts that, "[w]hile the immediate future is filled with hope for the disabled, cyborg technology may soon spread, giving ordinary people extraordinary skills."[36] On the one hand, Baker's claim can be seen as erasing the disabled/nondisabled divide in assuming that everyone can benefit from these technologies. On the other hand, however, her "soon" reminds us that disabled people are the only immediate cyborgs; "ordinary" people will have to wait.[37] For the time being, then, "cyborg" is linked more directly to disabled bodies than to able-bodied ones.

This distinction between disabled people and "ordinary" people surfaces in the raft of news stories covering Oscar Pistorius's attempt to compete alongside nondisabled runners in the 2008 summer Olympics (rather than in the Paralympics). With his gleaming high-tech prosthetics, Pistorius perfectly embodied the cultural understanding of a cyborg; he was one with his machine. The fact that his prosthetics, coupled with his training and athleticism, enabled him to run at breathtaking speeds only strengthened this description. Leslie Swartz and Brian Watermeyer discuss the ways in which the responses of the International Association of Athletics Federations reveal a profound anxiety about disabled athletes;[38] what I want to highlight here is the way in which news writers presented Pistorius as a definitive cyborg and, therefore, almost of a different species than his fellow runners. Anna Salleh, writing for an Australian news outlet, described the Pistorius case as one involving "the competing rights of cyborgs and non-cyborgs."[39] Bloggers from both sports and technology sites described the case in terms of the arrival of the "cyborg athlete," an arrival that would change everything about how we understand athletics. Not only was Pistorius's cyborgization taken for granted in these stories, but so, too—and relatedly—was his difference. As Swartz and Watermeyer note, doping can also be seen as cyborg technology, but athletes accused of doping are not described in those terms; physical disability and its attendant technologies render one cyborgian in a way nothing else can.[40]

The cyborg/noncyborg distinction points to a problematic assumption underlying popular conceptions of the cyborg. Although Haraway intended the figure to critique dualistic understandings of nature and culture or of human and machine, too often it serves only to reify such binary logic. In these news stories, "cyborg" represents the melding of pure body and pure machine; there is an original purity that, thanks to assistive technology, has only now been mixed, hybridized, blurred. To return to the Pistorius case, the athlete is simply a body; when it gets mixed with the prosthetic machine, it becomes impure, mixed, cyborg. A nondisabled runner, in other words, is natural, unmixed, unadulterated; it is only the presence of the prosthetic that makes one impure, or no longer purely natural.[41] The "cyborg" concept thus serves to perpetuate binaries of pure/impure, natural/unnatural, and natural/technological; rather than breaking down boundaries, it buttresses them.

Heroic "Cyborg Citizens"

Science studies scholar Chris Hables Gray adheres to this binary logic—cyborg/not-cyborg, disabled/not-disabled—when casting quadriplegics as definitive cyborgs; their dependence on high-tech equipment obviously, in Gray's view, renders them true cyborgs. While he argues that "[a]lmost all of us are cyborged in some way," he repeatedly lifts up disabled people as particularly cyborgian.[42] Indeed, he opens his book *Cyborg Citizen* not with cyborgs from science fiction or computer wizards who describe themselves in cyborgian terms but with Christopher Reeve.[43] Under the title "The Crippling of Superman," Gray writes, "In 1995, Christopher Reeve, the actor famous for portraying Superman in the movies, fell from his horse Buck and became a quadriplegic. A sad story? Yes, certainly, but also a heroic cyborg tale."[44] Although I can find no instance of Reeve referring to himself as a cyborg, he apparently struck Gray as the most effective way to introduce the cyborg figure to his readers. As Gray explains in an earlier article (coauthored with Steven Mentor), "[T]he quadriplegic patient totally dependent on a vast array of high-tech equipment" is one of the best examples of a true cyborg.[45]

Gray frequently uses words like "invalid" and "patient" to refer to quadriplegics, terms that assume spinal cord injury to encompass the whole of one's identity. Right after introducing Reeve as the hero of a cyborg tale, Gray describes him as "a barely mobile creature, dependent on and intertwined with machines, a cybernetic organism trapped in power beds and wheelchairs."[46] This kind of language is directly related to Gray's depiction of quadriplegics as definitive cyborgs: if disability is all that is needed to render one cyborg, and disability is the sum of one's identity, then cyborg becomes one's identity. Quadriplegics, like Reeve, simply are cyborgs.[47]

This reduction of disabled people to their impairments, and their subsequent classification as cyborg, leads Gray to present disability politics in terms very different from those he uses in describing other political movements. Drawing on Haraway, Gray articulates the "cyborg citizen" as someone who recognizes the importance of crafting contingent alliances and engaging in dissent. Yet he praises Reeve for mobilizing a "united front of invalid cyborgs," describing how the late actor "catalyzed the unification" of disabled people in his quest for a cure.[48] This description is troubling for many reasons, perhaps most obviously for its implication that prior to Reeve's accident, people with mobility impairments were aimless, unconnected, and politically inactive, unable to participate in society. Gray's rhetoric suggests that not only is Reeve's quest for the cure the only appropriate response to disability, it is also a quest that is shared by all disabled people.[49] What I want to highlight, though, is that Gray discusses politics as a process of unification and universal agreement *only* in terms of disability; elsewhere in his book he describes cyborg politics as contentious, diverse, and complicated, where one achieves or participates in "cyborg citizenship" through one's political acts. He primarily describes Reeve and his fellow "invalid cyborgs," however, in terms of their bodies, not their contentious acts, and repeatedly highlights their "unification." Thus, disability activists in general and Reeve in particular disappear when Gray moves on to articulate his politics of shifting and contingent alliances. This disappearance suggests that Gray is concerned with disability only insofar as he can use the disabled body as an illustration of human-machine interactions; disability as a complicated lived experience, and disabled people as a diverse group encompassing a range of opinions, are apparently not political, not in the realm of cyborg politics.

I focus on Gray because he offers such a clear example of the deployment of the disabled body in cyborg theory, but he is not alone in drawing this cyborg–disabled person connection, or in using Reeve as the exemplary cyborg. Cultural studies scholar Annie Potts, for example, begins her "taxonomy of cyborgs" by including Christopher Reeve alongside a list of science-fiction characters. Even though she goes on to list a range of cyborg criteria—most of them, I should note, medical or diagnostic—Reeve is the only human cyborg she mentions by name in her taxonomy.[50] By grouping him with fictional characters, she implies that his disability has rendered him less than human, or at least more cyborg than human. Journalists have followed suit, also using Reeve to describe cyborg technologies or to illustrate cyborgism.[51] This pattern is likely due in part to Reeve's celebrity; most readers are familiar with Reeve, making him an ideal case for explaining specific medical developments. But it is also due to the fact that the imagined figure of the quadriplegic—someone who uses a power wheelchair and ventilator—seems the perfect embodiment of popular understandings of the cyborg.[52] "Obviously," here is someone who transgresses boundaries between machine and organism, someone whose body doesn't end at the skin, someone who is, indisputably, a cyborg.

Thus the term "cyborg," rather than entailing a critique of existing categories and ideologies, is used to perpetuate distinctions between "normal" and "abnormal" bodies, distinctions that have material consequences involving discrimination, economic inequalities, and restricted access. If nondisabled people are persuaded by the assertion that disabled people are real-life cyborgs, then cyborg status signals a distinction between nondisabled people and disabled people. Cyborg qualities become markers of difference, suggesting an essential difference between disabled people and nondisabled people. Any potential transgressive tendencies in the term are lost when these labels become locked to certain bodies. "Cyborg" itself becomes reified, reduced to a particular kind of body.

"Paraplegics and Other Severely Handicapped" Cyborgs

It doesn't take long to realize that Haraway is someone who loves words.[53] Puns, alliterations, and unexpected pairings appear throughout her writing, and she frequently invents and combines words to illustrate her arguments. She plays extensively with language, and she does so consciously, explicitly; she is always quick to remind us of the multiple meanings of the words at hand. This play is integral to her politics: "If we are imprisoned by language, then escape from that prison-house requires language poets," she asserts, and "cyborg heteroglossia is one form of radical cultural politics."[54] Given the importance Haraway attributes to words, language, and stories, I want to pay close attention to the exact way in which she names disabled people in the cyborg manifesto. In the essay's final section, she writes, "Perhaps paraplegics and other severely handicapped people can (and sometimes do) have the most intense experiences of complex hybridization."[55] With that parenthetical "sometimes," Haraway leaves open the possibility that some disabled people might not achieve cyborgian hybridization, but states that those who do reach it experience "the most intense" versions of it. In noting that intensity, Haraway positions disability as one of the best means of achieving cyborgian boundary-blurring, suggesting that people with disabilities are exemplary cyborgs. Indeed, disabled people are one of the few types of "real-life cyborgs" hailed in the text.

When Haraway names "paraplegics and other severely handicapped people," she draws on the outdated (at least in the United States) language of "handicap."[56] At first glance, this terminology might be seen as a symptom of its time. First published in 1985, five years before the passage of the Americans with Disabilities Act, the manifesto could simply bear the traces of a time before the disability rights movement became more mainstream. Although many disability rights activists began calling for "people-first" language in the 1970s ("people with disabilities" as opposed to "disabled people") and referring to "disability" rather than "handicap," we might assume that Haraway, like many Americans, was unaware of such shifts in 1983, when she began the piece.[57] Legislation passed in the 1970s, for example, employed the language of "handicap," while later laws used "disability."[58] Yet, in the footnote attached to that sentence, Haraway uses the language of "the disabled/differently abled" and makes a quick reference to "the always context-relative social definitions of 'ableness.'"[59]

Why the difference? If Haraway were aware of the usage of "disabled," why did she deploy "severely handicapped" in the text, and not once but twice? My suspicion is that she needed to evoke in her readers an image of a person completely dependent on technology, an image of a body that could not possibly exist without a technological intervention. "Severe" plays in to exactly this notion, suggesting the most disabled bodies, the bodies most in need of rehabilitation and intervention.[60] "Handicapped" serves a similar purpose. Unlike "disabled," which potentially has more political overtones, or even "differently abled," which can be seen as a (naïve and unsuccessful) attempt to break down able-bodied/disabled binaries, "handicapped" is thoroughly immersed in individual, medical, and charity models of disability. It is a label that makes it easier to see all disabled people as monolithically bound to their adaptive equipment and, relatedly, makes it harder to notice the lack of attention to the experiences or perspectives of disabled people.

It is useful here to note that the one example Haraway gives of such "severely handicapped people" is not a real person but a fictional character from Anne McCaffrey's *The Ship Who Sang*: a "severely handicapped child" who was so physically disabled that her only hope of survival was to have her brain removed from her body and placed inside a machine (the spaceship of the title). While Haraway celebrates the story for its challenge to assumptions about "[g]ender, sexuality, and embodiment," it certainly echoes longstanding ableist assumptions about the uselessness of physically disabled bodies and the necessity of the technological fix, even—or especially—one that destroys the disabled body altogether. But Haraway needed just such a figure to make her argument about the cyborg; she was relying on her readers having an idea of what "severe handicap" looks like, an idea as fictional as the one in the story. In other words, she needed the stereotyped assumption that "severe handicap" means "total dependence" in order to convince her readers of the existence of bodies that don't "end at the skin, or include at best other beings encapsulated by skin," the passage that immediately follows the reference to disability.[61]

Haraway's reference to disabled bodies serves as the bridge between her discussion of two groups of texts, the work of US women of color and feminist science fiction.[62] Although the disability passage makes reference to McCaffrey's fiction, it occurs before Haraway explicitly moves into her "very partial reading of the logic of the cyborg monsters" in feminist science fiction.[63] The "severely handicapped" girl in McCaffrey's story thus serves as the segue into that reading, but structurally, she remains apart from it. It is hard, then, to read disability or disabled bodies as active participants in the cyborg politics Haraway articulates. Disabled people serve neither as the creators of cyborg writing (they are not included in "women of color" or the authors of science fiction) nor as the subjects of feminist literary criticism. Nor, for that matter, as the active subjects in their own narratives: while Haraway uses the passive tense to describe the cyborg political work of *The Ship Who Sang* ("Gender, sexuality, embodiment, skill: all were reconstituted in the story"), she employs the active tense to describe the work of the characters in stories that do not hinge on the character's disabilities.[64] In other words, although Haraway recognizes the potential insights to be derived from the experience of living with disability technology, casting disability as a challenge to "organic holism," she presents disability in remarkably monolithic terms, as a single, universal experience. Moreover, it is one that can best be described by referencing a text of science fiction, one that presents disability as the site of spectacular technological fixing. Several paragraphs later, she mentions "[u]nseparated twins and hermaphrodites," other sites of disability, but only as the monsters of early modern France.[65] The disabled body, then, is figured within the manifesto as the creature of futuristic fiction or the monstrous past; disabled bodies are, once again, cast as out of time. Disability may be a site of "complex hybridization," and disabled bodies may exemplify the cyborg, but their cyborgization appears as a type apart from the rest of the cyborg politics discussed here.

Haraway's naming practices are one of the most troubling aspects of the manifesto, and not only in terms of disability. Looking carefully at which kinds of bodies, or which identities, get positioned as cyborg makes clear the universalizing assumptions that operate within the text. Early in the essay, Haraway pairs two groups of women as cyborgs: "Ironically, it might be the unnatural cyborg women making chips in Asia and spiral dancing in Santa Rita jail whose constructed unities will guide effective oppositional strategies."[66] (Spiral dancing, she explains in a note at the bottom of the page, is "a practice at once both spiritual and political that linked guards and arrested anti-nuclear demonstrators at the Alameda County jail in the early 1980s.") While Haraway does not explicitly explain her reasons for this naming, she does hint at the processes making these women cyborgs. The Asian factory workers can be called cyborg because of their place in globalized capitalism. It is through their work in the assembly line, and their location in a region where multinational corporations can cut labor and safety costs, that they participate in the global economy. Their "nimble fingers," a description indebted to colonialist and racist stereotypes, link their bodies to the machines they are building. Based on Haraway's stated preference for affinity politics, it can be inferred that the Santa Rita protestors are cyborg because their anti-nuclear activism is based on coalition politics and affinity groups. Haraway may also position the protestors as cyborgs to stress that there is no position outside of technology; even as they protest certain manifestations of the technological age, they are simultaneously implicated in those same technologies.

Haraway gestures toward the reasons behind this naming, but she does not provide them, and it is that lack I want to highlight. Why is the act of Asian women making chips seen as self-explanatory, while the spiral dance requires definition? Spiral dancing may not be common knowledge, but neither are the reasons why assembling computer chips makes one "cyborg." Moreover, are there not differences between the kinds of activities and subjectivities Haraway links here—protestor and worker, jail and factory, Asia and the United States—that need exploring? Or what about the layers of history and assumption that lead to the differences in scale in Haraway's parallel, a single jail in a town in California versus the much more general, and generalizable, "Asia"?[67] In the next paragraph, Haraway goes on to praise "transgressed boundaries, potent fusions, and dangerous possibilities," and it is exciting to imagine what progressive work might be made possible by drawing links between such seemingly disparate groups and situations. At the same time, I'm left to wonder about the different effects of naming such groups "cyborg," questioning the consequences of making a global generalization based on a concept that developed in a particular historical moment.

I am not alone in these questions. Malini Johar Schueller, for example, argues that simply pairing these groups of women, linking them with an undertheorized "and," fails to attend to the differences in their location. While an alliance between these two groups of women could be "energizing and powerful," Schueller argues that "it cannot be articulated without an acknowledgment of the spatio-political difference of the demonstrators that positions them, in however weak a fashion, as beneficiaries of globalization and with different interests than Asian women laborers who, in the interests of feeding their families, might not always join the protestors against multinationals."[68] Joan Walloch Scott worries that Haraway's naming of women of color as cyborg adheres to an all-too-familiar pattern of white women idealizing, and thus otherizing, women of color as repositories of wisdom; "What," she asks, "is the difference between Haraway's looking to these groups for the politics of the future and . . . the romantic attribution by white liberal or socialist women to minority or working-class women of the appropriate (if not authentic) socialist or feminist politics?"[69]

Haraway herself acknowledges this problem during an interview with Constance Penley and Andrew Ross, who also question her choice to illustrate cyborgism in these terms. Haraway agrees that her "narrative partly ends up further imperializing, say, the Malaysian factory worker," noting that if she were to rewrite the manifesto, she would be much more cautious about attributing cyborgism to others. She goes on to speak of the need for a whole range of boundary creatures, in the hopes that expanding the kind of figures in her imaginary would reduce the imperialist effects of the cyborg; "Could there be," she hopes, "a family of figures who would populate our imagination of these postcolonial, postmodern worlds that would not be quite as imperializing in terms of a single figuration of identity?"[70]

Many other theorists join Penley and Ross in challenging Haraway's assertion that "we" are all cyborgs, echoing Haraway's later remarks about the ways in which the manifesto romanticizes and imperializes Asian factory workers. From Scott (who still finds the manifesto compelling) to Schueller (who does not), a range of feminist theorists have challenged Haraway's use of these women to illustrate her theory. None of them, however, question Haraway's connection between disabled people and cyborgs, none see parallels between the use of "third world women" as illustrations in first-world theory and the use of disabled people.[71] This lack of recognition, in my view, is the result of the depoliticization of disability and disabled bodies. Many feminist theorists have the tools and the training to recognize the imperializing move behind Haraway's description of the cyborged factory workers (or at least have the tools to recognize it once it has been pointed out to them) but lack the familiarity with disability studies to recognize these characterizations of disability as equally problematic, equally contentious. And this positioning, this generalization about (and, indeed, construction of) a particular group of people is seen as unremarkable, as benign and disinterested statement of fact rather than partial and contested interpretation.

Thus, in stark contrast to the controversy generated by Haraway's assertion that Asian women factory workers are real-life cyborgs, identifying disabled people with cyborgs is widely accepted without question. Labeling disabled people "cyborgs" is apparently without troubling implications or effects; such a move, even by nondisabled theorists, is not seen to require any self-examination or critical analysis. In making this contrast, I do not mean to suggest that race has already been adequately addressed in cyborg theory, or that we have solved the "problem" of race. As the editors of *Race in Cyberspace* note, references to the gendered cyborg abound, but texts exploring the race of the cyborg are fewer and farther between.[72] Rather, I am simply drawing attention to the fact that even as the cyborg continues to be bandied about in feminist, queer, and disability theory, we as cultural critics have still to reckon with its unspoken assumptions about bodies and physical difference.

What stands out in Haraway's analysis, then, is its reliance on narrow understandings of disability. She offers disabled people as exemplary hybrids, but without any examination of what such hybridization might feel like or entail. Disability may be an excellent site for witnessing the blurring of human and technology, but not, apparently, for exploring actual experiences of such blurring. Indeed, such experiences are collapsed under the category of "paraplegics and other severely handicapped people," a category which is itself presented as coherent and monolithic. Moreover, moving beyond the human/machine interface seems to require leaving disability behind: once Haraway moves into discussions about political identification, or shifting affinities, or future formations, disability and the disabled figure drop away altogether. Disability and disabled people are decontextualized, removed from the realm of the political, and presumed to play no active role in the category breakdowns that animate both the cyborg and the manifesto.

Cyborg Attachments

Given all these problems with the cyborg figure, perhaps it is time to move on. Not only do some scholars find the figure "somewhat tired and tiresome from academic overuse," but even Haraway herself has turned her attention elsewhere.[73] The concept of "companion species" has become her focus of late, particularly the co-constitutiveness of dogs and humans. Although the cyborg continues to surface in her work, it serves more often as a contrast to the dog or dogs; as she puts it, cyborgs "no longer do the work of a proper herding dog to gather up the threads needed for critical inquiry."[74]

Although I share Haraway's enthusiasm for the possibilities of companion species, and think that disability studies has much to offer those conversations, "A Cyborg Manifesto" and the cyborg figure continue to entice. Calls for replacement or successor figures and tropes (e.g., Ingrid Bartsch, Carolyn DiPalma, and Laura Sells discuss the vampire, and Sara Cohen Shabot recommends the grotesque) seem to bring their own problems for disability studies; the work of Margrit Shildrick demonstrates that, at the very least, the monstrous and the grotesque require their own careful readings and cannot be simple substitutes.[75] Moreover, Haraway's recent focus on dog agility practices, a competition that insists on the able-bodiedness of its dogs if not its humans, leaves me looking back longingly at the cyborg.[76]

And this longing is not despite its gaps and oversights, but because of them. In other words, one of the things that most appeals to me about the cyborg figure is its multiple, and often contradictory, deployments. Its very unpredictability is precisely what makes it such an important and potentially useful concept; its fluidity and permeability make it difficult to lock it permanently in to any one set of meanings. As Christina Crosby argues, it is "dynamic, mobile, [and] programmable, which makes the cyborg incalculably dangerous in the form of a cruise missile, but also offers opportunities that haven't yet been calculated for forming new alliances, new affinity groups, new coalitions."[77]

What I find most promising about Haraway's cyborg figure is its history—and present—in feminist activism and scholarship. As Zoë Sofoulis maps, the manifesto has played an integral role not only in the development of feminist science and technology studies but also in theories of architecture, anthropology, and literary criticism.[78] The pervasiveness of the manifesto makes clear its continued influence on critical theory; for example, Susan Stryker and Stephen Whittle chose to include the piece in their *Transgender Studies Reader*, even though the manifesto never explicitly takes up trans identities, because of its examination of how "marginalized embodied positions" are "politically charged sites of struggle."[79] In its ubiquity, the manifesto, and the cyborg as figured in it, can serve as a resource for vital cross-movement work. It is easy to imagine the potent fusions and fruitful couplings that can result from a meeting of disability studies and transgender studies, for example, including examinations of how scholars in both fields have used and challenged the cyborg. It is exactly this kind of cross-pollination that I want disability studies to nurture and extend, and the manifesto facilitates such work because cross-pollination was key to its inception. Haraway derived the figure, at least in part, from her readings of women of color, and from their attempts to forge multi-issue coalitions and communities. Fiction writer Octavia Butler, essayist Cherríe Moraga, theorist Chela Sandoval: each influenced Haraway's articulation of the cyborg, offering insights into a feminist politics based on fluid identities, border crossings, and partialities.

As disability studies continues to wrestle with the figure, we have over two decades' worth of queer, feminist, and women of color criticism to draw on and learn from. Not only can we return to the manifesto itself, mining it for nuggets of antiracist feminism or coalition politics, but we can, and should, examine the wealth of feminist theory that has similarly pushed and extended the cyborg and its manifesto. For the remainder of this section, I want to offer a brief overview of some of these critiques, partly to acknowledge the ways in which my own thinking is indebted to them, partly to insist on their centrality to cyborg theory, and partly to recognize them as relevant and integral to disability studies.

Chela Sandoval traces this heritage in her own work, reminding Haraway's audience that the cyborg figure is a direct descendant of what Sandoval refers to as "US third world feminism." Cyborg conceptions of the fluidity between self and other, of the importance of transgressing boundaries and borders, are "analogous to that called for in contemporary indigenous writings where tribes or lineages are identified out of those who share, not blood lines, but rather lines of affinity. Such lines of affinity occur through attraction, combination, and relation carved out of and in spite of difference, and they are what comprise the notion of mestizaje in the writings of people of color." Too many cyborg theorists, Sandoval laments, ignore this aspect of the manifesto's genealogy, attributing the notion of "affinity-through-difference" to Haraway alone.[80]

While Sandoval addresses the ways in which the cyborg has been taken up by others, Malini Johar Schueller and Mariana Ortega focus their critiques directly on Haraway and her manifesto. For both authors, Haraway's treatment of the writings of women of color is troubling; although Haraway repeatedly lifts up "women of color" as a political position achieved through struggle not natural identity, they argue that she simultaneously homogenizes the writings of women of color. In their readings, Haraway is far too quick to assume that all chicanas feel the same way about *La Malinche* or engage in the same struggles over language and identity.[81]

By including these critiques alongside my disability reading, I am aware that I run the risk of presenting the critiques as analogical: disability functions "like race" in cyborg theory, or "just as" women of color have been marginalized within the manifesto, "so too" have disabled people. These kinds of analogical moves are all too common in disability studies (and beyond), and they unfortunately have the result of obfuscating the relationships between disability and race rather than illuminating them. But it is my hope that exploring these critiques together—the disability critique and the race critique (labels that are themselves part of the problem)—will enrich and extend existing readings of both disability studies and "A Cyborg Manifesto." As Abby Wilkerson explains, the manifesto raises questions about what it means to be an ally, questions that arise partly out of the manifesto's explicit framing, and partly out of the manifesto's unacknowledged gaps and erasures.[82] One of my goals in this chapter, then, is to use both the manifesto and its critics to think through how to do cross-movement work within disability studies and, relatedly, how to draw on the critiques of women-of-color theorists without merely analogizing race and disability or universalizing the experiences and categories of race and disability.

Continuing a crip engagement with the cyborg—a *critical* crip engagement—is a way for disability studies to participate in these discussions. Decades after its original publication, the manifesto remains a site of provocative, rich, creative feminist scholarship, work that can enrich disability studies in unexpected ways. Using the cyborg in disability studies, then, means not only reading Haraway and the manifesto but delving into the many critiques and retellings of the manifesto, not all of which are faithful to their origins.

Pushing the Cyborg: Cripping Cyborg Politics

Donna Haraway insists that the cyborg is about both pleasure and responsibility; she positions her manifesto as "an argument for *pleasure* in the confusion of boundaries and for *responsibility* in their construction."[83] Thinking through what it means to approach the cyborg from a disability studies or crip theory perspective requires this kind of dual move, this simultaneous holding of pleasure and responsibility. In her book-length interview with Donna Haraway, *How Like a Leaf*, Thyrza Nichols Goodeve asks Haraway if the pervasiveness of the cyborg figure disturbs her, if she feels it has been distorted by its many appropriations, gaps, and uses. Haraway responds,

> I think the cyborg still has so much potential. Part of how I work is not to walk away when a term gets dirty and is used in all these appropriate and inappropriate ways because of its celebrity. Instead such uses just make me want to push the reality of the cyborg harder. . . . So instead of giving it up because it has become too famous let's keep pushing it and filling it.[84]

Following Haraway, then, this section "pushes and fills" the cyborg in order to imagine feminist queer crip futures.

"Pushing" the figure from a disability perspective entails bringing a disability consciousness to the cyborg, attending to the specific benefits and dangers it harbors for disabled people. This shift requires an acknowledgment that human/machine interfaces are not always beneficial or pleasurable; an awareness that many disabled people lack access to the cybertechnologies so highly praised in cyborg writing; an accounting for the ways in which cybertechnologies rely on disabling labor practices across the globe; and a realization that not all disabled people are interested in technological cures or fixes. Each of these elements takes cyborgology away from its traditional use of disability as metaphor, and toward an understanding of disability in political and social context. In so doing, they also—and ironically—bring cyborg theory closer to the promise of Haraway's manifesto, a promise of a fully situated cyborg that refuses easy celebrations of human/technology connections.

A non-ableist cyborg politics refuses to isolate those of us cyborged through illness or disability from other cyborgs. Disabled people, in other words, can no longer be cast as modeling a cyborged existence that nondisabled people have yet to achieve. Such a move only strengthens the abled/disabled binary, suggesting that disabled people are fundamentally and essentially different from nondisabled people. If, as Haraway and others argue, technoculture is pervasive, then disabled people are not alone in the cyborgian realm. Cyborg theory could then turn itself to interrogations, for example, of why the very same technology is alternately described as "assistive" or "time-saving" depending on whether a disabled or nondisabled person is using it.[85] In this framework, "cyborg" becomes an opportunity for exploring or interrogating the abled/disabled binary.

We can still discuss medical cyborgs, but why not do so in a way that actually engages with the insights and experiences of such cyborgs? We could explore what such identifications or characterizations might mean to them, or how they might themselves frame cyborg discourse. These kinds of discussions can enrich our understandings of cyborg technology and, in turn, extend our theoretical framings of the cyborg. Tobin Siebers's reflections on the ways in which a leg brace increases both function and pain, for example, might serve to deepen our understanding of the cyborg's ambivalent relation to technology. A cripped cyborg theory would then warn against easy celebrations of the technological fix; it would require a more complex and ambivalent relationship with technology.

Or Nirmala Erevelles's insistence on attending to the material realities of those seen as cyborg can be a way of revisiting the figure's effectiveness for class analysis.[86] Gill Kirkup, one of the editors of *The Gendered Cyborg*, argues that few scholars have used the cyborg to address socialist feminism or engage in materialist analyses, even though the manifesto was explicitly written in the interest of both.[87] How might disability prompt a reexamination of the cyborg's ability to imagine a socialist-feminism in the early twenty-first century or to convince feminists (and disability studies scholars) of the need to attend more to issues of class in our work? Rather than simply repeat the "people with disabilities = cyborgs" equation, we might revisit Haraway's interrogation of the homework economy and the integrated circuit, using her critical frameworks to examine the ways in which disabled people are positioned in terms of efficiency, productivity, and ability to work, or lack thereof.

Or, to take yet another example, a disability studies approach can facilitate renewed attention to the cyborg as human-animal or human-human hybrid. To date, cyborg theorists have focused their energies almost entirely on technology, ignoring the possibilities of boundary transgression between human and organism, even though the latter was an integral part of Haraway's manifesto.[88] (It is this focus on the human-machine hybrid that prompted the fixation on disabled bodies.) A cyborged disability politics can provide astute theoretical insights into the boundary blurring that occurs between disabled people and our attendants, or between disabled people and our service animals, or among disabled people in community with each other and our allies: all experiences that point to a cyborgian understanding of interdependence, mutuality, and relationship.

Sociologist Rod Michalko writes about understanding the nature of blindness more fully through his relationship with his guide dog Smokie; he details how the boundaries of his body, of his awareness, shifted when working with Smokie, experiences that certainly could be productively mined by cyborg scholars.[89] Michalko describes a relationship not of straightforward instrumentalism or utility, but of integration and co-constitutiveness. Smokie is not mere tool but an opening into a new way or new understanding of "being in the world." As Cary Wolfe explains, the human–service dog relation is "neither *homo sapiens* nor *canis familiaris*, neither 'disabled' nor 'normal,' but something else altogether, a shared trans-species being-in-the-world constituted by complex relations of trust, respect, dependence, and communication."[90] Examining the nature of such relations can not only extend theoretical framings of the cyborg but enrich emerging analyses of animality and the human.

Laura Hershey and Loree Erickson openly discuss their negotiations with personal attendants—an openness Erickson describes as being "out as a body"—and their work could similarly enrich existing understandings of the cyborg.[91] Erickson draws on phenomenology, for example, to articulate her relationship with attendants: "[M]y personal attendant and I, and our bodies," she writes, "are functioning as a self and as a unit," thereby breaking down the "dualism of singular self/combined unit."[92] Erickson is both singular and plural, neither fully "she" nor "they." The cyborg figure can offer a "theoretical prototype" for recognizing the ways in which such relationships push our notions of self and other, of body and boundary, of agency and interdependency.[93]

In other words, it is high time to explore how best to discuss the relationship between disability and cyborgism without facile references to disabled bodies as self-evident cyborgs simply by virtue of their use of "assistive" or "adaptive" technologies. Doing so will benefit not only disability studies but also cyborg theory and feminist critical theory more broadly. What I want to do for the remainder of this chapter, then, is sketch out alternative approaches to the cyborg, ones that crip the cyborg while still recognizing its frequently ableist deployments, ones that push disability studies in more feminist and queer directions.

Cripping the cyborg, developing a non-ableist cyborg politics, requires understanding disabled people as cyborgs not because of our *bodies* (e.g., our use of prosthetics, ventilators, or attendants), but because of our *political practices*. In this framing, Erickson can be understood in terms of cyborgism not because she has a disability that requires her to utilize attendant care, but because she critically thinks through what such uses might mean. In her short film *Want*, for example, Erickson explains that she has collaborated with her friends, lovers, and community members to craft a network of attendants that operates outside of the larger health care system. In so doing, she offers a radical reinterpretation of what community can mean, of what living with a disability can mean. In both her film and her writings, Erickson seamlessly weaves together images of sex acts with other "activities of daily life," such as her attendants lifting her on and off the toilet; we move from scenes of Erickson sitting on the toilet to scenes of her having sex with her lover to scenes of her confronting inaccessible buildings. Again, her cyborgism is not so much about the fact that she needs attendants or uses a power wheelchair but rather that she uses her experiences with both technologies to force people—disabled and nondisabled—to confront our ableist assumptions about disability and sexuality.

Cripping the cyborg, in other words, means recognizing that our bodies are not separate from our political practices; neither assistive technologies nor our uses of them are ahistorical or apolitical. As anthropologist Steven Kurzman explains,

I see cyborg more as a subject position than an identity, and believe it is more descriptive of my position vis-à-vis the relationships of production, delivery, and use surrounding my prosthesis than my actual physical interface with it. In other words, if I am to be interpellated as a cyborg, it is because my leg cost $11,000 and my HMO paid for it; because I had to get a job to get the health insurance; because I stand and walk with the irony that the materials and design of my leg are based in the same military technology which has blown the limbs off so many other young men; because the shock absorber in my foot was manufactured by a company which makes shock absorbers for bicycles and motorcycles, and can be read as a product of the post–Cold War explosion of increasingly engineered sports equipment and prostheses; and because the man who built my leg struggles to hold onto his small business in a field rapidly becoming vertically integrated and corporatized. I am not a cyborg simply because I wear an artificial limb.[94]

In tracing this prosthetic history, Kurzman recognizes his leg and the cyborg figure as political; his relationship to both, the prosthetic and the cyborg, is a political relationship, one embedded in larger histories, rhetorics, and economies.

Take, for example, the exoskeletons developed by Berkeley Bionics for both military and medical purposes; their products and promotional videos make clear the link between disability and the militarized cyborg. eLEGS is an exoskeleton that enables some paralyzed people to walk under certain conditions; according to Eythor Bender, the company's CEO, eLEGS are "built on the platform, or the legacy, of HULC (Human Universal Load Carrier)," a military application they licensed to Lockheed Martin.[95] The video touting HULC features multiple scenes of a man in fatigues wearing a HULC while he carries heavy loads over mountainous terrain. Jim Ni, the HULC program manager, explains that HULC was designed to facilitate soldiers carrying heavy weapons (one frame shows the soldier attaching a bomb to the front of the exoskeleton), thereby preventing back injuries and other repetitive-stress injuries associated with contemporary warfare. The same technology that enables a paraplegic to walk allows a soldier to kill more efficiently and ergonomically; cyborg ironies, indeed.[96]

Extending Kurzman's analysis, and reading it alongside the work of Erevelles, Siebers, and other crip theorists grappling critically with the cyborg, I want to provide a reading of the cyborg that places it within the realm of the political, moving it away from more essentialist readings that reduce it to particular kinds of (medicalized) bodies. Disability activists, communities, and movements often embody the kind of ironic, even blasphemous, politics that Haraway cast as necessary characteristics of the feminist cyborg. As Judy Rohrer argues, "Irony can help build the future-oriented, multiple-identity politics" we need, and disability politics offers a rich archive of ironic approaches to illness, disability, and the body.[97]

Haraway peppers her manifesto with ironic political slogans from her feminist nonukes work, sharing the slogans of others as well as inventing her own: "Cyborgs for Earthly Survival!" and perhaps the most (in)famous, "I would rather be a cyborg than a goddess."[98] Her use of these phrases grounds her high theory in grassroots activism, making clear that she is invested in the practical implications of her theoretical travels, and highlights her adherence to an ironic politics of blasphemy. In that spirit, I want to add another grassroots saying, one that does this same kind of ironic, blasphemous work: "Trached dykes eat pussy without coming up for air." Connie Panzarino, a long-time disability activist and out lesbian, would attach this sign to her wheelchair during Pride marches in Boston in the early 1990s. Shockingly explicit, her sign refuses to cast technology as cold, distancing, or disembodied/disembodying, presenting it instead as a source and site of embodied pleasure.

"Trach" is an abbreviation of tracheotomy, a medical procedure in which a breathing tube is inserted directly into the trachea, bypassing the mouth and nose. Someone with a trach, then, can, in effect, breathe through her throat, freeing her mouth for other activities (another version of this sign is "Trached dykes french kiss without coming up for air"). From a cyborgian perspective, this sign is brilliantly provocative and productive. It draws on the pervasive idea that adaptive technologies grant superior abilities, not merely replacing a lost capacity but enhancing it, yet it does so in a highly subversive way. The message here isn't about blending in, about passing as normal or hypernormal, but about publicly announcing the viability of a queer disabled location. It's disnormalizing, adamantly refusing compulsory heterosexuality, compulsory able-bodiedness, and homonormativity. As Corbett O'Toole argues, it challenges the perceived passivity of disabled women, presenting them as actively pleasuring their partners, thereby graphically refuting stereotypes linking physical disability with nonsexuality.[99]

The context of the sign is as important as its content. In sharp contrast to the disabled people in cyborg texts, who are presented as isolated individuals communing only with their technology, the woman with the sign is in public, participating in a political and social community. She is actively involved in shaping that community, extending the notion of "pride" to apply not only to her sexuality but also to her disability; indeed, she presents the two as erotically and productively inseparable. Appearing in such a public context, the sign can be read as an aggressive rebuke of the discourses of charity, pity, and tragedy that circulate around disabled bodies; in a direct challenge to the infantilization of "Jerry's kids," this woman proclaims herself a sexually active and actively consenting adult.

And she does so with a blasphemous humor born of community. For those unfamiliar with queer crip culture, Panzarino's sign might fly under the radar; those unaware of the workings of a tracheotomy might not understand the sexual promise of such a procedure. For queer crips, however, the sign is a revelation, a locating of pleasure not only in the body-technology interface but in the disabled body itself. In a culture in which technological and medical advances are constantly being touted for their ability to eliminate disability, to reduce the numbers of disabled bodies in the future, Panzarino asserts the value of those bodies, of her body.

Similarly, Laura Hershey becomes a cyborg not simply because of her use of a power chair or a ventilator, but because of her commitment to coalition politics and transformative social practices. A poet, essayist, and longtime activist, Hershey served as a "poster child" for the Muscular Dystrophy Association (MDA) in 1973–74, appearing on posters and other promotional material encouraging (nondisabled) donors to contribute to the organization. The MDA's stated goal is to "conquer neuromuscular disease," and its primary means of meeting this goal is through the selection of poster children and an annual Labor Day telethon, long associated with Jerry Lewis. Hershey's body, and the bodies of other children like her, was used to advocate for a "cure," although "cure" is code here for a combination of prenatal testing, selective abortion, and/or prenatal therapy. Hershey, in other words, was expected to raise money for research into how to prevent children like her from ever being born. In a blasphemous irony befitting cyborg politics, Hershey has since become one of the leaders in the anti-telethon movement, condemning the poster-child rhetoric to which she was subjected as a child. Working with a network of ex–poster children, disability rights activists, and nondisabled allies, Hershey is a fierce and vocal opponent of Jerry Lewis's annual MDA telethon, lambasting Lewis and the organization for their ableist attitudes toward disabled people; when Lewis remarked in a 2001 interview that "cripple[s] in wheelchairs" should "stay in [their] house" if they want to avoid pity, Hershey and her comrades took to the streets, highlighting Lewis's remarks as indicative of the tragic model of disability that permeates charity organizations.[100] In 2009, when Jerry Lewis won the Jean Hersholt Humanitarian Award from the Academy of Motion Pictures Arts and Sciences, a group of activists, including Hershey, organized a protest of the Oscar ceremonies.[101]

From a cyborg perspective, I am enticed by Hershey's provocative relationship to medical technologies. On the one hand, her very survival relies on this technology, a technology made possible by the medical industrial complex that supports and is supported by organizations like the MDA. On the other hand, she uses this technology to make her activism possible, activism that is often committed to interrogating the very system that she relies on. Hershey, in other words, is well-positioned to recognize the complexities of technology and biomedicine. As Haraway made clear in the manifesto, simple technophilia or technophobia is untenable; what we need to do is to take responsibility for the social relations of science and technology.[102] By tracing the effects of cure ideologies and pity narratives, by highlighting the economic assumptions and mechanisms of the telethon, Hershey and her comrades push for exactly this kind of responsibility without naively abandoning such technology altogether. Yet if Hershey were to be described in cyborg terms, most theorists would ignore these savvy negotiations, focusing only on her position in a wheelchair. Reducing Hershey to a cyborg because of her wheelchair or breathing tube ignores her cyborg political practices, thereby perpetuating the depoliticization of disability and disabled people.

In common parlance, Hershey and Panzarino could be considered "severely disabled" (Haraway's "severely handicapped"). They rely on power wheelchairs; they employ personal attendants to assist them in their daily activities; and their chronic impairments occasionally lead to medical crises, particularly respiratory ones. For most cyborg theorists, the story would stop there, serving as a perfect illustration of the ways in which (certain) bodies don't end at the skin. Indeed, in this framework, the more severely disabled one is, the more cyborgian, because the more likely to be using high-tech medical equipment and adaptive technologies. A cripped cyborg politics, however, refuses to stop with this kind of recitation of diagnosis or condition. Following Robert McRuer, "severe" can be read as defiance, fierceness, critique; the "severity" of these women's impairments is due not to their perceived failures to adhere to normative expectations of movement, flexibility, or appearance, but to their public "call[ing] out [of] the inadequacies of compulsory able-bodiedness."[103] Rather than reduce these activists' experiences to the details of their impairment, let us focus instead on their complex and contradictory negotiations with technology, or on the ways in which such negotiations lead to questions about community, responsibility, pleasure, and complicity.[104]

Bradley Lewis draws on Haraway's cyborg theory for precisely these reasons, arguing that the cyborg can help us better understand Prozac and the domination of psychopharmacology. Critical science studies and, in particular, cyborg theory make it possible for us to recognize the stories we tell about Prozac *as* stories, as narratives, and thereby deserving of an attentive read. Cyborg theory, argues Lewis, enables us to ask "local political questions of *consequences* and *inclusion*."[105] The cyborg, in demanding responsibility and critique, pushes progressives to engage with technoscience, to inquire into the effects and assumptions of emerging technologies. Lewis urges attention to Haraway's mode of critique, her ability to challenge the simplistic binaries and dualisms that prevent a taking of responsibility. Prozac, he argues, "is not clearly oppressive or liberatory. It is a contradictory mixture of both—sometimes one more than another, but always both. This makes the problem not Prozac itself but the politics of representation surrounding the production and circulation of Prozac discourse."[106]

Michelle O'Brien echoes this contradictory approach, arguing for greater attention to the politics of prescription drugs. Just as Kurzman sees his prosthetic leg as a nexus of overlapping biomedical, military, and economic discourses, O'Brien positions her use of prescription medications as a practice demanding contextualization within a wider political economy.[107] She traces the manufacturer of each medication, discusses where she obtains the syringes she needs for injections (leading to a brief rumination on HIV/AIDS, the war on drugs, and needle-exchange programs in Philadelphia), and describes the politics of health care that lead her to purchase these medications out of pocket, online, and away from a "proper" provider. As a trans woman, she is "invisible" to her health insurance company yet dependent on her medications, and it is this contradictory stance that leads her to the cyborg.[108] Inspired by Haraway's manifesto, she describes her position within biomedicine as contradictory, ironic, subversive. She may be interfacing with corporate medicine, but she does so "improperly."[109] The cyborg, O'Brien argues, offers a way to approach the medical industrial complex that

does not privilege "isolation, purity, or refusal" but recognizes the potential to interact unfaithfully with the medical system. As she puts it, "If your survival depends on
substantially accessing global pharmaceutical industries, a politics of purity and non-
participation just doesn't get you that far."[110]

Like O'Brien, Dean Spade recognizes that many trans people's reliance on medical
institutions necessitates a contradictory politics. He explains that some transgender
advocates have turned to state disability laws as a potential site of relief from gender discrimination; filing such claims, however, requires that transgendered people
be diagnosed with and identify as having gender identity disorder, or GID.[111] GID is
controversial within trans communities, with many activists wary of its identification
of gender difference as pathology. As Spade writes, "I do not want to make trans rights
dependent upon GID diagnoses, because such diagnoses are not accessible to many
low-income people; because I believe that the diagnostic and treatment processes for
GID are regulatory and promote a regime of coercive binary gender; and because I
believe that GID is still being misused by some mental health practitioners as a basis
for involuntary psychiatric treatment for gender transgressive people."[112] At the same
time, because "many trans people's lives are entangled with medical establishments,"
their best hope is a medical diagnosis and the recognition and access to services it
entails.[113] In describing the strategic use of medical models of difference, Spade carefully maps the implications of such uses, challenging ableism within trans communities while detailing the risks of disability identification. Reading Lewis, O'Brien, and
Spade together reveals that neither medical technologies nor diagnoses can be characterized as purely oppressive or politically neutral. As Haraway's cyborg insists, cyborg
bodies are "maps of power," requiring ironic, doubled, contradictory responses.

"Cyborg" is not the only way to describe activists such as Hershey or Panzarino, nor
is it the only way to frame their political practices and activist alliances. Indeed, it is
highly unlikely that they would use it to identify themselves, finding other ways to
characterize coalition politics or permeable identities. I want to be clear that I am not
arguing that these activists are "real" cyborgs, or that "cyborg" is the best mode for
conceptualizing their activist strategies and theoretical standpoints. We can describe
the fluid nature of disability or articulate a disability politics that embraces contradiction and ambiguity without referencing Haraway or deploying the figure of the cyborg.
Moreover, the cyborg figure may be more useful in examining some disabilities than
others; it might be less effective in explorations of blindness than deafness, for example, or Down syndrome than amputation. At the risk of undercutting my argument, I
want to acknowledge that cyborg theory is not necessary.

It may not be necessary, but, at the same time, it can help us do necessary work.
Cyborg theory remains one of the few places that disabled people, and particularly disabled bodies, are present in contemporary critical theory, and I think it is essential for
disability studies scholars to attend to the specificities of those appearances. Moreover,

rather than simply allow these representations to talk about us, we can intervene directly in them, adhering to the tradition of critical intervention of Haraway's original manifesto. How can we, by intervening in cyborg theory, wage our own multiple, often contradictory, critical interventions in feminist theory, in queer politics, in radical reimaginings of the future?

As I have suggested here, for the cyborg to guide us elsewhere, to lead us toward a more livable space, we must look to the cyborg as a guide for political practice, not strictly as a description of our physical bodies. Pushing the cyborg into an anti-ableist politics means refusing its reduction to the disabled body, refusing to use the figure to shore up binaries of normate/other or abled/disabled. It means recognizing the transgressive political practices of activists such as Hershey, Panzarino, and Spade, recognizing their work in forging coalitions and actions.

Cyborg Histories, Cyborg Futures

Although many analyses of the cyborg begin with Haraway, she was not the first researcher to use the figure in imagining a desired future. In a 1960 issue of *Astronautics*, scientists Manfred E. Clynes and Nathan S. Kline offered up the cyborg, or "cybernetic organism," as a way to imagine human flourishing in space.[114] The two had been invited by NASA to address potential medical problems related to human space travel, and they explored the possibilities of biochemically, electronically, and physiologically modifying the human body.[115] They described their solutions as a mixture of "presently available knowledge and techniques" and "projections into the future."[116] What they imagined, based on experiments with rats, was the ability to implant humans with osmotic pumps that would permit "continuous injections of chemicals at a controlled slow rate."[117] The pumps would be implanted subcutaneously and programmed so as to require no effort or attention from the astronaut. They could then be stocked with medications appropriate for space travel; pumps might carry drugs preventing radiation sickness or fatigue, for example. One of Clynes and Kline's "future projections" involved the "strong possibility" that astronauts would experience psychotic episodes but be incapable of recognizing that anything was awry; what was needed, they argued, was the ability to "[trigger] administration of the medication remotely from earth or by a companion," medication that could include "high-potency phenothiazines together with reserpine."[118]

As this last scenario might suggest, Clynes and Kline both worked in psychiatric research; their work with NASA supplemented their jobs as researchers at Rockland State Hospital, in Orangeburg, New York. Kline founded a psychiatric research center at the hospital in 1952, and he spent most of his career building the center into a major site for drug research, development, and clinical trials. He hired Clynes to work in the hospital's Dynamic Simulation Laboratory in 1955, where the latter worked on physiological instrumentation and data-processing systems. Although Clynes eventually left Rockland, Kline remained there until his death in 1982, and the research facility now bears his name (the Nathan S. Kline Institute for Psychiatric Research). According to the institute's website, Kline is "best known for his pioneering work with psychopharmacologic drugs," particularly his success with tranquilizers and antidepressants.[119] Inspired by these successes, and eager to spread the word about the efficacy of psychopharmacology, Kline wrote a mass-market paperback titled *From Sad to Glad*; first published in 1974, the 1989 edition featured the tagline, "Depression: You can conquer it without analysis." Kline's faith in drugs is evident in the article he coauthored with Clynes, "Cyborgs and Space," in which their imagined osmotic pumps deliver medicine that cures everything from radiation sickness to fatigue to psychosis.

It is this last condition, psychosis, that brings me up short. In their article, Clynes and Kline suggest that astronauts are unlikely to recognize when they have had a psychotic break (explaining that delusion and denial are common symptoms of psychosis) and will need to be involuntarily medicated by remote control. I do not know enough about the mental or emotional effects of space travel to evaluate their concern, but I cannot read their recommendation without being reminded of the two scientists' location in a state mental institution, one where many, if not most, of the patients were placed indefinitely and heavily medicated. Moreover, some of them likely served as research subjects for Kline's drug trials, trials that appear to have been grueling for the patients. In his early research on reserpine as a treatment for schizophrenia, Kline noted that for the first two to three weeks of treatment,

> patients are frightened by the feeling that they have "no control" over their impulses. Some feel that they "do not know what they are going to do next," and in point of fact may begin screaming and throw themselves to the floor. . . . Delusions and hallucinations increase and behavior not infrequently becomes more disturbed than prior to the beginning of treatment.[120]

As the treatment continued, Kline apparently thought that the patients eventually showed improvement, but it is hard to read this description without questioning the ethics of drug trials on institutionalized patients.

Rockland was infamous for its poor and negligent behavior toward patients. Overcrowding was rampant in the 1940s and 1950s, and the institution was repeatedly charged with contributing to, if not causing, the deaths of numerous patients by giving them lethal amounts of tranquilizers—to keep patients "under control"—or prescribing drugs that, in combination, are fatal. Accusations of rape and malnourishment were also lodged against workers and group homes affiliated with Rockland.[121] Although state commissions and investigations consistently rejected these charges, the frequency of such claims gives me pause.

Indeed, this connection to the warehousing of people with mental illnesses and intellectual disabilities in state institutions—and all that entails, from medical negligence to medical experimentation to physical and sexual abuse—should be enough to give any cyborg theorist, especially one identified with disability studies, pause. Haraway makes clear from the start that the cyborg is dangerous, non-innocent, and complicit; the only way to approach the figure is in the spirit of ironic blasphemy, turning the figure against its very origins. And Bradley Lewis's use of the figure to critique the same psychopharmaceutical industry that originally birthed the cyborg seems the perfect illustration of such blasphemy. We need more such disability studies perspectives. Yet part of that work must include a reckoning, an acknowledgement, of the cyborg's history in institutionalization and abuse. Otherwise the irony, the blasphemy, the critique, is lost.

I close with this story to insist, alongside both Haraway and her critics, that the cyborg is not innocent. Our metaphors, our tropes, our analogies: all have histories, all have consequences. As Hiram Perez argues, part of the work of the critic is to explore the effects texts and images have on people's lives.[122] The blurring of boundaries, the permeability of bodies, the porousness of skin—all take on different meanings depending on whether they are viewed through the prism of institutionalization or as part of a strategy of feminist analysis. Arguing for the breakdown between self and other, body and machine, takes on a different hue in the context of coercive medical experimentation and confinement. The cyborg, in other words, can be used to map many futures, not all of them feminist, crip, or queer.

Haraway herself acknowledges this fact, warning us from the beginning of the cyborg's complicity in militarization, colonization, and control. Yet it remains a figure of feminist possibility, pointing toward a feminist futurity or, in Haraway's framing, "an elsewhere, not as a utopian fantasy or relativist escape, but an elsewhere born out of the hard (and sometimes joyful) work of getting on together."[123] To return to the epigraph that begins this chapter, "who cyborgs will be is a radical question; the answers are a matter of survival."[124] This question has political, ethical, and epistemic dimensions, and answering it will require grappling with the histories and futures described here. It is a question I urge us to ask. If, as Haraway claims, "cyborgs are the people who refuse to disappear on cue," then the cyborg may very well be a perfect figure for refusing the erasure of disability from our presents and futures.[125] But in the spirit, if not the practice, of Haraway's manifesto, I argue for responsibility in making such claims.

6 Bodies of Nature

The Environmental Politics of Disability

> The creatures that populate the narrative space called "nature" are key characters in scientific tales about the past, present, and future. Various tellings of these tales are possible, but they are always shaped by historical, disciplinary, and larger cultural contexts.
>
> —Jennifer Terry, "'Unnatural Acts' in Nature"

ALTHOUGH CONCERN WITH the environment has long been an animating force in disability studies and activism, "environment" in this context typically refers to the built environment of buildings, sidewalks, and transportation technologies. Indeed, the social model of disability is premised on concern for the built environment, stressing that people are disabled not by their bodies but by their inaccessible environments. (The wheelchair user confronting a flight of steps is probably the most common illustration of this argument.) Yet the very pervasiveness of the social model has prevented disability studies from engaging with the wider environment of wilderness, parks, and nonhuman nature because the social model seems to falter in such settings. Stairs can be replaced or supplemented with ramps and elevators, but what about a steep rock face or a sandy beach? Like stairs, both pose problems for most wheelchair users, but, argues Tom Shakespeare, "it is hard to blame the natural environment on social arrangements."[1] He asserts that the natural environment—rock cliffs, steep mountains, and sandy beaches—offers proof that "people with impairments will always be disadvantaged by their bodies"; the social model cannot adequately address the barriers presented by those kinds of spaces.[2] I, too, recognize the limitations of the social model and the need to engage with the materiality of bodies, but I am not so sure that the "natural environment" is as distinct from the "built environment" as Shakespeare suggests. On the contrary, the natural environment is also "built": literally so in the case of trails and dams, metaphorically so in the sense of cultural constructions and deployments of "nature," "natural," and "the environment."

Disability studies could benefit from the work of environmental scholars and activists who describe how "social arrangements" have been mapped onto "natural environments." Many campgrounds in the United States, for example, have been designed to resemble suburban neighborhoods, with single campsites for each family, clearly demarcated private and public spaces, and layouts built for cars. Each individual campsite faces onto the road or common area so that rangers (and other campers) can easily monitor others' behavior. Such spacing likely discourages, or at least pushes into the cover of darkness, outwardly queer acts and practices.[3] Environmental historians such as William Cronon document the displacement of indigenous peoples from parklands; indigenous people were removed and evidence of their communities was destroyed so that the new parks could be read as pristine, untouched wilderness.[4] Nature writers such as Carolyn Finney and Evelyn White explain that African Americans are much less likely than whites to find parks and open spaces welcoming, accessible, or safe; histories of white supremacist violence and lynchings in rural areas make the wilderness less appealing. Park brochures, wilderness magazines, and advertisements for outdoor gear have, in turn, tended to cater to overwhelmingly white audiences.[5] As these examples attest, the natural environment is also a built environment, one shaped by and experienced through assumptions and expectations about gender, sexuality, class, race, and nation. As Mei Mei Evans argues, "One way of understanding the culturally dominant conception of what constitutes 'nature' in the United States is to ask ourselves who gets to go there. Access to wilderness and a reconstituted conception of Nature are clearly environmental justice issues demanding redress."[6]

How might we begin to read disability into these formations? How have compulsorily able-bodiedness/able-mindedness shaped not only the environments of our lives—both buildings and parks—but our very understandings of the environment itself? One way to address these questions is by examining the deployment of disability in popular discourses of nature and environmentalism; another method would be to uncover the assumption of able-bodiedness and able-mindedness in writings about nature. I follow both paths in this chapter, unpacking the work of disability and able-bodiedness/able-mindedness in cultural constructions of nature, wilderness, and the environment. As with the visions of a "better" future found in discussions of reproduction, childhood, community, and cyborgs, visions of nature are often idealized and depoliticized fantasies, and disability plays an integral, if often unmarked, role in marking the limit of these fantasies. Whether we focus on nature writing or trail construction (the subjects of the first two sections of this chapter), disabled people are figured as out of place.

Given the often exclusionary dimensions of "nature" and "wilderness," it is important to explore how those considered out of place find ways of engaging and interacting with nature. As Evans argues, the "culturally dominant conception of what constitutes 'nature'" becomes more clear when we encounter the narratives of those who are not expected or allowed "to go there."[7] In the final section of this chapter, then, I explore the possibility of a cripped environmentalism, one that looks to disabled bodies/minds as a resource in thinking about our future natures differently. I argue that the experience of illness and disability presents alternative ways of understanding ourselves in relation to the environment, understandings which can then generate new possibilities for intellectual connections and activist coalitions.

Natural Exclusions

We tend to think of the definitions of terms such as "nature," "wilderness," and "environment" as self-evident, assuming their meanings to be universal, stable, and monolithic. However, as William Cronon argues, "'nature' is not nearly so natural as it seems."[8] On the contrary, our encounters with wilderness are historically and culturally grounded; our ideas about what constitutes "nature" or the "natural" and "unnatural" are completely bound up in our own specific histories and cultural assumptions. What is needed, then, is an interrogation of these very assumptions.[9] Instead of taking for granted the qualities we attribute to wilderness experiences, such as spiritual renewal or physical challenge, we can ask, as Linda Vance does, "[W]hose values are these? What do they assume about experience, and whose experience is the norm? What other social relations depend on or produce these values? What is their historical context?"[10] We can extend the scope of these questions to include an examination of ableism and compulsory able-bodiedness/able-mindedness: Whose experiences of nature are taken as the norm within environmental discourses? What do these discourses assume about nature, the body/mind, and the relationship between humans and nature? And how do notions of disability and able-bodiedness/able-mindedness play a key role in constructing values such as "spiritual renewal" and "physical challenge" in the first place?

In this section, I examine three sites of able-bodiedness/able-mindedness: a canonical environmental memoir, a controversial ad in a mainstream hiking magazine, and an autobiographical essay in ecofeminist philosophy. These are three vastly different texts, with different agendas and from different time periods. I bring them together in order to sketch out the role disability plays in constructions of the natural environment. In the first two selections, the figure of disability is explicitly invoked in order to be immediately disavowed, making clear that disability has no place in the wilderness. Both hail the able body, or the nondisabled body, as the proper denizen of the outdoors; they deploy the figure of disability to further cultural representations of nature as a rugged proving ground, making disability the dystopic sign of human failure, or potential failure, in nature. The final example, the ecofeminist essay, shares the presumption of able-bodiedness that runs through the first two representations, this time presenting the nondisabled body as the grounds through which we arrive at ecofeminist insight. Reading each of these examples through a critical disability lens reveals the ways in which we assume the environmental body to be a very particular kind of body.

One of the most explicit articulations of a compulsorily able-bodied/able-minded environmentalism is found in Edward Abbey's cult classic *Desert Solitaire: A Season in the Wilderness*, first published in 1968.[11] In this highly acclaimed memoir, Abbey offers a polemic against "industrial tourism" in national parks, a phenomenon which is destroying wilderness areas across the country and robbing all of us of our ability to access nature. Abbey repeatedly draws on disability metaphors to make his case, most notably when he refers to cars as "motorized" or "mechanized wheelchairs."[12] By equating cars with wheelchairs, Abbey presents automobiles as having a literally crippling effect on our ability to experience nature. The motorized wheelchair becomes the epitome of technological alienation, of technology's ability to alienate us from our own wild nature and the wilderness around us. Sarah Jaquette Ray calls this pattern the "disability-equals-alienation-from-nature trope,"[13] arguing that Abbey's text relies on disability as "the best symbol of the machine's corruption of . . . harmony between body and nature."[14]

This representation becomes even more clear later in the book, when Abbey exhorts everyone to get out of their cars/wheelchairs and walk: "Yes sir, yes madam, I entreat you, get out of those motorized wheelchairs, get off your foam rubber backsides, stand up straight like men! like women! like human beings! and walk—*walk*—WALK upon our sweet and blessed land!"[15] Although Abbey elsewhere allows for travel by bicycle and horse, he frequently hails walking as the only way to access "the original, the real" nature.[16] Abbey's assertion that we must get out and walk, that truly understanding a space means moving through it on foot, presents a very particular kind of embodied experience as a prerequisite to environmental engagement. Walking through the desert becomes a kind of authorizing gesture; to know the desert requires walking through the desert, and to do so unmediated by technology. In such a construction, there is no way for the mobility-impaired body to engage in environmental practice; all modalities other than walking upright become insufficient, even suspect. Walking is both what makes us human and what makes us at one with nature.[17]

Abbey's framing has been influential. As Ray notes, the environmental movement is deeply attached to the notion of "the solitary retreat into nature as the primary source of an environmental ethic."[18] It is common to find ecocritics making connections and deriving insight from hiking trips and other adventures in the wilderness. By implying that one must have a deep immersion experience of nature in order to understand nature, ecocritics create a situation in which some kinds of experiences can be interpreted as more valid than others, as granting a more accurate, intense, and authentic understanding of nature. They ignore the complicated histories of who is granted permission to enter nature, where nature is said to reside, how one must move in order to get there, and how one will interact with nature once one arrives in it.[19] (As we will see later in the chapter, these assumptions then play a huge role in struggles over increasing disability access in parks and public lands.)

This kind of exclusionary framing of nature is on full display in a provocative advertisement for Nike's Air Dri-Goat shoe. The advertisement ran in eleven different outdoor magazines in the fall of 2000, reaching a combined circulation of approximately 2.1 million readers. It featured a picture of the shoe against a hot-pink background, with this accompanying text:

> Fortunately, the Air Dri-Goat features a patented goat-like outer sole for increased traction, so you can taunt mortal injury without actually experiencing it. Right about now you're probably asking yourself, "How can a trail running shoe with an outer sole designed like a goat's hoof help me avoid compressing my spinal cord into a Slinky˙ on the side of some unsuspecting conifer, thereby rendering me a drooling, misshapen non-extreme-trail-running husk of my former self, forced to roam the earth in a motorized wheelchair with my name, embossed on one of those cute little license plates you get at carnivals or state fairs, fastened to the back?"
>
> To that we answer, hey, have you ever seen a mountain goat (even an extreme mountain goat) careen out of control into the side of a tree?
>
> Didn't think so.

In the first two days after publication, Nike received over six hundred complaints about the ad, and the company withdrew it from further circulation. Three public apologies followed, each one containing more cause for offense.[20] The perceived need for multiple apologies testifies to the blatant offensiveness of the ad. It is not surprising that the ad came under attack: it paints an incredibly negative portrait of people in wheelchairs, trivializes and mocks the experiences of those who have survived spinal cord injuries, and dehumanizes disabled people. Most important for my exploration of crip futures, however, are its assumptions about disability and nature, or, more to the point, its assumptions about the place of a disabled person in nature.

First, in running this advertisement, Nike has assumed that the readers of *Backpacker* and similar magazines are neither disabled nor allies of the disabled, casting outdoor enthusiasts and disabled people as two mutually exclusive groups.[21]

Second, the advertisement assumes that disability prohibits encounters with nature, dooming one to roam "carnivals or state fairs" rather than mountain ranges. It is perhaps no accident that Nike's advertisement conjures an image of disabled people at the fair or carnival, buying accoutrements for their wheelchairs. From the 1840s through the 1940s in the United States, disabled people were frequently exhibited in public at traveling sideshows and carnivals, cast as "freaks," "freaks of nature," and, in a blending of ableist, racist, and colonialist narratives, "missing links."[22] Freak shows were one of the few places where one could see disabled people in public, and the Nike advertisement extends this depiction of the carnival as the proper terrain of the disabled body. Conversely, it makes clear that once one becomes disabled, mountain ranges and wilderness areas are out of reach.

Third, it reminds nondisabled hikers that they must be ever vigilant in protecting themselves from disability, denying any trace of disability in or on their bodies. These last two assumptions are interrelated, in that nondisabled hikers must deny disability precisely because it (allegedly) prohibits encounters with nature. In other words, the advertisement is explicitly invoking a disabled body in order to reassure readers of their own able-bodiedness. As Rosemarie Garland-Thomson argues, the figure of disability "assures the rest of the citizenry of who they are not while arousing their suspicions about who they could become."[23]

Thus, two distinct bodies appear in this text. The first is the nondisabled body ostensibly shared by both Nike associates (the advertisement's "we") and Nike consumers ("you"). The text tells its readers little about this nondisabled body; it takes shape only when juxtaposed with the second body in the text. Unlike the first body, which is unmarked, the second, disabled body is described with utmost specificity: readers learn of its appearance ("drooling, misshapen," and "forced" into a wheelchair), its inabilities ("non-extreme-trail-running"), its quality of life (a "husk of my former self"), and its home ("carnivals or state fairs"). The disabled body appears in the text only as the specter of impending tragedy; one can allegedly ward it away by assertively and aggressively staking one's claim to nature, by "taunting mortal injury" and celebrating one's alleged hyperability. As Ray suggests, it is the "threat of disability" that makes "the wilderness ideal body meaningful"; part of the thrill of adventure is risking—yet ultimately avoiding—disablement.[24] Thus disability exists out of time, as something not-yet and, with the right equipment, not-ever. In order to belong to the text's "us," one must deny any physical limitations or inabilities, casting oneself as separate from and superior to the disabled figure. "We" are not drooling or misshapen disabled people, the text proclaims, we are hikers, and never the twain shall meet. Nike explicitly repudiates the disabled body, casting it as the antithesis of the hiker's body, which is the body "we" all have and want to preserve.

The hiker's body as imagined by both Nike and Abbey is necessary because it is only through it that we are able to truly experience nature (or to experience true nature). Nature, wilderness, mountain ranges: all are described as separate from "us," but we can bridge or transcend that separation by rugged, masculine individualism; disability serves both to illustrate that separation between human and nature and to exacerbate it. Although my third site, an ecofeminist essay, does not rely on this kind of explicit ableism, it, too, continues the narrative of separation from nature. Its reliance on this trope is harder to recognize, as it comes in the context of a much more critical approach to "nature" and "wilderness" than that found in Abbey or Nike.

In her essay "Ecofeminism and the Politics of Reality," Linda Vance traces her political and theoretical development as an ecofeminist. Vance weaves accounts of her own hiking experiences into the essay, revealing how her experiences in and through nature have played an important role in her journey toward ecofeminism. For most of the essay, Vance writes in the first person, describing her personal experiences with nature (e.g., "I hike through the Green Mountains"), but there is one passage in which she shifts to the third person, writing about "an ecofeminist":

> On a bad day, then, say when she's hiking through a spruce bog trying to convince herself that being a food source for mosquitoes and black flies is an ecologically

sound role, an ecofeminist can despair, and start to feel like she is the least loved cousin of just about everyone, and sister to no one. Except, of course—and here she pauses, a boot heavy with black muck arrested in mid-step, and she looks around— except, of course, nature. Sister. Sister Nature.[25]

In this passage, Vance's phrasing itself suggests that "hiking" and "being an ecofeminist" are related activities: by shifting from a description of her own particular experiences to the adventures of an unnamed ecofeminist, Vance positions the figure as a stand-in for all ecofeminists. Moreover, she suggests that it is *through* this kind of rugged activity that "an ecofeminist" comes to understand herself in relation to nonhuman nature. Vance's ecofeminist comes to a key realization as she hikes through the muck; indeed, the act of stepping through the bog is what spurs her insight. Hiking, according to this passage, is vital to an ecofeminist's development of her relationship with and understanding of nature; without such hikes, "an ecofeminist" will remain in some way separate from nature. Once again, able-bodiedness is necessary in order to bridge or transcend the essential separation between human and nature.

Ecofeminism, for Vance, is a complex theoretical and conceptual framework deeply invested in activist practices; she would likely oppose Abbey's assumption that cities are unnatural and impure while wilderness is not.[26] However, the passage under consideration here reflects an assumption not far from Abbey's that one must immerse oneself in nature in order to understand it and one's relationship to it. In describing "an ecofeminist's" hike through the mucky bog, Vance suggests that people need to have personal, physical experiences of the wilderness in order to understand, appreciate, and care for nature. But what kind of experiences render one qualified to understand and care about nature? Are all experiences of nature equally productive of such insights? And how do we define "experiences of nature" in the first place?

These questions lead me back to Shakespeare's assumption that the natural environment is completely separate from social arrangements. Each of the sites I have examined here—Abbey, Nike, Vance—operates under a similar assumption, at least when it comes to the body of the hiker. These accounts take for granted the existence of trails that accommodate one's body, presenting access to "nature" not only as necessary to personal growth or renewal but also as apolitical. Abbey is the extreme here, making clear that the hiker's access to parks and wilderness is natural, but everyone else's (those in "motorized wheelchairs," for example) is political, debatable, and ideally stoppable. To tell a tale of a lack of appropriate access—no trails wide enough for a wheelchair or level enough for crutches—would be to insert the all-too-human into "the wilderness," thereby violating the persistent dualisms between the human and the natural and the natural and the political.

Thus, what is needed in ecofeminism, ecocriticism, and environmentalism in general are the narratives of people whose bodies and minds cause them to interact with nature in nonnormative ways. How might a deaf ecofeminist understand her position within the natural world differently than a hearing one? What can narratives about negotiating trails on crutches reveal about the ways in which all trails—not just "accessible" ones—are constructed and maintained? How do concepts of "nature," "wilderness," and "ecofeminism" shift when elaborated by an ecofeminist who experiences nonhuman nature primarily through sound, smell, and touch rather than sight, or by an ecofeminist who draws more on sounds and sensations than on words? In what ways would "ecofeminist activism" be transformed by someone whose chronic fatigue and pain prevent her from traveling more than a few blocks from her house but do not hinder her environmental organizing, lobbying, and fundraising efforts? How might the use of a service dog affect an ecofeminist's understanding of his relationship with nonhuman nature?

One of my hopes in writing this essay is that nondisabled ecofeminists will supplement these questions with queries of their own: How might reflecting on her able-bodied status affect a nondisabled ecofeminist's understanding of the ecofeminist project? In what ways would he alter his concepts of "nature" and "politics" after thinking through his position in an ableist culture? Making space for these kinds of questions expands the domain of ecofeminism and environmental movements, challenging the representation of nondisabled experience as the only possible way to interact with nonhuman nature. Such challenges will necessarily entail expanding our understandings of nature as well, which will, in turn, affect the environments around us. Our conceptions of "nature" and the natural, in other words, play a direct role in how we shape parks and other public lands.

Accessible Trails and other (Un)Natural Disasters

Ableist assumptions about the body certainly influence the concrete realities of access, thereby affecting disabled and nondisabled people alike. Steep, narrow, and root-filled trails are barriers not just for people with mobility or vision impairments but also for some seniors and families with young children. Similarly, nature education has developed around the needs of the nondisabled, as attested by the dearth of interpretive materials available in alternate formats such as Braille, large print, or audiotape.[27] The lack of maps, guidebooks, park brochures, and explanatory markers in large print affects not only those who identify as disabled, however, but all people with low vision. Thinking through these issues can help deconstruct the ableist assumptions embedded in contemporary and historical ideas about nature. Ecofeminists can then begin the process of tracing the impact those assumptions have had on the design of trails and park materials, designs that, in turn, have determined who is able to use such resources. As Rob Imrie and Huw Thomas argue, "These contexts may be thought of as perpetuating forms of environmental injustice, in which inappropriate and thoughtless design means that disabled people cannot use significant parts of the environment."[28]

Mobility is one of the key issues in terms of trail access, and proposals to create wheelchair accessibility are often met with scrutiny, as if such access were inherently more damaging to the environment than access points for nondisabled people.

Plans to build an accessible canoe launch on Maine's Allagash Wilderness Waterway, for example, were met with opposition from environmental groups because such a launch would allegedly damage the waterway.[29] Although some critics were clear that they opposed any new access points on the waterway, regardless of their design, others seemed more concerned about the level of accessibility offered by this proposal; there was a sense that an accessible launch would be more damaging to the environment than an inaccessible one. But most canoe launches are created by clearing away brush, altering the gravel or sand levels near the water, and constructing parking areas and toilets, raising doubts as to whether accessible launches are really more detrimental than inaccessible ones. An accessible site may differ from an inaccessible site only slightly, having wider doors on the bathroom and a wider and more level path to the water, changes that are not necessarily more disruptive or damaging.

When I was visiting a wildlife refuge in Rhode Island in the spring of 2007, one of the staff recounted the recent outcry from the local community about making trails within the refuge wheelchair accessible. According to their complaints, both the materials used in such a trail (in this case, crushed asphalt) and the users of such trails (presumably people with wheelchairs or other mobility aids) would be too noisy; birds that nested in the area would be scared away by the trail's imagined new inhabitants. However, given how frequently hikers use cellphones, talk loudly with their companions, or yell after a child, it is hard to believe that noise is the real fear here. While birders may dislike those interruptions as well, they were not advocating for barriers to keep them out; children were permitted in the park without having to undergo some kind of silencing or muting practice. (Moreover, I would imagine a crushed asphalt trail or, especially, a paved trail would be much quieter than one made of thick gravel or covered in dry, brittle leaves and branches).

Or, to take yet another example, in 2000, when a group of disabled and nondisabled hikers made a trek to the newly accessible hut at Galehead in the White Mountains, they were met with derision on the trail by a nondisabled hiker who accused them of taking up too much room and harming the terrain. In a letter to the editor of the *New York Times*, Dan Bruce condemned those involved with the hike, charging them with "selfishness": "Wheelchairs do incredible damage to trails in these fragile areas. Did anyone in the group do an environmental assessment before attempting the exploit or consider that the damage done to the trail by their wheeled equipment may take years for nature to repair?"[30] What interests me about Bruce's letter, and the comments from the hiker on the trail, is the presumption that wheelchair users inevitably damage trails more than other hikers do.

It was not just the disabled hikers' presence on the trail that garnered criticism, however, but the very idea that a backcountry cabin would be retrofitted with a wheelchair ramp and accessible bathroom. Challenging the need for the ramp, one reporter asked "why people in wheelchairs could drag themselves up the trail and not drag themselves up the steps to the hut?"[31] If the hikers were able to complete such an arduous hike, in other words, surely they were capable of crawling up the steps to the cabin. This challenge to the appropriateness of the Galehead ramp exemplifies the ways in which nondisabled access is made invisible while disabled access is made hypervisible. Steps are themselves an accommodation, just one made for a different kind of body; as Jill Gravink notes, rather than focus on ramps as being out of place, the reporter could have just as easily focused on stairs, demanding of nondisabled hikers, "Why bother putting steps on the hut at all? Why not drag yourself in through a window?"[32]

Those who protest the development of accessible trails and services consistently use the language of protection in making their claims; in their view, increasing disability access and protecting the environment are irreconcilable. But the fact that it is often only *disability* access that comes under such interrogation suggests an act of ableist forgetting. As the steps/ramp question shows, the development of trails and buildings that suit very particular bodies goes unmarked as access; indeed, it is only when atypical bodies are taken in to account that the question of access becomes a problem. The rhetoric of ecoprotection then seems to be more about a discomfort with the artifacts of access—ramps, barrier-free pathways—and the bodies that use them. Trails, which are mapped, cut, and maintained by human beings with tools and machinery, are seen as *natural*, but wheelchair accessible trails are seen as *unnatural*. The very phrasing of these sentences reveals the differences in valence: trails, by definition (or, more to the point, *naturally*), are not wheelchair accessible; they need no modifier. Reading for disability, then, opens up these assumptions, making visible the ways in which the constructedness of *all* trails is covered over by focusing on the constructedness of *some* trails.

Some disability organizations, such as California-based Whole Access, have countered these assumptions, stressing that, while all trails affect the land, well-designed trails can both minimize that impact and maximize accessibility for all people, including those with mobility disabilities.[33] For example, installing boardwalks over fragile land, as has been done in the Florida Everglades, Cape Lookout National Seashore, and Yellowstone National Park, promotes access for people with mobility impairments and people with small children while also protecting delicate terrain from direct traffic. People are less likely to step off the boardwalk and walk through prohibited/protected areas than they are on a trail. In collaboration with California State Parks, Whole Access documented how trails that follow the natural contours of the land (as opposed to steeper trails that cut vertically through a slope) tend to reduce erosion, require less maintenance, and increase accessibility because of their more gentle slopes and inclines.[34]

Access to the wilderness, as many disability activists and advocates argue, is not an all-or-nothing endeavor. Some accessible trails and entry points are better than none, and trails that cannot be brought into full compliance with accessibility guidelines can often be easily modified to permit some disability access. Don Beers, a district supervisor with California State Parks, explains, "The big thing was changing my mindset that [accessibility] had to be all or nothing. . . . The thought now is, let's look at every trail to make it as accessible as possible."[35] Beers's instruction to make every trail "as accessible as possible" can be interpreted narrowly; like the call for "reasonable" accommodation under the Americans with Disabilities Act, it can potentially be used as a way to rule out some changes as too extreme (as "unreasonable"). But, read radically, making every trail "as accessible as possible" means that every trail needs to take every kind of body and way of movement into account. That doesn't mean that every single trail will actually accommodate every single body—there will be terrain too rocky or too steep for some bodies and modalities. But this is true for all bodies, disabled and nondisabled. What shifts in this view is that trails are no longer designed only for one single body, and that decisions about trails are recognized *as* decisions, ones that can be changed, extended, modified.

Moreover, making every trail as accessible as possible disrupts the long-standing pattern of making visitors' centers and very short nature trails accessible, while ignoring disability access everywhere else. Such a model of access, argues Ann Sieck, a wheelchair hiker who has long been involved in attempts to improve wheelchair access in Bay Area parks, sends "the alienating—if unintended—message that for disabled people the outdoors is available only at 'special' facilities. It is hard to describe how painful it is to be excluded through simple indifference, or through the ignorance of planners who see no need to maximize the usability of trails that are not designated 'whole access.'"[36]

Yet, as Laura Hershey recounts, even when wheelchair hikers discover trails for themselves, their experiences are often not incorporated into official park literature. Hiking in Yosemite with her lover and their attendant, Hershey came upon a sign with "a red circle and bar canceling out the universal wheelchair access symbol." After much discussion, Hershey and her companions chose to continue, and after a difficult and bumpy ride they arrived at a magnificent view of a waterfall. Hershey included a description of the hike in "Along Asphalt Trails," an essay for *National Parks*, the magazine of the National Parks Conservation Association. Prior to publication, however, an editor cut that section of the essay because it might encourage readers to ignore posted signs.[37] Yet, as Hershey's story demonstrates, such signs are based on ableist assumptions about what "accessible" trails look like. I have hiked on the trail Hershey describes, and it was more rugged than I could handle in my manual chair; I made it to the waterfall only with generous help and my willingness to crawl on the ground. It *is* inaccessible to many folks with mobility impairments (and perhaps also to adults traveling with small children, or elderly hikers, or those uninterested in such a strenuous hike), but not all. What seems important in Hershey's story is its insistence that disabled hikers have the same opportunities as nondisabled hikers to make their own decisions about access, including unsuccessful (or even risky) ones.

Thus, the problem of assuming access to be an all-or-nothing endeavor extends beyond the construction and maintenance of trails to the training given park rangers and wildlife docents. As long as they are talking to nondisabled hikers, park rangers are full of detailed information about hiking trails in the area. I have often observed rangers asking hikers what kind of terrain they want, how long they want to hike, and what level of difficulty best suits their needs. As a wheelchair user, however, I am seldom asked these kinds of questions, as if my desired level of difficulty were self-evident. As Sieck notes, "park rangers are also unable to answer questions about a trail's usability—it's either designated as accessible or not, end of discussion."[38] This lack of information is mirrored in park maps and other material that make no mention of accessible facilities, or, more often, that assume accessible facilities to mean only one kind of experience.

Scrambling, Climbing, Touching, Holding: How to Crip the Trail Map

Loss is a topic disabled people are typically reluctant to discuss, and for good reason. Disability is all too often read exclusively in such terms, with bitterness, pity, and tragedy being the dominant registers through which contemporary US culture understands the experiences of disabled people. Why encourage such attitudes by speaking publicly about our inabilities, frustrations, and limitations? Yet loss is undeniably one of the motivations behind this chapter, behind my concern with trails and beaches and access. Prior to my injuries, I was a runner, and running was an activity I loved largely for its solitude. Running gave me the adrenaline high of physical exertion, but more importantly it served as a meditative practice, as a way to be outside alone in nature. I ran along the beach in eastern North Carolina, through the woods in upstate New York, next to farmland in northern California; I used these experiences to clear my head, to make sense of my thoughts, to maintain my mental and physical health. When Linda Vance writes about discovering herself in nature, feeling at one with the ecosystem, or developing relationships with nonhuman nature by wading through a bog, I know exactly what she is talking about; I feel it in my bones. Although I agree with environmental critics in their deconstruction of the "nature" experience, and their insistence that there is no bright line between nature and culture, I cannot deny that I feel different "outside," away from traffic and exhaust pipes and crowds of people. That I have been conditioned to feel this way does not change the fact that I feel more at peace in my body when perched on the side of a cliff, or gazing over a meadow, or surrounded by sequoias.

Loss factors into all of this because such experiences are made much more difficult by the body I have now, the body that relies primarily on a wheelchair for mobility. It is hard to find an isolated yet accessible trail that will grant me the solitude I seek; it is hard to get down to the water's edge or up the cliff's peak. Part of this difficulty is due to the histories of trail development and access discussed earlier—the assumption that only certain kinds of bodies need to be accommodated in parks and on trails—but it is also due to the terrain itself. There simply are hills too steep, creeks too rocky, soil too sandy for a wheelchair; or, rather, ensuring access to some locations would mean so drastically altering those locations that the aesthetic and environmental damage to the area would be profound. (The same is true, of course, for *nondisabled* access to some areas.)

Thus, this kind of project entails reckoning with loss, limitation, inability, and failure. Indeed, I long to hear stories that not only admit limitation, frustration, even failure, but that recognize such failure as ground for theory itself. What might Vance's ecofeminist have learned about her connection to nonhuman nature if she had fallen in that mucky bog? How might her framing of nature shift if she had turned around that day, finding the bog too slippery for her loping gait? Moving outward from eco-feminism, we can occasionally find disability in popular nature writing, but almost always as something to be overcome, and overcome spectacularly. The story of Eric Weihenmayer's blind ascent of Mount Everest, for example, relies on disability to hold our interest, but the narrative's very structure assumes that our interest is dependent on disability eventually being vanquished.

Weihenmayer's memoir, *Touch the Top of the World*, suggests that successfully hiking Everest was a way for him to "transcend" his blindness. His story would lose its thread if it ended not with the successful ascent but with Weihenmayer discovering that the peak was simply too high, or the climb too dangerous, or the risks too great. Weihenmayer does mention two instances when he and his climbing partner turned back, failing to reach the summit of Humphrey's Peak in Arizona, and, later, of Long's Peak in Colorado. But these two stories appear in the first few pages of the book, and only in passing; their function in the narrative is to make Weihenmayer's later successes all the more remarkable.[39]

Weihenmayer's climb—not to mention his career as a motivational speaker—exemplifies the narrative of the "supercrip," the stereotypical disabled person who garners media attention for accomplishing some feat considered too difficult for disabled people (depending on the kind of impairment under discussion, supercrip acts can include anything from rock climbing to driving a car). Weihenmayer is familiar with the supercrip narrative, and at times seems wary and tired of it, but his book cannot easily be read through any other lens. Its narrative structure repeats the overcoming tale over and over again, both within and between chapters, and everything about the marketing of the book, from its cover images to its promotional blurbs, reiterates this interpretation of Weihenmayer. Supercrip stories rely heavily on the individual/medical model of disability, portraying disability as something to be overcome through hard work and perseverance. And a disabled person accomplishing an amazing adventure in the wilderness is one of the most pervasive supercrip narratives; such stories are popular because of their twinned conquests: both disability and wilderness are overcome by individual feats of strength and will. As Petra Kuppers notes, "[T]he same language of overcoming used traditionally in relation to nature conquests also informs much writing about disability: conquest and vanquishing, lording over or being lorded over, climbing the mountain or perishing on its slopes."[40] Indeed, it is the very combination of these barriers that makes the stories work.

To return to my earlier questions, then, what stories get effaced by this focus on the supercrip's achievements? Can we imagine a crip interaction with nature, a crip engagement with wilderness, that doesn't rely on either ignoring the limitations of the body or triumphing over them? In asking these questions, I am motivated by a desire to write myself back into nature even as I unpack the binary of nature and self, nature and human. Discussions about the practicalities of access—such as Whole Access's advocacy for universally designed trails—is certainly a necessary part of this work; the sooner we recognize that all trails are built interventions on the landscape, and as such can be reimagined or reconceived, the sooner we can make room for a fuller range of bodies, including but not limited to disabled people. Equally important, however, is a willingness to expand our understanding of human bodies in nonhuman nature, to multiply the possibilities for understanding nature in and through our bodies. If, as Catriona Sandilands argues, queer ecology means "seeing beauty in the wounds of the world and taking responsibility to care for the world as it is," then perhaps a feminist/queer/crip ecology might mean approaching nature through the lenses of loss and ambivalence.[41]

There are disabled people and disability studies scholars doing exactly this kind of reimagining. In *Exile and Pride: Disability, Queerness, and Liberation*, poet Eli Clare provides a moving reflection on the diverse ways human bodies interact with nonhuman nature. He begins with a tale of hiking New Hampshire's Mount Adams:

> The trail divides and divides again, steeper and rockier now, moving not around but over piles of craggy granite, mossy and a bit slick from the night's rain. I start having to watch where I put my feet. Balance has always been somewhat of a problem for me, my right foot less steady than my left. On uncertain ground, each step becomes a studied move, especially when my weight is balanced on my right foot. I take the trail slowly, bringing both feet together, solid on one stone, before leaning into my next step. . . . There is no rhythm to my stop-and-go clamber.[42]

Clare scrambles up and down the mountain, climbing on all fours when he cannot trust his feet. As do other ecocritics and ecofeminists, Clare uses his experiences as a ground for theory, in his case moving from this particular hike to a longer meditation on the politics of bodies, access, and ableism. In other respects, however, Clare's narrative of the mountain stands in stark contrast to the prevailing narrative of moving through nature without any difficulties. In Clare's ascent of Mount Adams, he must eventually reckon with the limitations of his own body. As the afternoon wears on, Clare and his friend realize that they will probably need to turn around before reaching the summit, given Clare's slow pace and the remaining hours of daylight. Such a decision doesn't come easily, however, and Clare shares his frustrations with his reader:

> I want to continue up to treeline, the pines shorter and shorter, grown twisted and withered, giving way to scrub brush, then to lichen-covered granite, up to the sun-drenched cap where the mountains all tumble out toward the hazy blue horizon. I want to so badly, but fear rumbles next to love next to real lived physical limitations,

and so we decide to turn around. I cry, maybe for the first time, over something I want to do, had many reasons to believe I could, but really can't. I cry hard, then get up and follow Adrianne back down the mountain. It's hard and slow, and I use my hands and butt often and wish I could use gravity as Adrianne does to bounce from one flat spot to another, down this jumbled pile of rocks.[43]

Clare goes on to discuss his ambivalence with this decision, an ambivalence stemming from his own internalized ableism. He cannot help but feel that he should have gone on, he should have overcome his limitations:

I climbed Mount Adams for an hour and a half scared, not sure I'd ever be able to climb down, knowing that on the next rock my balance could give out, and yet I climbed. Climbed surely because I wanted the summit, because of the love rumbling in my bones. But climbed also because I wanted to say, "Yes, I have CP [cerebral palsy], but see. See, watch me. I can climb mountains too." I wanted to prove myself once again. I wanted to overcome my CP. . . . The mountain just won't let go.[44]

Clare uses this experience to reflect on the ways in which disabled people hold ourselves up to norms that we can never achieve, norms that were based on bodies, minds, or experiences unlike our own. We want to believe that if we accomplish the right goals, if we overcome enough obstacles, we can defend ourselves against disability oppression.[45] The mountain, both literal and metaphorical, becomes a proving ground rather than a site of connection or relation, and it is this characterization that Clare challenges throughout the book.

The mountain as proving ground is a terrain of fierce independence; "In the wilderness myth, the body is pure, 'solo,' left to its own devices, and unmediated by any kind of aid."[46] Cripping this terrain, then, entails a more collaborative approach to nature. Kuppers depicts human-nonhuman nature interactions not in terms of solo ascents or individual feats of achievement, but in terms of community action and ritual. Describing a gathering of disabled writers, artists, and community members, she writes,

We create our own rhythms and rock ourselves into the world of nature, lose ourselves in a moment of sharing: hummed songs in the round, shared breath, leanings, rocks against wood, leaves falling gentle against skin, bodies braced against others gently lowering toes into waves, touch of bark against finger, cheek, from warm hand to cold snow and back again.[47]

In this resolutely embodied description, the human and nonhuman are brought into direct contact, connecting the fallen leaf to the tree, or the breath to the wind. What entices me about this description is that it acknowledges loss or inability—she goes on to describe the borders of parking lots and the edges of pathways as the featured terrain, not cliff tops and crevices—and suggests alternative ways of interacting with the worlds around us. Rather than conquering or overcoming nature, Kuppers and her comrades describe caressing it, gazing upon it, breathing with it. Such forms of interaction are made more possible by recognizing nature as (and in) everything around us. The edges of the park, the spaces along its borders, are a part of nature, too.

Moreover, Kuppers's "we" is an acknowledgement of the ways in which our encounters with nature include and encompass relations with other people. Humans are interdependent, and our relationships with each other play a role in our understanding of the nonhuman world. Samuel Lurie, who is nondisabled, hints of this interdependence in an essay about his relationship with Clare:

> On one of our first hikes in Vermont, on a steep, slippery trail, the kind where Eli moves especially slowly—he was shrugging off my outstretched hand, not wanting any help. But I was only offering it in part to provide balance. "We're lovers out on a hike," I reasoned, "you're supposed to want to hold my hand." He laughed, relaxing, the tension breaking. . . .
>
> We hike more easily now, Eli referring to my hand serving as that "third point of contact"—stabilizing and comforting.[48]

How might this story of interdependence, of moving through nonhuman nature in relationship, expand the realm of ecofeminism? How might it bolster the claims of ecocritics who reject popular distinctions between humans and nature by presenting other humans as part of our encounters with nature? What happens to theory when it is no longer based primarily on tales of individuals' encounters with nature, but on experiences of interdependence and community? Hiking with a small child, assisting an elderly relative through the woods, or sitting with a neighbor in a city park—all activities we might be doing already—can transform our ideas about nature and about ourselves. Recognizing our interdependence makes room for a range of experiences of human and nonhuman nature, disrupting the ableist ideology that everyone interacts with nature in the same way.

In her video "In My Language," A. M. (Amanda) Baggs offers a visual and aural description of her interactions with the world around her, a description that radically expands econormative conceptions of both nature and interaction. To be clear, the video is not "about" nature and the environment but is, rather, an autobiographical account of living with autism. Yet, in this self-portrait, Baggs interacts fully with her surroundings, challenging implicit assumptions that nature only exists "out there" as opposed to in the everyday spaces around us. In the first half of the video, the only sounds we hear are Baggs's wordless songs and noises; the second half features a script Baggs wrote that is voiced by her computer. Throughout, we watch Baggs touch, smell, listen to, look at, and tap objects around her. In one scene, Baggs runs her fingers under a faucet, gently moving her fingers through the water. These images are accompanied by text scrolling across the bottom of the screen, and Baggs's computer voices the words she has typed: "It [my language] is about being in a constant conversation with every aspect of my environment. Reacting physically to all parts of my surroundings. . . . The water doesn't symbolize anything. I am just interacting with the water as the water interacts with me."[49] The images confirm Baggs's syntax: the water spills across her fingers, shifting its flow in response to her movements. In foregrounding this mutual interaction between fingers and water, between self and stream, Baggs pushes us to expand our conceptions of both language and nature; indeed, the two are intimately related. Language is about interaction with our environments, a mutual interaction that does not, cannot, occur only in spoken words or written text.

Yet, as Baggs reminds us, spoken words and written text are almost always the only forms of communication recognized and valued as language. Similarly, only certain kinds of interactions with the environment are recognized as such; swimming in the ocean and wading in mountain streams are more likely to be understood as meaningful ways to interact with water, while running one's fingers under a faucet is not. But why not? The answer lies partly in long-standing assumptions that nature and the environment only exist "out there," outside of our houses and neighborhoods; the answer lies, too, in long-standing—and even less visible—assumptions that only certain ways of understanding and acting on one's relation to the environment (including other humans) are acceptable. These assumptions have significant material effects. Seeing nature as only "out there," or faucet water as categorically different from ocean water, makes environmental justice work all the more difficult. And, as Baggs argues in her video, seeing her diverse interactions with her environment as strange or abnormal makes it all too easy to ignore the institutionalization and abuse of people on the autism spectrum or people with intellectual disabilities.

Artist Riva Lehrer offers more visual images of crip approaches to nature, representations that argue for human-nonhuman relationships based on the very limitations or variations of the body that are typically ignored in environmental literature. In *In the Yellow Woods* (fig. 6.1), a woman kneels on the ground, peeling the bark from a branch with her knife. She looks down, concentrating on her work, completely focused on the task before her. On the ground around her are scattered bones, bones she has carved herself from tree branches and trunks. A perfect pelvis, a rib cage, random bits of leg and spine—all lie next to her on the ground. She is literally carving a body from the trees. The painting, and the woman, seem inhabited by loss; the intensity of her concentration suggests the necessity of these new bones, these bones untouched by pain or surgery or breakage. And yet the scattered placement of the bones suggests that this work is not about creating some wholeness, not about finding the cure in this forest; she has not arranged the bones in the shape of a body, and she is not inserting them into her skin. Rather the bones seem to sink into the fallen leaves, to become part of the autumn landscape.

Bones become roots, linking this woman—her body, her self—to the landscape, literally grounding her in space and time. And time itself is in play here, as these bones vary in their coloration, marking time across their surfaces. The pelvis gleams white, new, untouched by rain and storm, while some of the longer bones—rib, clavicle, femur—bear the marks of time, calling to mind fossils of previous generations, suggesting that these bones are not only for her. By the same token, the dress pattern

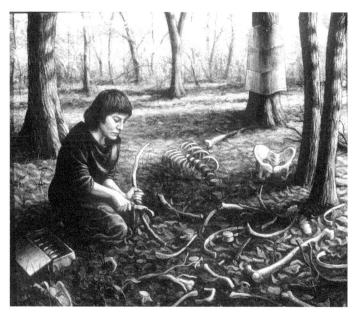

Figure 6.1. Riva Lehrer, *In the Yellow Wood*, 1993, acrylic on panel.

tacked to the tree in the background suggests a future project, a sign of additional work to come, a guideline for other bodies. Although depicted alone in this forest, signs of other bodies, other figures, echo around the woman.

It is the process captured in the painting that captures me, that draws me in to the figure's meditative practice. How does this painting simultaneously offer a new map of the body and a new map of nature? How might it open up new avenues of understanding ourselves in relationship to nonhuman nature? Indeed, how does it blur the very line between the human and the nonhuman? Reading this painting from a cripped ecofeminist perspective, I see a woman making a connection between caring for the body and caring for the earth, suggesting an expanded view of health that looks beyond the boundaries of the body. This is not a supercrip story of triumphing over disability, and it's not an ableist story of bodies without limitation. It's a story of recognizing ourselves in the world around us, recognizing common structures of bone, flesh, oxygen, and air.

These connections manifest again in Lehrer's portrait of Eli Clare, part of her *Circle Stories* series of paintings chronicling the lives of disability artists, activists, and intellectuals. In this 2003 painting (fig. 6.2), Clare crouches on the ground, one knee touching the sandy soil, the other bracing his body. In the background is a river lined by trees, trees that are reflected in the surface of the water. The detail with which the flora is represented is telling, making clear that the plants are as important as the person. In fact, "person" and "plant" are not so easily distinguished, as evidenced by the young sapling emerging out of Clare's chest. The tree is rooted firmly in the ground

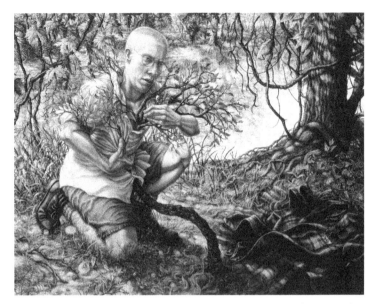

Figure 6.2. Riva Lehrer, *Circle Stories/Eli Clare*, 2003, acrylic on panel.

before Clare, and it curves to snake through his shirt. It's not clear if Clare has buttoned his shirt around the tree, clutching it to his chest, or if the tree made its own way onto Clare's skin, the two figures moving upward together. The painting is breathtaking in its conjuring of an entire ecosystem, one that recognizes human as inextricably part of nature. Its power also lies in its mythology, in its blending together of environmental, disability, and gender politics.

As Lehrer makes clear in her artist's statement, her *Circle Stories* paintings are intensely collaborative. She meets repeatedly with her subjects, studying and discussing their work, and brainstorming potential imagery. Lehrer's work with Clare coincided with his transition from butch female to genderqueer to transman (the collaboration lasted approximately two and one-half years), and it seems no accident that this young tree explodes from the site of Clare's changed chest. The image implicitly challenges easy depictions of technology as bad, as encroaching on the alleged purity of nature. This tree is healthy, vibrant; advanced biomedicine hasn't stunted its growth. On the ground before Clare are long locks of red hair, even a piece of a braid, suggesting that Clare has shed traces of femininity just as the trees around him will drop their leaves. The site of nature serves as a site of transformation in this painting, the clutched tree rooting Clare in his history but also exploding outward in new directions.

These tales of the gendered body intertwine with tales of the crip body. Clare writes poignant prose and poetry about living in a body marked by tremors and an uneven gait, signs of his cerebral palsy. Knowing these histories of Clare's body, I can't help but notice that it is Clare's right hand that clutches the tree to his chest, his right hand that pulls the shirt closed around his sapling. In an essay titled "Stolen Bodies, Reclaimed Bodies," Clare writes, "Sometimes I wanted to cut off my right arm so it wouldn't shake. My shame was that plain, that bleak."[50] This image serves as an antidote to that memory, a reclaiming of that right arm. The steady sureness of the sapling—rooted, curving into Clare's body without breaking or splintering—becomes linked to the sure shaking of Clare's body, so that the tremors become rooted in both the body and the place. Like with the bone woman in the forest, Clare isn't connecting with nature in order to be cured of his allegedly broken body, but rather is solidly locating that body in space and time. He's not getting rid of the tremor but locating it, grounding it; it's as much a part of his body as the tree. As in her self-portrait *In the Yellow Wood*, Lehrer again presents a model of embodied environmentalism, of a concern with how we can get on together, earth, bone, and body.

I bring these paintings into my exploration of disability and environmentalism because they conjure images of nature-human relationships that not only allow for the presence of bodies with limited, odd, or queer movements and orientations, but they literally carve out a space for them, recognizing them as a vital part of the landscape. The content of Clare's and Lehrer's work as activists encourages my paying attention to these images, facilitates my placing them within the discourse of ecological feminism and environmentalism. Both of them are longtime advocates for environmental causes: *Exile and Pride* is a complex meditation on relationships among race, class, poverty, labor politics, gender, and environmental destruction/conservation in the Pacific Northwest, and Lehrer is a longtime supporter of animal rights movements.[51] Moreover, they both make explicit connections between these environmental projects and their location in disability communities. Clare writes poignantly about the disabling effects of logging on bodies and ecosystems, and of coming to understand his crip body on the rural roads and creeksides of rural Oregon. His book, which bears the subtitle *Disability, Queerness, and Liberation*, is dedicated "to the rocks and trees, hills and beaches," suggesting a direct link between his understanding of queer disability and the landscapes around him. Similarly, Lehrer's paintings often combine landscapes with portraits, and nonhuman animals are a common presence in her paintings and drawings. In two of her most recent series, *Family* and *Totems and Familiars*, she showcases relationships between human and nonhuman animals; in the latter, she depicts crip artists such as Nomy Lamm alongside their animal familiars, animals that serve as alter egos or sources of strength. The cultural productions of artists such as Clare and Lehrer enact alternate versions of nature and of humans' position within it. They are imagining and embodying new understandings of environmentalism that take disability experiences seriously, as sites of knowledge production about nature. Their future visions, because grounded in present crip communities, recognize disability experiences and human limitations as essential, not marginal or tangential, to questions about "nature" and environmental movements.

7 Accessible Futures, Future Coalitions

> A vital moment in coalitional political rhetoric is its ability to construct connections among struggles that may be not only diverse, but opposed to one another in many respects.
>
> —Catriona Sandilands, *The Good-Natured Feminist*

WHEN DESCRIBING DISABILITY studies to my students, I often draw on Douglas Baynton's insight that "disability is everywhere in history once you begin looking for it."[1] For Baynton, "looking for it" entails not only recovering the stories of disabled people or tracing histories of disability discrimination but also exploring how notions of disability and able-mindedness/able-bodiedness have functioned in different contexts. Baynton issues his provocation to historians, but disability studies scholars in other fields have extended its reach, pushing their own colleagues to recognize disability as a category of analysis. Deeply influenced by and indebted to this work, I use this final chapter to read Baynton's assertion differently. Rather than direct his insight outward, to those not currently working in disability studies, I turn inward, directing it to the field itself. If "disability is everywhere . . . once you begin looking for it," where do we, as disability studies scholars and activists, continue *not* to look? Where do we find disability and where do we miss it? In which theories and in which movements do we recognize ourselves, or recognize disability, and which theories and movements do we continue to see as separate from or tangential to disability studies?

These questions, and potential answers to them, have surfaced in previous chapters, but in this final chapter I address them more directly. In imagining what accessible futures might look like or might include, I find myself thinking about the possibilities of cross-movement work, both intellectually and politically. If disability is everywhere once we start looking for it, then why not look for it in the other social justice movements at work in contemporary culture? My understanding of disability rights, justice, politics, culture, and scholarship has always been informed by my investments in feminist and queer theories and practices. Reading disability into and alongside those investments is one way to imagine disability differently. In other words, looking within disability studies for the traces of other movements while simultaneously looking for disability in places it has gone unmarked is one way of moving us toward accessible futures.

I begin "looking for disability" in a canonical feminist studies text—Bernice Johnson Reagon's influential essay on coalition politics—that is not widely recognized as being "about" disability. Reading disability into it not only allows for an expansion of feminist and disability studies genealogies but also offers a framework for imagining future work. I then move outward from Reagon's text to explore three potential areas of growth for feminist, queer, crip theory and activism: bathroom politics and contestations over public space; environmental justice; and reproductive justice. Zeroing in on each of these sites allows us to think through how different formulations of disability encourage (and discourage) unexpected but generative alliances. I close by invoking still more connections and coalitions, making clear the multiple and overlapping possibilities for feminist, queer, crip futures.

Reagon's text serves as an apt introduction to this chapter because of her frank acknowledgment of and engagement with practices of dissent and strife. Throughout the essay, she encourages us to recognize that the *benefits* of coalition politics are bound up in the *difficulties* of such politics. Disagreement pushes us to recognize and acknowledge our own assumptions and the boundaries we draw around our own work; without such disagreement, and the ways it compels us to reexamine our positions, we can too easily skim over our own exclusions and their effects. I have chosen each of the sites I highlight here—trans/disability bathroom politics, environmental justice movements, and reproductive justice movements—in large part because they, too, are contentious. They force our attention to the formation of the identities, positions, and practices we name as feminist and/or as queer and/or as crip. They also offer contradictions that are not easily resolvable, contradictions that make difficult any facile claims to "unity" or sameness.

I am influenced here by the work of feminist theorists such as Audre Lorde, Chantal Mouffe, and Ranu Samantrai, each of whom argues for the value, and necessity, of dissent. Samantrai explains that "dissenters draw attention to the border zones where . . . norms are negotiated," subjecting "the terms of membership" in a political community to "continual revision."[2] Indeed, rather than "expelling conflicts and suppressing their annoying reminders," a coalition politics that embraces dissent can begin to ask "how we can take advantage" of such conflicts.[3] Thus, in using the language of "coalition," I am less interested in imagining coalition politics "as a process of dealing with already-constituted interests and identities"—women as discrete group working with disabled people as discrete group—than in thinking through coalitions as a process in which the interests and identities themselves are always open to contestation and debate.[4] How does "disabled" shift, expand, or contract in these various movements and theories? In other words, part of what excites me about the coalitions I examine here is that they often trouble the boundaries of the constituencies involved. Thinking through trans/disability bathroom politics, then, means not only accounting for "disabled people" working alongside "trans- people," or even people who are both trans and disabled, but also questioning the very categories of "disabled people" and "trans- people."

Finding Disability: Feminist Texts, Disability Theory

I teach in a feminist studies program at a small liberal arts college, and my courses are marked "feminist studies" far more often than "disability studies." The productive overlaps between the two fields, however, allow me to insert disability studies insights and analyses into conversations that are not marked as such; disability often surfaces in our conversations even though we were not explicitly looking for it. In that spirit, I want to offer here a rereading of a text familiar, even canonical, to feminist studies audiences, but one that is not widely recognized as a "disability studies text." Reading it again, through the lens of disability, opens up additional possibilities for overlap and critique between disability and feminist studies. As my understandings of crip futurity and feminist cross-movement work have been deeply influenced by this essay, it feels fitting to explore it in this final chapter.

"Coalition Politics: Turning the Century," by Bernice Johnson Reagon, was published in Barbara Smith's *Home Girls: A Black Feminist Anthology* in 1983.[5] Reagon reflects on the process of coalition building, asserting that forming coalitions across difference is both necessary and terrifying: necessary, in that in order to create political change we need to recognize the interrelations among different issues and identities; terrifying, in that we often are working with people unlike us, people who might frame the issues in different ways or to different effects, people who come from different perspectives or with different histories, people who might challenge our founding assumptions.

Reagon's essay is based on a presentation she gave at the 1981 West Coast Women's Music Festival in California's Yosemite National Forest. As many scholars have noted, her piece bears the traces of this location; her focus on coalitions, and on the limitations of monolithic constructions of "woman," was clearly based on contemporary conversations about racism and classism within the women's movement and the role (and composition) of women-only spaces.[6] I want to highlight, however, the ways in which her essay bears the traces not only of the women's music festival but also of the Yosemite National Forest.

Reagon begins the essay with this paragraph:

I've never been this high before. I'm talking about the altitude. There is a lesson in bringing people together where they can't get enough oxygen, then having them try to figure out what they're going to do when they can't think properly. I'm serious about that. There probably are some people here who can breathe, because you were born in high altitudes and you have big lung cavities. But when you bring people in who have not had the environmental conditioning, you got one group of people who are in a strain—and the group of people who are feeling fine are trying to figure out why you're staggering around, and that's what this workshop is about this morning.[7]

Reagon is undoubtedly speaking metaphorically here. She uses this story of being out of breath as a way of talking about how coalitions are hard, uncomfortable, stressful places where we can never fully let go and relax; in coalition, as on the mountain, we can never fully catch our breath. As she explains in the next paragraph, "I feel as if I'm gonna keel over any minute and die. That is often what it feels like if you're *really* doing coalition work. Most of the time you feel threatened to the core and if you don't, you're not really doing no coalescing."[8] Coalition politics, for Reagon, entails working beyond the limits of one's comfort zone, being pushed into dangerous territory, engaging with people or practices or principles that frighten because of their difference.

But to read this anecdote solely as metaphor is to erase the specificities of Reagon's experience.[9] Immediately before stating that she feels like keeling over, Reagon explains that she "belong[s] to the group of people who are having a very difficult time being here" because of the high altitude; she is *literally* having a difficult time catching her breath.[10] Thus, for Reagon, "coalition politics," both the eponymous essay and the practice, begin with a focus on the body. And not just any body, but a limited body, an impaired body. Reagon is theorizing from the disabled body, using her embodied experience of disability—having a physical limitation in a sociopolitical setting that acts as if that limitation were nonexistent, or at least irrelevant—as a springboard for thinking about difference, relation, and politics. She illustrates the ways in which experiences of disability can be useful not only in informing our understandings about bodies but also our understandings of ethical relations and political practice.

Part of this analysis, on both the literal and metaphorical level, means reckoning with the bodies that cannot survive, let alone thrive, in particular settings. Reagon's breathing difficulties at this altitude, combined with her reflections on whose bodies are absent from this "women's" space, raises questions about the assumptions that undergird feminist practice. Whose bodies, whose experiences, whose desires, and whose identities shape the issues that get framed as feminist, and who does the framing? How accessible—financially, culturally, intellectually, physically—are feminist spaces, spaces in and through which feminist futures are imagined? In other words, Reagon calls feminism to task for creating spaces, both literally and metaphorically, in which certain bodies/minds play no role, or can participate only at great personal risk. She offers a powerful illustration of how the kinds of spaces we imagine often determine the kinds of bodies/minds that can inhabit those spaces. As a result, the conversations that occur in those spaces are dramatically—and all too often invisibly—diminished by the absence of those folks who, for reasons of inaccessibility or exclusion or ignorance, cannot participate.

Reagon explicitly directs her critique to feminism and the women's movement, but we can read her text as offering a challenge to disability studies and disability movements as well. Although the word "disability" appears only in passing in Reagon's text, and she does not identify herself as disabled or describe her breathing difficulties in those terms, we can easily read her essay as a narrative of inaccessibility or as an illustration of the insights to be gained from disability.[11] Recognizing this text as a crip text then allows for a whole set of necessary questions: In focusing so intently on disability identity, how have disability studies and disability rights movements overlooked the crip insights of people like Reagon? How might her formulation of coalition politics, of the need for feminism to acknowledge and grapple with racialized differences, inform a disability studies marked by whiteness, or disability rights movements slow to deal with issues of race and ethnicity? Or how might her focus on breathing difficulties inspire disability analyses of asthma, perhaps even prompting the field to recognize itself in or ally with environmental studies and environmental justice movements? In other words, what can disability studies and disability movements learn from our own exclusions?

Reading Reagon as a crip theorist is one way to begin answering these questions. Such a reading, and the expansive approach to disability politics it entails, means locating the subject of disability studies not just in bodies identified as disabled but in minds and bodies surviving inaccessible spaces, with both "access" and "spaces" defined broadly. It means recognizing contestations over whiteness, or economic disparity, or heteronormativity as part of disability studies and disability activism, not merely side projects or subdisciplines. It means challenging the homophobia and transphobia that lurk within the disability rights movement, marginalizing the experiences of queer- and trans-identified people with disabilities. It requires a continued examination of the whiteness and ethnocentrism of disability studies and disability activism in the United States, as well as committed engagement with the work of disability rights, antiglobalization, and antipoverty activists around the globe.

Like Reagon, however, we can pair our internal criticisms of our own positions and movements with engaged critiques of our partners and allies. Thinking through accessible spaces and accessible futures means addressing the exclusions of feminist and queer political visions of the future, highlighting these theories' reliance on ideologies of wholeness, complicity in compulsory able-bodiedness/able-mindedness, and marginalization of disabled people. What is needed, then, is not only a trenchant critique of ableism but also a desire to think disability otherwise.

This kind of robust combination of future dreams and present critique is essential to politics, and it requires leaving open the parameters of our political visions. Our animating questions could then include the following: Who is included or excluded in our political imaginaries? How are "disability" and "disabled person" (or "woman" or "queer" or "race" or . . .) being defined in these dreams of the future? Who has access to these imaginaries, and how is access being described? Which issues are being marked as feminist or queer or crip? And, to return to my earlier questions, where are disability studies or disability movements going to look for disability? Where does disability studies see or recognize itself?

The rest of this chapter profiles sites where answers to these kinds of questions are happening. Each of the following sections offers a snapshot of coalitions in progress, and I include them here as stories of disability told, or being told, otherwise. These stories are necessarily incomplete, but in their incompleteness they provide examples of how to imagine disability differently: finding it in unexpected places, using it to make connections to other social justice movements, and recognizing in it the possibilities of desire. These are, potentially, more accessible futures.

"Calling All Restroom Revolutionaries!" Coalescing around Bodies in Space

Reagon's text bridges feminist and disability concerns by drawing our attention to the political implications of space, and questions of access and inaccessibility continue to be productive points of overlap across multiple movements for social justice.[12] Public toilets, in particular, have long been sites of exclusion and activism; as Judith Plaskow explains, because "access to toilets is a prerequisite for full public participation and citizenship . . . almost all the social justice movements of the last century in the United States have included struggles for adequate toilet facilities."[13] Women moving into traditionally male spaces often discover the bathroom, or lack thereof, to be a key site of sexual harassment and discrimination; the toilet serves as an indicator of the kinds of gendered bodies expected in particular spaces.[14] In response, women have turned public restrooms into sites of political agitation and activism, challenging the architectural and political assumption of the male body as the ideal citizen.[15] Of course, this ideal citizen is not only male but white, and bathrooms have created not only gender dyads but racial ones: for much of the twentieth century, "urinary segregation" taught users powerful lessons about the intertwining of gender and race in public spaces, particularly in the south. There, too, public restrooms were made into contentious sites of struggle and citizenship, and Elizabeth Abel notes that African American men living under Jim Crow were violently punished for refusing to use restrooms marked "colored."[16] Public toilets continue to be heavily policed for inappropriate behavior or inappropriate users. Homeless people are frequent targets of attempts to "clean up" public restrooms, as are those practicing public sex, with cities doing everything from locking "public" facilities to refusing to build or install new public restrooms. Private businesses and restaurants typically designate their restrooms as "for customers only," a restriction that affects not only the homeless but also people who enter public spaces for reasons other than shopping or consumption.[17]

Given these practices of exclusion and resistance, it is not surprising that the toilet has also been a site of intellectual exploration and scholarly engagement, and there has been a vast expansion of toilet talk in the past few years.[18] This work clearly supports Plaskow's observation that toilets are sites of intersectional study and activism, but gender is heavily foregrounded here; histories of gender segregation, policy analyses of "potty parity," and speculations about nonsexist bathrooms dominate these discussions. This focus on gender, especially on gender presentation and identity, often feels absolutely necessary given that using the "wrong" bathroom for one's perceived gender can lead to harassment, arrest, and violence; moves to create unisex or gender-neutral restrooms continue to meet ridicule and hostility, even as more and more groups lobby for their creation.[19]

Two clear exceptions to the strict gender segregation of toilets (and to the hostility greeting attempts to desegregate such toilets) are the "family" restrooms increasingly popular in airports and the single-stall restrooms marked with a wheelchair.[20] The notion that people of one gender might need to assist a child or elder of another gender is much more readily accepted and accommodated than the notion that people with different gender presentations or identities might use the same restroom (even if, as in the case of single-stall toilets, at different times).[21] Similarly, we are more willing to accept people of all gender identities and sexes using the same space if those people are already seen as separate from the body politic because of their disabilities.[22] Simply put, unisex/gender-neutral bathrooms are neither threatening nor ridiculous as long as gender nonconformity is not the main reason for their use or creation.

Once they are created, however, such bathrooms are easily taken up for other purposes. In a queer expansion of the meanings of both "family" and "accessible," these spaces are increasingly recognized as options for genderqueer and trans users. Women's rooms, Sally Munt explains, are sites of uncomfortable and often threatening exchanges with those who cast her butch body as dangerously out of place. In this context, the third space of the accessible stall offers a much-needed "stress-free location, a queer space in which I can momentarily procure an interval from the gendered public environment, and psychically replenish."[23] Munt's pleasure is tempered, however, by her feelings of trespass; she sees herself as "treading on another borderline, not worthily disabled."[24] Yet cripping her account—not to mention cripping the disabled stall itself—leads to the recognition that gender-segregated spaces are not any more accessible to her than narrow doorways are to me, although the forms such inaccessibility takes are different.[25] The solution to this issue is not to assign more "worthiness" to my use than Munt's (or vice versa) but rather to recognize the possibility for queercrip alliances in the space of the toilet. If, as Munt suggests, the disabled toilet is a "room set aside for the disjunctive, ungendered and strange," then we can use the potential openness of those terms as grounds for coalition.[26]

PISSAR (People in Search of Safe and Accessible Restrooms) offers one example of this kind of collaboration. Founded at the University of California–Santa Barbara in 2003, PISSAR explicitly linked disability access with gender access, creating a bathroom checklist that assessed a restroom's disability-accessibility (e.g., door width, dispenser heights, Braille signage) right alongside its genderqueer-accessibility (e.g., functioning door locks, gender-specific signage, location) (see Appendix A).[27] "PISSAR

Patrols," which featured activists carrying clipboards and wearing "free 2 pee" shirts, used the checklist to rate and map campus restrooms. In so doing, they brought people together around the issue of access, regardless of whether or how they identified in terms of disability and gender. More recently, TransBrandeis, part of the GLBT/Queer Alliance at Brandeis University, expanded their mapping and survey project to include attention to disability access, and disability activists at the University of Washington have included attention to trans and genderqueer needs in their own access activism.[28]

It remains rare, however, for issues of disability access and trans access to be raised concurrently on GLBTQ organizational websites or in the (often sensationalized) news coverage about trans campus activism.[29] The frequency with which activists, administrations, and reporters use the language of "gender-blind," as opposed to "gender-neutral," "unisex," or "nongendered," suggests that critical disability perspectives are not at play here.[30] By the same token, my own experiences with PISSAR suggest reluctance on the part of some disability activists to engage with trans and genderqueer issues: one of the disabled students initially opposed forming PISSAR for fear that addressing trans access would dilute the struggle for disability access. The annual conference of the Society for Disability Studies has yet to consistently include gender-neutral restrooms as a required component of access, and too few disability studies scholars include attention to the relationship between trans and disability in our work on access, sexuality, stigma, or medicalization, only a few potential areas of overlap.[31] Trans essayist and activist Eli Clare is widely cited in disability studies, but scholars usually treat his writings on transphobia or on transgender experiences in general as an aside to his work on disability (as if the two were not intimately, and often explicitly, intertwined).

In his introduction to *Toilet: Public Restrooms and the Politics of Sharing*, Harvey Molotch points to the political dilemma facing disability communities as we look to the loo: "Should disabled people demand to be part of the convention [of gender segregated bathrooms]? Or should they be the leaders of a movement to combat it?"[32] One could certainly make the argument that, given the link between access to public spaces and access to the body politic, not to mention the link between hegemonic gender identities and cultural intelligibility, we should lean toward the former. Disabled people should have access to gendered restrooms just as nondisabled people do. The problem with that answer, though, is that it fixes—in both senses of the word—the problem of access too narrowly; rather than transform existing structures, both physical and political, it merely argues for including more people within them (by excluding others). Not only does it overlook the reality that some disabled people are also, simultaneously, trans and genderqueer people (a possibility similarly erased in Molotch's framing of the question), it also forecloses on the possibility that disability studies and activism could ally with other movements.

Thus, I argue for the latter response, with disabled people and disability movements working to undo the gendered conventions of the toilet as part of our larger struggles for access to public space. Such a move feels all the more necessary given that transgender and transsexual people were explicitly excluded from coverage under the ADA.[33] We can treat the public toilet as a site for undoing this exclusion, recognizing public inaccessibility as a problem that connects both those authorized to claim disability and those who are not. Thinking through access can then become a way of thinking through questions of disability identity, analyzing when it is deployed, and by whom, and to what effects. As Tanya Titchkosky argues, "[A]ccess [is] not . . . a synonym for justice but a beginning place for critical questioning."[34]

Recognizing bathroom access as a site for coalition building can potentially move us beyond the physical space of bathrooms, turning our critical attention to the acts of elimination that occur *beyond* the socially sanctioned space of the toilet, public or private. As Carrie Sandahl explains, "Our society cannot tolerate incontinence; once beyond infancy, incontinence divides the human from the non-human."[35] Not only is there profound shame and disgust directed toward those who "cannot control themselves," as the common colloquialism puts it, but the inability to control oneself is often what drives elderly or disabled people into nursing homes and other institutions. Indeed, this link between continence and full citizenship is too often written into policy and practice: Sandahl condemns the fact that often "Medicare and Medicaid will pay for these products [adult diapers and other incontinence products] if you're in a nursing home, but not if you're living at home."[36] Coalitions of feminists, queers, and crips lobbying not only for broadly accessible toilets but also affordable and accessible diapers may not yet be familiar, but I hope it is starting to sound necessary. We should not limit the "restroom revolution" to the four walls of the restroom.

Indeed, part of the pleasure and possibility of restroom revolutions is that they offer the opportunity to expand the terms of our movements and our theories. As Lisa Duggan notes in her praise of *Toilet*, "Peeing is political"—and so are the places where peeing happens (or doesn't) and the bodies doing the peeing. Attending to the space of the toilet not only makes room for coalitions between trans and disability concerns, it continues the crip theory move of keeping the meanings and parameters of disability, access, and disability studies open for debate and dissent.

Finding Disability in Environmental Justice

Typing "environmentalism" or "environmental justice" into databases alongside "illness" or "disability" brings up hundreds of hits, but the majority of them are public health articles describing conditions linked to environmental exposure (e.g., asthma, cancers, and skin rashes). These pieces map disease clusters, detail specific exposures, record pollutant levels, and/or track chemicals and other pollutants suspected of being carcinogenic or teratogenic ("teratogenic" is from *terata*, or monster, and refers to birth "defects" or "malformations").[37] Finding illness or disability in these texts means finding stories of error and aberration; illness and disability appear almost exclusively as tragic mistakes caused by unnatural incursions into or disruptions of the natural body and the natural environment. These were not the kind of pieces I had in mind when I began researching links between disability and environmentalism.

These were not the kind of pieces I had in mind, but that is not to say that they play no role in this book or in disability studies more broadly. On the contrary, such questions of body/environment interaction belong squarely within the purview of disability studies, as do public health analyses of toxic neighborhoods and sick buildings. We need a disability studies and disability activism that can challenge the siting of power plants or waste dumps in neighborhoods already overburdened by toxic industries; we need disability analyses that condemn the poisoning of bodies (human and otherwise) by both catastrophic spills and explosions as well as the "everyday" pollution of dry cleaners, contaminated water, and landfills. Disability and environmental movements can find common cause in their concern with the built environment; lead paint and cracked or missing sidewalks create disabling environments for everyone living around them.[38]

The essays I tracked down, then, are essential *to* disability studies, but most of them have yet to be influenced *by* disability studies (much as disability studies has yet to engage fully with this literature). What is needed, then, are analyses that recognize and refuse the intertwined exploitation of bodies and environments without demonizing the illnesses and disabilities, and especially the ill and disabled bodies, that result from such exploitation. As Valerie Ann Johnson argues in "Bringing Together Feminist Disability Studies and Environmental Justice," one of the few essays explicitly doing this kind of bridge work, "We [in the environmental justice movement] tend to conflate disability, disease and environmental injustice. What is needed is to disaggregate the possible results of environmental injustice (i.e., exposure to toxic substances emanating from landfills or hog operations that injure the body) from the *person*, however they are embodied."[39]

This kind of disaggregation requires a more complex and interconnected understanding of disability than is currently circulating in both disability studies and environmental studies. In terms of disability studies, the continued reliance on the social model (and its corollary assumption that there can be no room for medical approaches) makes it difficult to engage with antitoxics movements that work to eliminate or at least decrease disability. My own reluctance to recognize articles warning of birth defects and deformities as part of my project is an example of this difficulty. Yet, as Stacy Alaimo argues, disability studies and activism would "be enriched by attending not only to the ways in which built environments constitute or exacerbate 'disability,' but to how materiality, at a less perceptible level—that of pharmaceuticals, xenobiotic chemicals, air pollution, etc.—affects human health and ability."[40] Similarly, environmental studies and activism could benefit from a more critical approach to disability, one that recognizes disability as a cultural, historical, and political category, rather than simply a medical one. We need environmental analyses that do more than cast disability and disabled bodies/minds as tragedies or aberrations, in part because focusing exclusively on disabled people as the signs of environmental injustice effaces the ways in which we are all affected by toxic pollution and contamination, not just those of us with visible or diagnosed "abnormalities."

Moreover, by relying on the specter of disability to motivate public response, environmental movements rely on what Giovanna Di Chiro calls "eco(hetero)normativity."[41] Making connections across disability, environmental, and queer studies, Di Chiro offers a model for the kind of coalitional thinking that can lead to more accessible futures. She documents how environmentalists "mobilize socially sanctioned heterosexism and queer-fear" by creating and circulating sensationalized accounts of "sexual abnormalities" in fish, animals, and humans. In so doing, mainstream environmentalists reify hegemonic ideals of gender and sexuality, thereby foreclosing on the possibility of cross-movement work. Rather than relying on uncritical concepts of "normal" bodies and orientations, Di Chiro argues that antitoxics activists should focus on more "serious health problems associated with POPs [persistent organic pollutants]," such as "breast, ovarian, prostate, and testicular cancers, neurological and neurobehavioral problems, immune system breakdown, heart disease, diabetes, and obesity."[42]

We can extend Di Chiro's concern about the normalizing strains of antitoxic environmentalism by questioning not only the queer fear embedded within these discourses but also the disability fear.[43] How can we continue the absolutely necessary task of challenging toxic pollution and its effects without perpetuating cultural assumptions about the unmitigated tragedy of disability? How can we attend to "serious health problems" while also deconstructing the stigma attached to those problems or even historicizing the very construction of such conditions as problems? One way is to challenge environmental representations of disability that are completely removed from the experiences of people living with those very disabilities. Or, to put it differently, disability scholars and activists can work to ensure that descriptions of the possible impairments linked to toxic exposures do not replicate ableist language and assumptions. Surely we can find ways to protest lead and mercury poisoning without resorting to warnings about how "developmental delays, learning disabilities, ADHD, and behavioral disorders extract a terrible toll from children, families, and society. . . . The costs associated with caring for these children can be high for families and society. Special education programs and psychological and medical services drain resources."[44] These statements, posted on the website of the Collaborative on Health and the Environment, not only perpetuate long-standing fears about the economic burden of disabled people but, more disturbingly, imply that disabled people—*rather than polluting industries*—are the ones responsible for draining resources. Disability studies and activism can be a resource here, helping environmental movements avoid this kind of misdirection and create broader coalitions against pollution.

Breast cancer lends itself to these kinds of complex, tangled, and ambiguous reckonings, and feminist theorists and activists continue to produce rich work analyzing its connections. Audre Lorde's *The Cancer Journals* has found a home in disability studies, with scholars pointing to Lorde's searing indictment of prosthetics and passing; Lorde's refusals to become a compliant patient and, relatedly, to hide her mastectomy behind puffs of wool have been a welcome resource for disability movements searching for models of how to refuse medicalized silence. Environmental studies has found the book useful as well for "its insistence on the interconnections between body and environment, which poses cancer as a feminist, antiracist, and environmental justice issue."[45] As Alaimo's reading of the text makes clear, the book serves as a bridge between these various movements. Lorde refuses breast prosthetics in order to transform silence not only about illness and the body but also about the environmental causes of illness. "Lorde displays her scars against the cancer establishment," explains Alaimo, challenging its denial of "the environmental causes of cancer."[46]

Environmental and disability studies and activisms can find common cause in critically examining the medical industrial complex and its current approach to cancer. Organizations such as Breast Cancer Action (BCA) can be understood as simultaneously deploying disability and environmental analyses. Breast Cancer Action offers a strong challenge to cancer rhetorics that present breast cancer as primarily a problem of individual bodies, a challenge that echoes critiques of the medical model of disability. In insisting that we attend to both voluntary and involuntary exposures to carcinogens, BCA moves away from individualized models of cancer to more structural ones; similarly, in arguing that it is "not just genes, but social injustices—political, economic, and racial inequities—that lead to disparities in breast cancer outcomes," BCA argues for a more political/relational model of illness and, by extension, disability.[47]

The Disability Rights Education and Defense Fund (DREDF) is one of the pioneers in this work, laying the groundwork for environmental justice projects informed by disability rights. Silvia Yee, one of the staff attorneys at DREDF, is positioning the organization as a resource for people living in communities overburdened by toxic industries and emissions. The Disability Rights Education and Defense Fund understands that those living in such communities may not have accurate information about the availability of disability protection laws and social services; even though many of the people living in overburdened communities are already ill or disabled, or may become so because of their exposure to toxins, they may not identify themselves as disabled or recognize themselves within disability rights movements. Yet, as Yee explains, federal and state disability laws could potentially be used to

> reduce environmental hazards for the entire community. For instance, children with respiratory disabilities in a public school using chemical pesticides could potentially bring a cause of action that will reduce pesticide exposure for all their classmates as well as the surrounding community. These litigation ideas have been largely unexplored, both theoretically and in practice.[48]

Recognizing the links between disability and environmental justice opens the door to such explorations. Yee and DREDF position disability laws as a way to protect entire communities; "disability rights" thus becomes a tool used not only on behalf of disabled people, and affecting not only disabled people, but for all people.

Activism by and on behalf of people with multiple chemical sensitivities (MCS) provides another example of deploying categories of disability to do environmental justice work. As with trans and genderqueer folks using the language of access to disrupt gender segregation, MCS activists discuss their need for scent- and chemical-free spaces as a component of accessibility. "How and Why to Be Scent-Free," a flyer distributed to attendees of the Queer Disability Conference (held in San Francisco in 2002), offers one such example (see Appendix C); the flyer first details the physical and cognitive effects of toxic exposure in order to testify to the necessity of safer spaces:

> Symptoms of chemical exposure include dizziness, nausea, slurred speech, drowsiness, irritation to mouth, throat, skin, eyes, and lungs, headache, convulsions, fatigue, confusion, and liver and kidney damage. As you can imagine, these symptoms constitute serious barriers for people with chemical sensitivities in work, life, and of course, conference attendance. Promoting scent-free environments is very much like adding ramps and curb-cuts in terms of the profound difference in accessibility it can produce.[49]

Reading the work of scholars and activists with MCS makes this point abundantly clear, as they describe feeling trapped in their homes, or forced out of their homes, or made ill by their encounters with other bodies and environments.[50] Disability studies scholars and activists, with their experience linking *access to spaces* with *access to the body politic*, can serve as useful allies here; these stories of chemically disabling environments are also stories of inaccessibility. Both disability studies and environmental justice disrupt what Mel Chen calls "the fiction of independence and of uninterruptability"; we can see in this shared disruption the possibility for coalition.[51]

Meet Reproductive Justice

Women of color have been at the forefront of struggles to shift the focus of reproductive rights movements and public discourses about reproduction away from a single-issue focus on abortion.[52] Without denying the importance of legal abortion (and especially *access* to legal abortion), activists have long argued for a much broader approach, one that takes into account the widespread social and economic disparities among women. Andrea Smith explains that "the pro-life versus pro-choice paradigm reifies and masks the structures of white supremacy and capitalism that undergird the reproductive choices that women make."[53] As Smith and other activists and scholars detail, the language of choice presents women more as consumers than citizens, opening the door for some women to be cast as bad decision makers and for some choices to be deemed bad or inappropriate. Moreover, the language of choice fails to take into account how different women have different access to different choices; it removes from analysis the conditions under which women and families make decisions about reproduction. Indeed, choice rhetoric can easily be deployed to cover over sterilization abuses:

informed consent policies, which would seem to support women's "choices," have often been compromised by racism, classism, ableism, and xenophobia.[54] As a result of these histories and practices, many activists within these movements use the language of "reproductive justice" to "emphasize the relationship of reproductive rights to human rights and economic justice."[55]

I offer this brief overview of reproductive justice for three reasons. First, I want to highlight that both reproductive justice activists and disability activists interrogate the rhetoric of choice found in reproductive rights movements. Much as the experiences of women of color, immigrant women, poor women, and indigenous women exceed the notion of "free choice," the language of choice fails to account for the ableist context in which women make decisions about pregnancy, abortion, and reproduction in general. As Marsha Saxton notes, only certain choices are recognized as valid choices, and only certain choices are socially supported; "Our society profoundly limits the 'choice' to love and care for a baby with a disability."[56] Shelley Tremain echoes Saxton, warning that ableist notions of "prenatal impairment" "increasingly limit the field of possible conduct in response to pregnancy."[57] Disability studies scholars and activists also argue that the continued commodification of pregnancy, a process enabled and perpetuated by the framework of choice, facilitates ableist rhetoric of fetuses, babies, and children as "defective"; positioning women as consumers and babies as products makes possible conversations about and practices toward "selecting" the baby one wants (and deselecting or terminating the babies one doesn't want). A critique of choice, then, bridges both movements.

Second, I want to encourage a greater familiarity with, and support of, reproductive justice movements and frameworks on the part of disability studies and activism. As the definitions above suggest, reproductive justice insists upon a cross-movement approach to reproductive issues, recognizing that questions of reproduction cannot be disentangled from those of race, class, and sexuality, not to mention poverty, welfare, health care, social services, environmental justice, and so on. Disability is an essential piece of this assemblage, and reproductive concerns about disability cannot be untangled from these other factors. Thinking about disability and reproduction requires the kind of cross-movement analysis promised by reproductive justice. Even if reproductive justice movements do not always live up to this promise in terms of disability (as when a major reproductive justice text relegates disability to a single footnote), the possibilities remain.[58] In fact, I think reproductive justice frameworks offer the possibility not only of cross-movement analyses that fully integrate disability but also of fuller *cross-disability* analyses. Physical disabilities and intellectual disabilities are often construed differently in debates about prenatal testing and selective abortion, and disability movements need to acknowledge (even as we interrogate) those distinctions.

Third, thinking about reproductive politics only in terms of abortion and the pro-choice/pro-life binary makes coalition building among disability and reproductive rights and justice activists more difficult. As Smith argues, the pro/anti binary fosters "simplistic analyses of who our political friends and enemies are," which can lead us to "lose opportunities to work with people with whom we . . . have sharp disagreements, but who may, with different political framings and organizing strategies, shift their positions."[59] Smith's warning strikes me as especially salient for the disability and reproductive rights relationship. Within the logic of the pro/anti abortion binary, anyone who expresses concern about particular abortion practices or rhetorics can too easily appear as an enemy of feminism and an opponent of reproductive rights. Reproductive rights activists are then wary of engaging with disability critiques of prenatal testing and selective abortion; within this context, to take up these critiques, seriously wrestling with the ableist implications of prenatal testing, feels dangerously close to dismantling abortion rights. Similarly, disability rights activists are wary of engaging with reproductive rights groups who continue to use disability as a justification for abortion; it can be hard to find common ground with organizations that take for granted the undesirability of disability. Reproductive justice approaches, which insist as much on the right to continue a pregnancy (and be supported in doing so) as the right to terminate one, offer one possible means of connection.[60]

This kind of connective work is necessary as antireproductive rights activists increasingly use progressive rhetoric for their own purposes.[61] Capitalizing on the eugenic and ableist histories of the reproductive rights movement, opponents of abortion are moving steadily to present themselves as the better ally to disability movements. Feminists for Life (FFL), for example, explicitly defines abortion as a form of discrimination against disabled people, appropriating the rhetoric of disability movements in their campaign against abortion.[62] This deployment of disability rights is evident in their poster series, "It's time to *question abortion*," which includes a poster equating abortion to eugenics. The black-and-white poster features a photograph of an unsmiling dark-skinned man sitting in his manual wheelchair; he has his arms crossed and a defiant expression. "Would you say that to my face?" appears in handwritten script across the photograph, while the following text appears below the picture: "Would you tell me that I never should have been born? That is the message sent when people talk about aborting 'gross fetal anomalies.' People who overcome adversity inspire, challenge and enrich our world." I have often heard disability activists respond to ableist abortion rhetoric with that very question: "Would you tell me that I never should have been born?" Debates about the proliferation of prenatal testing often draw similar responses, with disabled people wondering aloud whether they would have been aborted if their mothers had had the chance.[63] In making space for this line of thinking, the FFL presents itself as more aligned with the interests of disability communities than the pro-choice movement is; according to this logic, advocates for abortion and other reproductive rights are too closely tied to eugenic practices and histories to support disabled people.

Yet working with reproductive rights and justice organizations can be a way for disability movements to make progress on long-held goals, as seen with the Prenatally and Postnatally Diagnosed Conditions Awareness Act of 2008 (also known as the Kennedy Brownback Act). The legislation requires doctors, genetic counselors, and other medical professionals to provide current, accurate, and comprehensive information about disability when they consult with women about their pregnancies. Its purpose is to ensure that women are adequately informed before they make any decisions about continuing or terminating their pregnancies; covered information includes available social services, support groups, and the experiences of disabled people and families with similarly-disabled children. Although it is still too early to evaluate the law's efficacy in terms of the quality of information parents receive, the very passage of the law is significant. By stressing parents' need for information prior to decision making, the Kennedy Brownback Act underscores the fact that there is a decision to be made; it begins to unravel the assumption that abortion is the only viable, rational response to a positive test. Indeed, by focusing on the right to true informed consent, the act acknowledges that women have typically been given inaccurate or incomplete information about disability, information that both reflected and perpetuated cultural fears and stereotypes about disability.[64]

The law is also significant in that it was supported by both disability and reproductive rights and justice organizations. Generations Ahead, recognizing in the bill the potential for cross-movement collaboration, fostered a partnership among the World Institute on Disability, the Disability Rights Education and Defense Fund, the National Women's Health Network, and the Reproductive Health Technologies Project. Together the five organizations disseminated an information sheet about the bill, urging their allies to support the legislation.[65] It was, admittedly, an easier sell for disability rights groups. Reproductive rights organizations were wary of the bill, worried that it was another sideways attempt to restrict women's access to abortion; then Senator Sam Brownback's cosponsorship of the bill fueled these fears because of his longstanding and vocal opposition to reproductive rights. The coalition of disability and reproductive rights groups eventually convinced their allies not to oppose the bill, making the argument that everyone would benefit from more and improved information about disability. They posed the problem not in terms of abortion per se, thereby sidestepping the entrenched pro-choice/pro-life binary, but rather in terms of eliminating the ableist bias in genetic counseling and improving the information and supports given to women expecting a disabled baby.

Two seemingly disparate events in early October 2010 set the stage for another moment of coalition building between disability and reproductive rights and justice movements: Robert Edwards was awarded the Nobel Prize in medicine for his work developing in vitro fertilization; and Virginia Ironside, a British advice columnist, generated controversy over her comments about the alleged suffering of disabled children. Both figures publicly promoted the use of reproductive technologies to select against disability. Edwards argued that it would be a "sin of parents to have a child that carries the heavy burden of genetic disease. We are entering a world where we have to consider the quality of our children."[66] Several pro-life and antiabortion groups seized upon this quote in their condemnation of Edwards's award, but his position on disability was otherwise ignored in the media coverage; it was unremarkable.[67] Ironside's position on disability, on the other hand, is precisely what generated media coverage, but there, too, the assumption that disability is best met with abortion went largely unchallenged. In a televised debate about abortion, Ironside described the abortion of "a baby [that] is going to be born severely disabled" as the "act of a loving mother"; she then offered that, faced with such "a deeply suffering child," she would not hesitate to "put a pillow over its face," as would "any good mother."[68] Although Ironside's comments about infanticide were quickly condemned, her assumption that abortion was the best response to disability generated little discussion.[69] More to the point, her decision to use the specter of disability as a justification for abortion continued a long pattern of pitting disability rights against reproductive rights.

In response to these events, which happened within a couple of days of each other, a group of six scholars and activists (including myself) drafted a statement articulating a disability and reproductive rights and justice position; it currently has over 150 signatories, both organizations and individuals (see Appendix D).[70] Titled "Robert Edwards, Virginia Ironside, and the Unnecessary Opposition of Rights," the statement presents reproductive rights and justice as fully intertwined with the rights of and justice for people with disabilities:

> As people committed to both disability rights and reproductive rights, we believe that respecting women and families in their reproductive decisions requires simultaneously challenging discriminatory attitudes toward people with disabilities. We refuse to accept the bifurcation of women's rights from disability rights, or the belief that protecting reproductive rights requires accepting ableist assumptions about the supposed tragedy of disability. On the contrary, we assert that reproductive rights includes attention to disability rights, and that disability rights requires attention to human rights, including reproductive rights.

In drafting the statement, we rehearsed familiar debates over terminology and affiliation: Were we discussing human rights or women's rights? Did we want to refer to ourselves as feminists or leave such identifications more open? Should we use the language of disability rights or disability justice? Would it be accurate to describe current practices as eugenic or would that be too inflammatory? On each count, we opted to use the broadest and most familiar terms and frames possible; although some of us might individually make different decisions, we wanted a critical mass of "people committed to both disability rights and reproductive rights" to recognize themselves in our call. Indeed, it is these kinds of questions that can, we hope, lead to further articulations, coalitions, and conversations.

What seemed key to any document was a refusal of the bifurcation of disability rights and justice from reproductive rights and justice. We knew that disability activists, particularly those less directly engaged with reproductive justice movements and frameworks, desperately needed a clear statement from reproductive rights activists and organizations that they would not accept "the rhetorical use of disability as an argument for abortion rights."[71] Similarly, reproductive rights groups needed a signal that a significant number of disability activists and scholars were willing to articulate their support for women's reproductive rights. As with the Prenatally and Postnatally Diagnosed Conditions Awareness Act, the statement in no way condemns or limits individual women's choices but rather speaks to the widespread cultural disparagement of disability and disabled people. In identifying shared values between disability and reproductive movements, the statement explicitly calls for continued collaboration:

> We hope, with this statement, to support other activists and scholars who are equally committed to both reproductive rights and disability rights. We hope that as advocates in movements that share similar values around civil and human rights we can continue to speak out against the use of reproductive rights to undermine disability rights and the use of disability rights to undermine reproductive rights.

This statement was made possible by the work of feminist and disability studies scholars who have been steadfastly refusing the bifurcation of reproductive rights and disability rights for decades.[72] Adrienne Asch, Anne Finger, Rayna Rapp, Dorothy Roberts, Marsha Saxton: all demonstrate that challenging ableism, even within the context of reproductive politics, is not necessarily the same as challenging or limiting women's access to abortion.[73] Perhaps to make that point clear, especially in a context in which disability is being deployed to undermine abortion rights, those trying to bridge the two movements have often been very explicit about their allegiances. In "Abortion and Disability: Who Should and Who Should Not Inhabit the World?" Ruth Hubbard states four separate times that she supports a woman's right to abortion, whatever her reasons.[74] The fact that she felt compelled to repeat this belief over and over again testifies to the difficulty facing those who want to question the ableist underpinnings of the system of prenatal testing without questioning access to abortion. Yet these very scholars, as well as those involved in the actions I describe here, argue that having to make decisions about reproduction in the face of ableist representations of disability and in a culture "that promises much grief to parents of children it deems unfit" harms everyone.[75] To put it plainly: critically examining the reasons why women choose to terminate pregnancies based on disability, challenging reproductive rights movements for using disability as a justification for legal abortion, and deconstructing the assumptions about disability built into prenatal testing policies and practices—none of these necessarily translate into denying women's access to abortion.

In fact, failing to do these things may in fact undermine women's access; at the very least, it makes it more difficult for reproductive rights and justice movements to support and be supported by disability rights and justice movements. I close this section with a provocation, one that also appears in one of the founding texts of feminist disability studies. In their contribution to their anthology *Women with Disabilities: Essays in Psychology, Culture, and Politics*, Adrienne Asch and Michelle Fine argue for the right to abortion "for any reason [women] deem appropriate."[76] Following Asch and Fine, rather than "presume or prescribe any reason (for example, 'the tragedy of the defective fetus')," we should defend women's right to make their own decisions about reproduction, fully supporting them in having or not having a child.[77] Abortion for any reason and under any circumstance must then be accompanied by accessible and affordable prenatal care for all women, as well as reliable and affordable child care, access to social services, and the kind of information about and supports for disability mandated in the Kennedy Brownback Act.

I know that I am arguing for an impossibility, at least in the current political climate. We are moving farther and father away from the radical feminist call of "abortion on demand," seeing more and more burdens on abortion as acceptable rather than unduly prohibitive. Yet when we force women (and reproductive rights, health, and justice movements) living in an ableist culture to prove that their abortions are "justifiable," disability remains a convenient and effective justification for preserving at least a minimal right to abortion. Even those who are uncomfortable with seeing disability as the grounds for abortion may find themselves in the untenable situation of deciding which conditions are grounds for abortion and which are not. When the legality of abortion hinges on some pregnancies being seen as "abortable," drawing lines between impairments becomes inevitable: it is acceptable to abort for blindness but not for deafness; it is permissible to abort for Down syndrome but not for an atypically-formed hand; this condition is too severe but that one is not. Disability movements cannot win in these conversations; I agree with Adrienne Asch and others who argue that casting some impairments as justification for abortion harms those currently living with those impairments.[78] Making disability do the work of defending abortion may be effective in securing abortion rights in the short term, but it does so by trafficking in discriminatory stereotypes about disability. Moreover, its long-term effectiveness is doubtful, as it opens the door to a continued interrogation of individual women's reasons and decisions.

It is still true that "neither the pro-choice nor the disability rights movement has consolidated around a position on 'choice' and disability," and neither have reproductive rights and justice movements more broadly.[79] Even in arguing for unrestricted access to abortion, I am not calling for such consolidation, at least not consolidation around a single position. I offer this provocation, one that has been offered many times before by others, in order to continue the process of articulating feminist disability positions on reproduction. We need to expand the terrain of dialogue, moving away from such a limited focus on suffering, quality of life, and unlivable disabilities—notions that often perpetuate ableist assumptions—and toward creating opportunities to support reproductive justice for all, including for and by disabled people. Continuing to accept disability as the reason to keep abortion legal, and casting abortion as the only reasonable choice when dealing with disability, is a narrowing of both abortion rights and the terms of debate. So, too, is the assumption that the meaning of "suffering" or "quality of life" is self-evident and monolithic; rather than using these concepts as if they "obviously" led us to only one conclusion, we could attend instead to their shifts in meanings across different registers, contexts, or bodies/minds. As Sujatha Jesudason argues in her description of Generations Ahead's methodology, coalitions around genetic and reproductive technologies require a willingness to take risks and have frank dialogue about the issues that divide us. Having these kinds of difficult conversations can help different movements discover and articulate their shared values while also laying the groundwork for future conversations as values, identifications, and goals change.[80]

Accessible Futures

In presenting these three possibilities of crip coalition as accessible futures, or as feminist/queer/crip futures, I have focused on only a few possibilities out of many. I could have discussed antiwar protests, for example, and the need to speak out against the disabling effects of the US war on terror. The military-industrial complex causes illness, disability, and death on a global scale, and there is much work to be done in theorizing how to oppose war violence and its effects without denigrating disability and disabled people in the process. (We can see still further links here with environmental justice movements, as the US military is one of the world's worst polluters.)

Or what of potential links between the prison abolition movement and deinstitutionalization movements? There certainly is much to be gained in critically examining the prisons, nursing homes, and asylums of the past and present. The prison industrial complex serves as the primary source of (inadequate) health care for increasing numbers of poor people and people of color, notes Dorothy Roberts, who offers as an example the fact that the psychiatric wing of the Los Angeles County Jail "is the largest mental health facility in the country."[81] Prisons, moreover, not only house disabled people but *produce* them: violence, isolation, and inadequate and inconsistent access to medicine and health care have a disabling effect on the bodies and minds of inmates and prisoners.[82] How might probing these links allow us to recognize the problem Liat Ben-Moshe describes as "trans-incarceration" or "the move from one carceral edifice such as a psychiatric hospital to another such as a jail"?[83]

Or I could have explored connections between disability movements and movements for the rights of domestic workers. At a 2009 protest in Oakland challenging state budget cuts to health care, I watched a group of disabled people and union workers not trade but share chants: "We are the union, the mighty, mighty union!" they all shouted, followed by "We're out, we're loud, we're disabled, and we're proud!" As I watched these interactions, and participated in both sets of chants, I kept thinking about Robert McRuer's concept of "the nondisabled claim to be crip" and his reminder that it is often useful, "for the purposes of solidarity, to come out as something you are—at least in some ways—not."[84] Yet we can also see these union workers' claiming of disability not only as an act of solidarity or affiliation but also as a recognition of what McRuer calls "the disability to come." Some of these women (and they were mostly women) are themselves sick or disabled, and many more will become so through this hard work.[85] In other words, not only are there overlaps between those communities (many care workers are disabled or will become so), there are also overlaps between their needs: both groups will benefit in a system that values attendant care and the workers who provide it.[86]

Or, to turn a critical eye on my own coalitional imaginings, we can trace how each of the issues and movements I have discussed separately in this chapter are themselves intertwined. These imaginings are, in Donna Haraway's framing, "partial": I have selected moments that I myself am involved in and partial to, and they are necessarily incomplete. Not only could we add still other coalitions to this list, we could also complicate, extend, critique, refute, and enrich the cases I have included here.

Indeed, these coalitional moments will be known to many of you; my provocations may feel more familiar than provocative. Yet that possibility is part of my motivation for including them here. Not only am I interested in pushing the parameters of disability studies to include these not-really-so-disparate sites, I am also invested in making clear that this work is happening. In other words, I mention these various coalitional moments not because they currently are absent but because they are present, vibrant, and ongoing. There is rich disability (and feminist, and queer, and environmental, and racial justice, and reproductive, and . . .) work happening in each of these locations; alternative political imaginaries are being debated and discussed in and through these various political practices. Disabled people have more than a dream of accessible futures: we continue to define and demand our place in political discourses, political visions, and political practice, even as we challenge those very questions and demands. More accessible futures depend on it.

Appendices

The disability to come . . . will and should always belong to the time of the promise. . . . It's a crip promise that we will always comprehend disability otherwise and that we will, collectively, somehow access other worlds and futures.

—Robert McRuer, *Crip Theory*

Activist Presents

I titled this project *Feminist, Queer, Crip* because I wanted to acknowledge the possibilities—past, present, and future—for such alliances. To that end, in lieu of a conclusion per se, I offer instead various documents from the organizations and actions described in chapter 7. These documents are not "conclusions" but rather answers-in-progress, partial attempts to think disability otherwise.

I include these materials for three reasons. First, they provide concrete details about how to engage in access activism, offering information about creating scent-free spaces and assessing the accessibility of public restrooms. They also offer language for efforts to link disability movements with reproductive rights and justice movements. Second, my project was directly inspired by the work of these various activists and organizations, and including these documents here allows me to highlight that connection. Although I was involved in organizing the events that spawned these documents and/or in the writing of these texts, I cannot and do not claim ownership over them; rather, I include them as signs of the collaborative nature of this entire project. Finally, I offer them here, intact and separate from analysis, as primary sources for other readings and interpretations. Neither these documents nor (especially) my readings of them are definitive statements on feminist, queer, crip politics, and I offer them up as fodder for continued discussion and debate. It is my hope that the explorations featured here might be of some service to theorists and activists both now and in the future. Indeed, part of my interest in moving back and forth among past, present, and future crip imaginings is in sparking other conversations about these relationships, generating alternate histories and futures, and making space for multiple activist and theoretical trajectories.

Appendix A: Pissar Checklist

Type of bathroom (circle one): Men's   Women's   Unisex
Location of Bathroom: Bldg_____ Floor_____ Wing (east, west)_____ Room #_____
Does the bathroom open directly to the outside, or is the entry inside the building?
_____

If the bathroom is inside a building, please give the closest entrance or elevator to the bathroom_____

Your Name & Email Address_____

Disability Accessibility

1 Is the door into the bathroom wide enough? Give width. (ADA = 32 in.)_____
2 What kind of knob does the door have? Circle one: Lever / Round knob / Handle
   Automatic push-button / Other (specify)_____
3 Are there double doors into the bathroom? (i.e., do you have to open one door and then open another door to enter the bathroom?) Yes / No
4 Is the stall door wide enough? Give width. (ADA = 32 in.)_____
5 What kind of latch is on the stall door? Sliding latch / Small turn knob / Large turn knob with lip / Other (specify)_____
6 Does the stall door close by itself? Yes / No Is there a handle on the inside of the door to help pull it closed? Yes / No
7 Measure the space between the front of the toilet and the front wall_____. If the stall is wide, with open space next to the toilet, measure the space between the side of the toilet and the farthest side wall_____. If the stall is a skinny rectangle, measure the width of the stall in front of the toilet._____
8 Are there grab bars? Yes / No First side bar is ___long, ___high, begins ___ from rear wall, and extends ___ in front of the toilet. Second side bar is ___ long, ___high, begins ___ from rear wall, and extends ___ in front of the toilet. Back bar is ___long and ___high.
9 Facing the toilet, is the grab bar on the right side or the left side of the toilet? Right Left / Both sides
10 How accessible is the toilet paper holder? Height___ Is it too far from the toilet to reach without losing one's balance? Yes / No
11 Describe the flush knob. (Is it a lever? If yes, is it next to the wall or on the open side of the toilet? Is it a center button?)_____
12 How high is the toilet seat? (e.g., is it raised or standard?) (ADA = 17–19 in.)___
13 Is the path to the toilet seat cover dispenser blocked by the toilet? Yes / No How high is the dispenser?
14 How high is the urinal?_____How high is the handle?_____
15 If a multi-stall bathroom, how many stalls are accessible?_____
16 Is there a roll-under sink? If so, are the hot water pipes wrapped to prevent burns? (ADA = counter top no higher than 34 in.)
17 What kind of faucet handles does the sink have? Lever / Automatic / Separate turn knobs / Other (specify)
18 Is there a soap dispenser at chair height (ADA = you have to reach no higher than 48 in.)?_____ A dryer / paper towel dispenser?

19 Is the tampon / pad dispenser at chair height? (ADA = you have to reach no higher than 48 in.)__
20 Is there a mirror at chair height? (ADA = bottom of mirror no higher than 40 in.)__
21 Is there an audible alarm system? Yes / No A visual alarm system (lights)? Yes / No
22 Is the accessible stall marked as accessible?_____
23 Is the outer bathroom door marked as accessible?_____
24 Are there any obstructions in front of the sink, the various dispensers, the accessible stall, the toilet, etc.? Please specify. __

Gender Safety

25 Is the bathroom marked as unisex? Specify._____
26 Is it in a safe location? (i.e., not in an isolated spot)_____
27 Is it next to a gender-specific restroom so that it serves as a de facto "men's" or "women's" restroom?
28 Does the door lock from the inside? Does the lock work securely?_____

Aunt Flo and the Plug Patrol

29 Type of machine in the bathroom (circle one): Tampon / Pad / Tampon & Pad
30 Does it have a "this machine is broken" sticker? Sticker / No Sticker
31 Does it look so rusty and disgusting that even if it works, you doubt anyone would use it? Yes / No
32 Is the machine empty? (look for a little plastic "empty" sign) Yes / No
33 Does it have a new full-color "Aunt Flo" sticker? Sticker / No Sticker

Child Care

34 Does the bathroom have a changing table? (Specify location)

Created in spring 2003 at the University of California, Santa Barbara, by the members of PISSAR: People in Search of Safe and Accessible Restrooms.

Appendix B: Statement on Bathrooms and Gender

Part of making this conference accessible is recognizing that sex-segregated bathrooms are limiting for people who do not fit easily into Men's and Women's rooms. Please support making this conference safe for everyone by recognizing that there may be people choosing a bathroom that doesn't "match" the one others might think they should use. A gender-variant person using the bathroom that feels safest to them is not there to "look at" other people in the bathroom, but to go about their business.

Thanks for supporting the gender-variant folks at this conference by supporting everyone's right to use the bathroom.

Created for the Queer Disability Conference held at San Francisco State University in June 2002.

Appendix C: How and Why to Be Scent Free

If you are not accustomed to going "scent-free," it is important to think carefully about all the products you use in your day. You can either not use shampoo, soap, hair gel, hair spray, perfume/scented oils, skin lotion, shaving cream, makeup, etc., or use fragrance-free alternatives for at least a whole day before attending an event that is "scent-free." Suggestions for scent-free products are on the other side of this page.

What Will It Do for My Health, and the Health of Others, to Go Scent-Free?

Becoming scent-free is an important step toward access for people with disabilities. Plus you be surprised to find that you feel better as well!

People with Multiple Chemical Sensitivities (also called Environmental Illness) experience serious and debilitating physical and neurological symptoms when exposed to the chemicals used in most scented products. Often the damage caused by these chemicals causes an individual to react to other intensely volatile substances, such as essential oils, tobacco smoke, and "natural" fragrances. The process by which we smell something actually involves microscopic particles of that substance being absorbed through mucous membranes and entering the nervous system.

Because no government agency regulates the ingredients of household and personal care products, the last several decades have seen a huge increase in the number of harmful chemicals added to these products. Many of these chemicals are banned for use in industrial settings because of their known toxic effects. According to a 1986 US House of Representative study: "95% of chemicals used in fragrances are synthetic compounds derived from petroleum. They include benzene derivatives, aldehydes, and many other known toxics and synthesizers—capable of causing cancer, birth defects, central nervous system disorders, and allergic reactions."

Symptoms of chemical exposure include dizziness, nausea, slurred speech, drowsiness, irritation to mouth, throat, skin, eyes, and lungs, headache, convulsions, and liver and kidney damage. As you can imagine, these symptoms constitute serious barriers for people with chemical sensitivities in work, life, and, of course, conference attendance. Promoting scent-free environments is very much like adding ramps and curbcuts in terms of the profound difference in accessibility it can produce. We appreciate all participants in the Queer Disability Conference cooperating with the No-Scent Policy to make our conference as accessible as possible.

If You Smoke

Please smoke only in the designated smoking area outside of the conference center and away from the entrances. Please also keep in mind that many chemically sensitive people will also get sick from the smoke clinging to your clothing and hair. If you smoke OR hang out with people who are smoking, please sit or stand as far away as possible from the areas designated as "MCS Safer Zones." Also, keep in mind that smoking is banned in virtually all buildings in California, including the conference housing, bars, and restaurants. Thank you!

Product Suggestions

> SOAP: Tom's of Maine unscented, Kiss My Face Pure Olive Oil, Neutrogena unscented, Dr. Bronner's Aloe Vera Baby Mild, Simple, Body Shop unscented shower gel
> LAUNDRY DETERGENT: Arm & Hammer Free, Tide Free, Wisk Free, Planet, 7th Generation fragrance-free, Granny's, any other fragrance-free brands
> SHAMPOO AND CONDITIONER: Pure Essentials fragrance-free, Magick Botanicals fragrance-free, Simple, Granny's
> SKIN LOTION: Eucerin, Simple, any other fragrance-free variety
> DEODORANT: Almay fragrance-free, Tom's of Maine fragrance-free, Simple, Jason Natural unscented, Kiss My Face fragrance-free, any other fragrance-free variety
> HAIR GEL: Magick Botanicals, or make your own with gelatin (really works!)
> HAIR SPRAY: Magick Botanicals, Almay
> MAKEUP: Almay (in all drugstores), Clinique (in department store cosmetic sections and online)
> SHAVING CREAM: Ray Ban hypoallergenic, Kiss My Face fragrance-free, Simple

Many fragrance-free products can be bought in your local drugstore. For hard-to-find products (especially hair products), check out your local health food store or the NEEDS catalog: www.needs.com. If you are unable to find "fragrance-free" at a store, often the hypo-allergenic version of a product is scent-free. Simply read the ingredients on the label and see if the word "fragrance" appears. If not, you're OK. In a pinch, you can use baking soda to wash your hair (it really works!) and clothes.

Created for the Queer Disability Conference held at San Francisco State University in June 2002.
*Please note that the product suggestions list contains inaccuracies (e.g., Tide Free and Wisk Free are not safe for many people with MCS). I have reproduced the original document without changes.

Appendix D: Robert Edwards, Virginia Ironside, and the Unnecessary Opposition of Rights

As people committed to both disability rights and reproductive rights, we believe that respecting women and families in their reproductive decisions requires simultaneously challenging discriminatory attitudes toward people with disabilities. We refuse to accept the bifurcation of women's rights from disability rights, or the belief that protecting reproductive rights requires accepting ableist assumptions about the supposed tragedy of disability. On the contrary, we assert that reproductive rights includes attention to disability rights, and that disability rights requires attention to human rights, including reproductive rights.

We offer the following statement in response to two recent events that promote eugenic reproductive decision making, and that further stigmatize disabled people by presenting disability exclusively in terms of suffering and hardship. Although seemingly disparate events, they share the presumption that disability renders a life not worth living and that people with disabilities are a burden on society. Moreover, they seem to imply that the only appropriate response to disability is elimination, thereby limiting women's reproductive choices; they suggest that all women must either abort fetuses with disabilities or use IVF to deselect for disability.

The awarding of the 2010 Nobel Prize for medicine to Dr. Robert Edwards demands a more considered response. He has made no secret about promoting reproductive technologies to prevent the birth of disabled children, arguing that it would be a "sin of parents to have a child that carries the heavy burden of genetic disease. We are entering a world where we have to consider the quality of our children." We protest any recognition of Dr. Edwards that also fails to acknowledge his discriminatory statements, and we dispute the notion that his political views should be isolated from his medical accomplishments. It is precisely this separation that pits reproductive rights against disability rights.

Edwards's work has assisted in the birth of four million babies worldwide and has helped single people, people struggling with infertility, and gays, lesbians, and transgender people to have biologically related children. However, we can celebrate Edwards's accomplishments and also call out his controversial advocacy against disability. In the same way that most of the articles celebrating his achievements acknowledge the religious and ethical controversies of his techniques, we can recognize his problematic disparagement of disability. The role he has played in increasing the reproductive options for women and families does not need to be justified or substantiated by arguing for an elimination of disability. It can be marked as an important reproductive option and means of creating families without denigrating disability or people with disabilities.

We also protest any use of disability by antiabortionists in their criticism of Edwards and his work in developing assisted reproductive technologies. Many people with disabilities have used such technologies in creating their own families and recognize that IVF has made their families possible. Although we share the concern that women and families do not always have the information they need to make reproductive decisions about disability, and that stereotypes about disability persist, we do not think the response to that situation is to oppose assisted reproductive technologies or limit women's rights.

The recent statements by British advice columnist Virginia Ironside about the "suffering" of disabled children similarly require a challenge from disability and reproductive rights supporters. In arguing for the right to abortion, Ironside stated that knowingly giving birth to a child with disabilities is cruel, and that in such cases abortion is the "moral and unselfish" response. She added that if she had a sick or disabled child, she would not hesitate to "put a pillow over its face," as would "any loving mother." Although Ironside's comments about infanticide have been rightly condemned, her assertion that abortion is the only proper response to disability has prompted little controversy, as has her assumption that advocacy for abortion rights requires accepting the construction of disability as unrelenting tragedy. As reproductive rights advocates who are committed to disability rights, we refuse to accept the rhetorical use of disability as an argument for abortion rights. Reproductive rights demands not only access to abortion but also the right to have children, including children with disabilities, access to information about parenting, and the social and economic supports to parent all children with dignity.

In other words, we hold both disability rights and reproductive rights together, refusing arguments for women's reproductive autonomy that deny disability rights, and refusing arguments for the human rights of people with disabilities that deny the right of women and families to make the best reproductive decisions for themselves.

Although our statement is motivated by these events, we recognize that these are only the most recent manifestations of long-standing prejudices against people with disabilities and of the use of disability stereotypes to undermine women's and families' reproductive autonomy and access to abortion. We hope, with this statement, to support other activists and scholars who are equally committed to both reproductive rights and disability rights. We hope that as advocates in movements that share similar values around civil and human rights we can continue to speak out against the use of reproductive rights to undermine disability rights and the use of disability rights to undermine reproductive rights. Reproductive rights and disability rights are intertwined.

In solidarity,
    Julia Epstein
    Laura Hershey
    Sujatha Jesudason
    Alison Kafer
    Dorothy Roberts
    Silvia Yee

        October 15, 2010

Notes

Introduction

1. Michael Gerson, "The Eugenics Temptation," *Washington Post,* October 24, 2007, A19.

2. I have borrowed my phrasing here from Ruth Hubbard. See her "Abortion and Disability: Who Should and Who Should Not Inhabit the World?" in *The Disability Studies Reader,* ed. Lennard J. Davis (New York: Routledge, 2006), 93–103. For an overview of Watson's career by one of his former assistants, see Charlotte Hunt-Grubbe, "The Elementary DNA of Dr. Watson," *Sunday Times* (UK), October 14, 2007. In that article, Watson laments that "all our social policies are based on the fact that [Africans'] intelligence is the same as ours—whereas all the testing says not really." He has been quoted elsewhere as supporting the abortion of fetuses that contain "the gay gene," if such tests eventually become possible, although he later claimed he was simply defending women's right to choose under any circumstances. V. MacDonald, "Abort Babies with Gay Genes, Says Nobel Winner," *Telegraph* (UK), February 16, 1997; Steve Boggan and Glenda Cooper, "Nobel Winner May Sue over Gay Baby Abortion Claim," *Independent* (UK), February 17, 1997; and Richard Dawkins, "Letter: Women to Decide on Gay Abortion," *Independent* (UK), February 19, 1997. Watson is often described as a provocateur, willing to put things in the most shocking way to make a point, and, as a result, it is tempting to dismiss his comments as extreme and isolated. But his personal penchant for the outrageous doesn't change the fact that many of his assumptions, particularly about disability, are quite pervasive. The filing of wrongful birth suits would be another manifestation of this notion that no one wants disabled children; in these suits, parents sue their doctors for failing to catch disabling conditions in utero and thereby preventing them from aborting the fetus. I discuss the issue of disabled children and reproduction in chapters 3 and 7.

3. In his deployment of "crazy," Watson employs the same kind of "common sense" logic he uses regarding Down syndrome: in this framework, "obviously" both conditions are undesirable and irredeemable. Part of my project in this book, then, is to work to counteract this assumption about both mental illness and cognitive disabilities. That work occasionally involves occupying and reimagining epithets like "crazy."

4. Monica J. Casper and Lisa Jean Moore, *Missing Bodies: The Politics of Visibility* (New York: New York University Press, 2009), 4.

5. Although disability theorist Tom Shakespeare and journalist Norah Vincent hold opposing views about the worth and need for disability studies (with Shakespeare "for" and Vincent "against"), they share the belief that casting disability as desirable leads, logically, to the belief that we can intentionally disable other people. Vincent suggests, for example, that adhering to such a position must mean that one is opposed to giving pregnant women access to folic acid because it decreases the incidence of certain impairments. Shakespeare argues that "if impairment were just another difference"—not negative but neutral—"there would be nothing wrong with painlessly altering a baby so they could no longer see, or could no longer hear, or had to use a wheelchair." Contrast their position with that of Nirmala Erevelles, who argues that a critical disability response to the question of desiring disability is not to deny such a possibility but rather to explore the social and material conditions under which such desire is possible. Nirmala Erevelles, *Disability and Difference in Global Contexts: Enabling a Transformative Body Politic* (New York: Palgrave Macmillan, 2011), 29. Tom Shakespeare, *Disability Rights and Wrongs* (London: Routledge, 2006), 64; Norah Vincent, "Enabling Disabled Scholarship," *Salon,* August 18, 1999, http://www.salon.com/books/it/1999/08/18/disability/index.html.

6. For an account of disability as human biodiversity, see Rosemarie Garland-Thomson, "Welcoming the Unbidden: The Case for Preserving Human Biodiversity," in *What Democracy Looks Like: A New Critical Realism for a Post-Seattle World*, ed. Amy Schrager Lang and Cecelia Tichi (New Brunswick, NJ: Rutgers University Press, 2006), 77–87. See also Kenny Fries, *The History of My Shoes and the Evolution of Darwin's Theory* (New York: Carroll & Graf, 2007).

7. Although most simulation exercises focus on mobility-impairment/wheelchairs and blindness/blindfolds, I have heard of exercises employing deafness/noise-canceling headsets and, astonishingly, speech impairment/marbles (i.e., asking students to try to speak with marbles in their mouths). Other disabilities, however, seem beyond the reach of these exercises. There are not simulations, for example, of chronic illness, pain, or fatigue, perhaps because people assume they already know what those sensations feel like. I suspect simulations are limited to those conditions that sound fun to experience because they come with props or accoutrements, e.g., canes and wheelchairs. Mental disability and multiple chemical sensitivities are less visible and perhaps therefore more frightening; it would be harder to know when the simulation was beginning and ending, thereby interrupting the distancing dynamic on which these exercises ultimately rely. Some impairments are harder to take on and off.

8. Tobin Siebers, *Disability Theory* (Ann Arbor: University of Michigan Press, 2008), 29. For another critique of disability simulation exercises, see Art Blaser, "Awareness Days: Some Alternatives to Simulation Exercises," *Ragged Edge Online*, September/October 2003, http://www.ragged-edgemagazine.com/0903/0903ft1.html.

9. Simi Linton, *Claiming Disability: Knowledge and Identity* (New York: New York University Press, 1998), 11.

10. Nor do all medical professionals employ an individual/medical model of disability; service providers are also often allies and activists, and there certainly are medical professionals who themselves have disabilities. Thus, as Leslie J. Reagan notes, "[t]he disabilities critique of the medical model . . . perhaps may be best understood as a critique of the entire society, rather than of the medical profession alone, for prioritizing medicine and medical solutions over social reconstruction." Leslie J. Reagan, *Dangerous Pregnancies: Mothers, Disabilities, and Abortion in Modern America* (Berkeley: University of California Press, 2010), 65.

11. Denis Dutton, "What Are Editors For," *Philosophy and Literature* 20 (1996): 551–66, accessed September 24, 2009, http://www.denisdutton.com/what_are_editors_for.htm; emphasis in original.

12. To clarify this point, Dutton provides a list of the symptoms of cretinism: "The bodily symptoms (including limb stunting, enlarged lips, open, drooling mouth, broad, flat face, sallow skin, etc.), and intellectual subnormality to the level of imbecile or moron, are actual medical conditions." Dutton, "What Are Editors For."

13. Rosemarie Garland-Thomson, "Integrating Disability, Transforming Feminist Theory," in *Gendering Disability*, ed. Bonnie Smith and Beth Hutchison (New Brunswick, NJ: Rutgers University Press, 2004), 77.

14. For one of the most well-known examples of this phenomenon, see Susan Wendell, *The Rejected Body: Feminist Philosophical Reflections on Disability* (New York: Routledge, 1996).

15. Jim Swan, "Disabilities, Bodies, Voices," in *Disability Studies: Enabling the Humanities*, ed. Sharon L. Snyder, Brenda Jo Brueggemann, and Rosemarie Garland-Thomson (New York: Modern Languages Association, 2002), 293.

16. Shakespeare suggests that the focus on the medical model as the main site for disability critique is misguided; "when closely analyzed, it is nothing but a straw person" because no one actively and explicitly argues for such an approach to disability. Although I agree that a notion of "the" medical model is unnecessarily simplistic and reductionist—medical approaches to disability are not monolithic, and many service providers support social change on top of any medical treatments—medical constructions and definitions of disability, impairment, and disabled bodies/minds remain the most culturally pervasive frameworks. Shakespeare, *Disability Rights and Wrongs*, 18.

17. Janet Price and Margrit Shildrick, "Uncertain Thoughts on the Dis/abled Body," *Vital Signs: Feminist Reconfigurations of the Bio/logical Body*, ed. Margrit Shildrick and Janet Price (Edinburgh: Edinburgh University Press, 1998), 243, 246.

18. B. J. Gleeson, "Disability Studies: A Historical Materialist View," *Disability and Society* 12, no. 2 (1997): 193. See also Shakespeare, *Disability Rights and Wrongs*.

19. Wendell, *Rejected Body*, 14. See also Shelley Tremain, "On the Subject of Impairment," in *Disability/Postmodernity: Embodying Political Theory*, ed. Mairian Corker and Tom Shakespeare (New York: Continuum, 2002), 32–47.

20. See, for example, Adrienne Rich, "Notes Toward a Politics of Location," *Blood, Bread, Poetry: Selected Prose, 1979–1985* (New York: W. W. Norton, 1994): 210–31.

21. Nor, suggests Michael Bérubé, can the social model adequately address cognitive or intellectual impairments; although social and structural changes are both necessary and long overdue, "it's possible that [a] cognitively impaired person . . . would be impaired by any built environment." Michael Bérubé, "Term Paper," *Profession* (2010): 112. For other recent critiques of the social model, particularly its foreclosure of certain questions from debate, see Julie Livingston, "Insights from an African History of Disability," *Radical History Review* 94 (Winter 2006): 111–26; Anna Mollow, "'When *Black* Women Start Going on Prozac': Race, Gender, and Mental Illness in Meri Nana-Ama Danquah's *Willow Weep for Me*," *MELUS* 31, no. 3 (2006): 67–99; Anna Mollow and Robert McRuer, introduction to *Sex and Disability*, ed. Robert McRuer and Anna Mollow (Durham, NC: Duke University Press, 2012), 1–34; and Shakespeare, *Disability Rights and Wrongs*.

22. Liz Crow, "Including All of Our Lives: Renewing the Social Model of Disability," in *Encounters with Strangers: Feminism and Disability*, ed. Jenny Morris (London: The Women's Press, 1996), 210. For sharp analyses and moving insights on the importance of trauma and depression to radical projects—what Heather Love calls "feeling backward"—see Ann Cvetkovich, *An Archive of Feelings: Trauma, Sexuality, and Lesbian Public Cultures* (Durham, NC: Duke University Press, 2003); and Heather Love, *Feeling Backward: Loss and the Politics of Queer History* (Cambridge, MA: Harvard University Press 2007).

23. Tom Shakespeare, "The Social Model of Disability," in *The Disability Studies Reader*, 2nd ed., ed. Lennard J. Davis (New York: Routledge, 2006), 199.

24. Dutton uses race as his primary example, arguing that there can be no disability equivalent to the "Black is Beautiful" movement of the 1960s.

25. Simone Chess, Alison Kafer, Jessi Quizar, and Mattie Udora Richardson, "Calling All Restroom Revolutionaries!" in *That's Revolting! Queer Strategies for Resisting Assimilation*, ed. Matt Bernstein Sycamore (New York: Soft Skull, 2004), 189–206. I discuss PISSAR in more detail in chapter 7.

26. Chantal Mouffe, *The Return of the Political* (London: Verso, 1993), 3.

27. Jodi Dean, "Introduction: The Interface of Political Theory and Cultural Studies," in *Cultural Studies and Political Theory*, ed. Jodi Dean (Ithaca, NY: Cornell University Press, 2000), 6.

28. Dean, "Introduction: The Interface of Political Theory," 4; emphasis mine.

29. For an examination of ableism, see Fiona Kumari Campbell, *Contours of Ableism: The Production of Disability and Ableness* (New York: Palgrave Macmillan, 2009). On compulsory able-bodiedness, see Robert McRuer, "Compulsory Able-Bodiedness and Queer/Disabled Existence," in *Disability Studies: Enabling the Humanities*, ed. Sharon L. Snyder, Brenda Jo Brueggemann, and Rosemarie Garland-Thomson (New York: Modern Language Association, 2002): 88–99; and Alison Kafer, "Compulsory Bodies: Reflections on Heterosexuality and Able-bodiedness," *Journal of Women's History* 15, no. 3 (2003): 77–89.

30. Susan M. Schweik, *The Ugly Laws: Disability in Public* (New York: New York University Press, 2009), 280.

31. For other critical accounts of disability identity, see Gloria Anzaldúa, "Disability and Identity," in *The Gloria Anzaldúa Reader*, ed. AnaLouise Keating (Durham, NC: Duke University Press,

2009), 298–302; Robert McRuer, *Crip Theory: Cultural Signs of Queerness and Disability* (New York: New York University Press, 2006); Anna Mollow, "Identity Politics and Disability Studies: A Critique of Recent Theory," *Michigan Quarterly Review* 43, no. 2 (2004): 269–96; and Mollow and McRuer, introduction to *Sex and Disability*.

32. Ben Pitcher and Henriette Gunkel, "Q&A with Jasbir Puar," *darkmatter Journal*, accessed December 3, 2009, http://www.darkmatter101.org/site/2008/05/02/qa-with-jasbir-puar/.

33. Joan W. Scott, "Cyborgian Socialists?" in *Coming to Terms: Feminism, Theory, Politics*, ed. Elizabeth Weed (New York: Routledge, 1989), 216.

34. Linton, *Claiming Disability*, 4, emphasis mine.

35. The field of philosophy has a fair number of texts dealing with cognitive impairments, partly because of the importance of, and discourses around, rationality in the field. Disability studies approaches to these topics within the field, however, remain quite rare. For exceptions, see, for example, Licia Carlson, "Cognitive Ableism and Disability Studies: Feminist Reflections on the History of Mental Retardation," *Hypatia* 16, no. 4 (2001): 128–33; Licia Carlson, *The Faces of Intellectual Disability* (Bloomington: Indiana University Press, 2010); and Sophia Isako Wong, "At Home with Down Syndrome and Gender," *Hypatia* 17, no. 3 (2002): 89–117. There is also a critical set of historical texts addressing cognitive impairments through a disability studies lens. See, for example, Martin S. Pernick, *The Black Stork: Eugenics and the Death of "Defective" Babies in American Medicine and Motion Pictures since 1915* (New York: Oxford University Press, 1996); and James W. Trent, Jr., *Inventing the Feeble Mind: A History of Mental Retardation in the United States* (Berkeley: University of California Press, 1995).

36. Margaret Price, *Mad at School: Rhetorics of Mental Disability and Academic Life* (Ann Arbor: University of Michigan Press, 2011); Ellen Samuels, "My Body, My Closet: Invisible Disability and the Limits of Coming-Out Discourse," *GLQ: A Journal of Lesbian and Gay Studies* 9, nos. 1–2 (2003): 233–55; and Susan Wendell, "Unhealthy Disabled: Treating Chronic Illnesses as Disabilities," *Hypatia: A Journal of Feminist Philosophy* 16, no. 4 (2001): 17–33.

37. Signorello et al. explain that "[r]easons for racial disparities in diabetes prevalence are not clear, but behavioral, environmental, socioeconomic, physiological, and genetic contributors have all been postulated." Their findings suggest that these differences cannot be attributed to "race" per se, but to other established risk factors including socioeconomic status. L. B. Signorello et al., "Comparing Diabetes Prevalence between African Americans and Whites of Similar Socioeconomic Status," *American Journal of Public Health* 97, no. 12 (2007): 2260. For a critique of race-based medicine, see Dorothy Roberts, *Fatal Invention: How Science, Politics, and Big Business Re-create Race in the Twenty-first Century* (New York: The New Press, 2011).

38. Chris Bell, "Introducing White Disability Studies: A Modest Proposal," in *The Disability Studies Reader,* 2nd ed. (New York: Routledge, 2006): 275–82. Nirmala Erevelles and Andrea Minear offer a productive reading of theories of intersectionality through the lens of disability studies; they work in both directions, interrogating the whiteness of disability studies and the inattention to disability in critical race studies. Nirmala Erevelles and Andrea Minear, "Unspeakable Offenses: Untangling Race and Disability in Discourses of Intersectionality," *Journal of Literary and Cultural Disability Studies* 4, no. 2 (2010): 127–45. See also Corbett Joan O'Toole, "The Sexist Inheritance of the Disability Movement," in *Gendering Disability*, ed. Bonnie G. Smith and Beth Hutchison (New Brunswick, NJ: Rutgers University Press, 2004), 294–95.

39. Carrie Sandahl, "Queering the Crip or Cripping the Queer: Intersections of Queer and Crip Identities in Solo Autobiographical Performance," *GLQ* 9, nos. 1–2 (2003): 27; Robert McRuer, *Crip Theory: Cultural Signs of Queerness and Disability* (New York: New York University Press, 2006), 36.

40. Robert Hoffmeister, "Border Crossings by Hearing Children of Deaf Parents: The Lost History of Codas," in *Open Your Eyes: Deaf Studies Talking*, ed. H-Dirksen L. Bauman (Minneapolis: University of Minnesota Press, 2008), 189–215; see also Lennard J. Davis, *My Sense of Silence:*

Memoirs of a Childhood with Deafness (Champaign: University of Illinois Press, 2000). Brenda Jo Brueggemann offers a productive examination of deaf identity and the space between identities. Brenda Jo Brueggemann, *Deaf Subjects: Between Identities and Places* (New York: New York University Press, 2009).

41. McRuer, *Crip Theory*, 36–37.

42. Linton, *Claiming Disability*, 13. See also Carlson, *Faces of Intellectual Disability*, 192–94.

43. Drawing on her work on disability in Botswana, Julie Livingston suggests the term "debility" as an alternative to disability because it encompasses chronic illness, aging, and a wide range of impairments, not just "disability per se." Livingston, "Insights," 113.

44. Ladelle McWhorter, foreword to *Foucault and the Government of Disability*, ed. Shelley Tremain (Ann Arbor: University of Michigan Press, 2005), xv.

45. For a discussion of the inclusion of women who do not identify as feminists in feminist political activism and coalition work, see Sohera Syeda and Becky Thompson, "Coalition Politics in Organizing for Mumia Abu-Jamal," in *Feminism and Antiracism: International Struggles for Justice*, ed. France Winddance Twine and Kathleen M. Blee (New York: New York University Press, 2001), 193–219.

46. In some of his recent work on disability and identity politics, Lennard J. Davis provides a progress narrative of theories of identity in which he consigns the work of feminist and queer theorists to earlier, problematic stages, with disability—a disability apparently separate from feminist and queer theory—offering a solution to the problems of identity politics. See *Bending Over Backwards: Disability, Dismodernism, and other Difficult Positions* (New York: New York University Press, 2002), 9–32. For a brief critique of Davis's representation of feminist and queer theory and activism, see McRuer, *Crip Theory*, 202.

My desire to make these links explicit echoes the work of Gayatri Gopinath, who, in her study of queer diasporas, "challenges the notion that these fields of inquiry [queer and feminist scholarship] are necessarily distinct, separate, and incommensurate." Gayatri Gopinath, *Impossible Desires: Queer Diasporas and South Asian Public Cultures* (Durham, NC: Duke University Press, 2005), 16.

47. Nancy Mairs, *Plaintext: Essays* (Tucson: University of Arizona Press, 1992), 9.

48. On the dynamic of staring, see Rosemarie Garland-Thomson, *Staring: How We Look* (New York: Oxford University Press, 2009).

49. Eli Clare, *Exile and Pride: On Disability, Queerness, and Liberation* (Boston: South End Press, 1999), 70.

50. Sandahl, "Queering the Crip," 53n1; McRuer, *Crip Theory*, 35.

51. "Critical disability studies" is another term describing this orientation toward disability and disability studies; as Margrit Shildrick describes it, critical disability studies is the frame favored "by those . . . for whom the original challenge of the social model of disability no longer provides an effectively dynamic model." Margrit Shildrick, *Dangerous Discourses of Disability, Subjectivity, and Sexuality* (New York: Palgrave Macmillan, 2009), 15.

52. Sandahl, "Queering the Crip," 27.

53. Part of my reluctance to articulate a strict boundary between feminist disability studies (or queer disability studies) and crip theory stems from an awareness that contradictory strategies and epistemologies often circulate under the same name. Merri Lisa Johnson explains, for example, that some work marked "feminist disability studies" refuses all medical terminology while other feminist disability studies approaches do not; similarly, some "disability studies" texts deconstruct the disabled/nondisabled binary while others reify it. Moreover, I worry about the possibility of "crip theory" being positioned as a successor narrative to disability studies, as if all the problems with the field could be solved with this one shift in approach. (After all, crip theory could also be critiqued, in Bell's terms, as *white* crip theory.) I hasten to add that neither McRuer nor Sandahl have positioned crip theory this way, and both continue to practice and claim "disability studies"; I believe their

distinction invites a contestatory approach to both disability and disability studies while remaining invested in the promises of the field as a whole. For an example of a theorist who is interested in mapping the differences between feminist disability studies and crip feminism, see Merri Lisa Johnson, "Crip Drag Swan Queen: Two Readings of Darren Aronofsky's *Black Swan*," National Women's Studies Association Conference, Atlanta, GA, November, 2011.

54. "Compulsory able-mindedness" is a way of capturing the normalizing practices, assumptions, and exclusions that cannot easily be described as directed (exclusively) to *physical* functioning or appearance. Kristen Harmon suggests, for example, that "able-bodiedness" cannot sufficiently address what she calls "compulsory hearing." Kristen Harmon, "Deaf Matters: Compulsory Hearing and Ability Trouble," in *Deaf and Disability Studies: Interdisciplinary Perspectives,* ed. Susan Burch and Alison Kafer (Washington, DC: Gallaudet University Press, 2010), 42. For extensive analyses of compulsory able-mindedness in terms of mental disability, see Andrea Nicki, "The Abused Mind: Feminist Theory, Psychiatric Disability, and Trauma," *Hypatia* 16, no. 4 (2001): 80–104; and Margaret Price, *Mad at School: Rhetorics of Mental Disability and Academic Life* (Ann Arbor: University of Michigan Press, 2010).

55. Anna Mollow makes a similar argument in her discussion of depression and mental illness; to engage fully with questions of mental illness, disability studies will need to shift its guiding frameworks and terminologies. Mollow, "'When *Black* Women Start Going on Prozac.'" See also Elizabeth J. Donaldson, "Revisiting the Corpus of the Madwoman: Further Notes toward a Feminist Disability Studies Theory of Mental Illness," in *Feminist Disability Studies*, ed. Kim Q. Hall (Bloomington: Indiana University Press, 2011), 91–113.

56. Judith Butler, *Bodies That Matter: On the Discursive Limits of "Sex"* (New York: Routledge, 1993), 223.

57. Carrie Sandahl expresses the same hope, and concern, noting that queer theory (and, I would add, disability studies) has a "tendency to absorb and flatten internal differences, in particular to neutralize its constituents' material and cultural differences and to elevate the concerns of gay white men [or middle-class white male wheelchair users] above all others." Sandahl, "Queering the Crip," 27.

58. Mattilda suggests that it is in the "messiness" of intersectional work that "the possibility for a rigorous analysis emerges." Jason Ruiz, "The Violence of Assimilation: An Interview with Mattilda aka Matt Bernstein Sycamore," *Radical History Review* 100 (Winter 2008): 239.

59. Jasbir K. Puar, *Terrorist Assemblages: Homonationalism in Queer Times* (Durham, NC: Duke University Press, 2007), 212.

60. Of course, this lack is even more pronounced in the other direction; papers on disability studies topics or drawing on disability theory remain few and far between at many cultural studies and critical theory conferences.

61. Puar, *Terrorist Assemblages*, 209; emphasis in original.

62. Janet Price and Margrit Shildrick play with this desire for and practice of disability identification in some of their collaborative work, as do Robert McRuer and Anna Mollow. See Price and Shildrick, "Uncertain Thoughts"; and Mollow and McRuer, introduction to *Sex and Disability*.

63. John B. Kelly's analysis of quad rugby offers a potent reminder that ableism or, in his framing, the ideology of ability, affects relationships *between* disabled people. John B. Kelly, "'It Could Have Been Worse': Quadriplegic Athletes and the Ideology of Ability," Society for Disability Studies Annual Meeting, Chicago, June 2000.

64. Eve Kosofsky Sedgwick, *Tendencies* (Durham, NC: Duke University Press, 1994), xiv. See also Margaret Price, "'Her Pronouns Wax and Wane': Psychosocial Disability, Autobiography, and Counter-Diagnosis," *Journal of Literary and Cultural Disability Studies* 3, no. 1 (2009): 11–33.

65. Robert McRuer and Abby L. Wilkerson, "Introduction," *GLQ: A Journal of Lesbian and Gay Studies* 9, nos. 1–2 (2003): 13.

Chapter 1

1. David Penna and Vickie D'Andrea-Penna, "Developmental Disability," in *Encyclopedia of U.S. Disability History*, ed. Susan Burch (New York: Facts on File, 2009), 261–62.

2. As I noted in the introduction, *disabled* can also be a temporary category. Some people have illnesses or disabilities whose manifestations come and go repeatedly over the course of their lives; others may see their illnesses or disabilities cured, either through medical intervention or "over time." Moreover, the meanings of *disabled* shift significantly by and in context, such that determining a timeless definition is both futile and, I would argue, misguided. As Margrit Shildrick reminds us, part of the work of critical disability studies is to trouble the distinction between disabled and able-bodied, or between disabled and nondisabled. Margrit Shildrick, *Dangerous Discourses of Disability, Subjectivity, and Sexuality* (New York: Palgrave Macmillan, 2009); Janet Price and Margrit Shildrick, "Uncertain Thoughts on the Dis/abled Body," in *Vital Signs: Feminist Reconfigurations of the Bio/logical Body*, ed. Margrit Shildrick and Janet Price (Edinburgh: Edinburgh University Press, 1998), 224–49.

3. In the same volume, Michael Bérubé urges an accounting "of temporality in our theories of identity," including disability. Sharon Snyder, Brenda Brueggemann, and Rosemarie Garland-Thomson, "Introduction: Integrating Disability in Theory and Scholarship," in *Disability Studies: Enabling the Humanities*, ed. Sharon Snyder, Brenda Brueggemann, and Rosemarie Garland-Thomson (New York: Modern Language Association of America, 2002), 2; Michael Bérubé, "Afterword: If I Should Live So Long," in *Disability Studies: Enabling the Humanities*, ed. Sharon Snyder, Brenda Brueggemann, and Rosemarie Garland-Thomson (New York: The Modern Language Association of America, 2002), 339.

4. Donald McNeil, Jr., "Broad Racial Disparities Seen in Americans' Ills," *New York Times*, January 14, 2011. Researchers note similar health disparities between straight people and gays, lesbians, and bisexuals, particularly as they age. Roni Caryn Rabin, "Disparities: Illness More Prevalent among Older Gay Adults," *New York Times*. April 1, 2011.

5. Irving Kenneth Zola, "The Language of Disability: Problems of Politics and Practice," *Australian Disability Review*, 1988, accessed January 6, 2011, http://www.disabilitymuseum.org/lib/docs/813.card.htm; Carol J. Gill, "A Psychological View of Disability Culture," *DSQ: Disability Studies Quarterly* 15, no. 4 (1995): 16–19.

6. Some readers will recognize similarities to "people of color time" and "queer time."

7. *Dictionary of American Slang*, "crip time," accessed January 6, 2011, http://www.diclib.com/cgi-bin/d1.cgi?base=amslang&page=showid&id=2159.

8. Kate Bornstein suggests that some trans-identified folks might find themselves with similar temporal needs: "[A] newly transgendered person . . . moves just a bit slower than most people; he or she is unlearning old ways of moving, and picking up new ways of moving. So one of the first things you try to do is to move at a normal pace." Kate Bornstein, *Gender Outlaw: On Men, Women, and the Rest of Us* (New York: Vintage, 1995), 87.

9. Margaret Price, *Mad at School: Rhetorics of Mental Disability and Academic Life* (Ann Arbor: University of Michigan Press, 2011), 62. See also Margaret Price, "Access Imagined: The Construction of Disability in Conference Policy Documents," *DSQ: Disability Studies Quarterly* 29, no. 1 (2009), http://www.dsq-sds.org/article/view/174/174.

10. For examples of queer approaches to temporality, see Judith Halberstam, *In a Queer Time and Place: Transgender Bodies, Subcultural Lives* (New York: New York University Press, 2005); and Elizabeth Freeman, ed., "Queer Temporalities," special issue of *GLQ: A Journal of Gay and Lesbian Studies* 13, nos. 2–3 (2007). Lee Edelman's polemic against the future and José Esteban Muñoz's articulation of a queer futurity can also be seen as part of the larger queer exploration of temporality, as can Elizabeth Freeman's and Heather Love's engagements with queer history and queer

historiography. Lee Edelman, *No Future: Queer Theory and the Death Drive* (Durham, NC: Duke University Press, 2004); José Esteban Muñoz, *Cruising Utopia: The Then and There of Queer Futurity* (New York: New York University Press, 2009); Elizabeth Freeman, *Time Binds: Queer Temporalities, Queer Histories* (Durham, NC: Duke University Press, 2010); and Heather Love, *Feeling Backward: Loss and the Politics of Queer History* (Cambridge, MA: Harvard University Press, 2009).

The 2009 Society for Disability Studies Conference referred to temporality in its general theme—"It's 'Our' Time: Pathways to and from Disability Studies: Past, Present, Future"—but few of the papers at the conference engaged with queer temporality (or with theories of futurity and temporality in general); similarly, the special issue of *DSQ: Disability Studies Quarterly* that showcased several papers from the conference featured no such engagement with queer approaches to temporality. Jim Ferris, ed., "In (Disability) Time," *DSQ: Disability Studies Quarterly* 30, nos. 3–4 (2010).

11. As Carrie Sandahl puts it, "Cripping spins mainstream representations or practices to reveal able-bodied assumptions and exclusionary effects." In turning my attention to "queer time," I propose expanding the terrain of cripping to include not only "mainstream representations or practices" but also *queer* representations and practices. How do they, too, "reveal able-bodied assumptions and exclusionary effects"? Carrie Sandahl, "Queering the Crip, or Cripping the Queer? Intersections of Queer and Crip Identities in Solo Autobiographical Performance," *GLQ: A Journal of Lesbian and Gay Studies* 9, nos. 1–2 (2003): 37.

12. For an incisive queer reading of rehabilitation, see Robert McRuer, *Crip Theory: Cultural Signs of Queerness and Disability* (New York: New York University Press, 2006), especially 103–45.

13. Much as an individual's desire for a cure does not necessarily signal an adherence to a curative imaginary but can, instead, be felt alongside a strong crip affiliation, so, too, can these questions exist apart from a curative temporality. Indeed, such questions can be used to animate a *crip* temporality if they serve to trouble the abled/disabled binary or to disrupt the assumed stability of disability categories and diagnoses. I refer here only to the more common framing of these questions.

14. Carla Freccero, "Fuck the Future," *GLQ: A Journal of Gay and Lesbian Studies* 12, no. 2 (2006): 332–34.

15. Edelman, *No Future*, 11. See also Lauren Berlant, *The Queen of America Goes to Washington City: Essays on Sex and Citizenship* (Durham, NC: Duke University Press, 1997).

16. Ibid., 11, 3.

17. Ibid., 3.

18. Patrick McCreery, "Save Our Children/Let Us Marry: Gay Activists Appropriate the Rhetoric of Child Protectionism," *Radical History Review* 2008, no. 100 (2008): 186–207.

19. Testing "positive" is not a guarantee that a child will have a certain disability, and most tests are unable to determine the extent of a child's impairment; children with Down syndrome, for example, differ widely in their level of function. For extended analyses of prenatal testing practices, see Rayna Rapp, *Testing Women, Testing the Fetus: The Social Impact of Amniocentesis in America* (New York: Routledge, 1999); and Janelle S. Taylor, *The Public Life of the Fetal Sonogram: Technology, Consumption, and the Politics of Reproduction* (New Brunswick, NJ: Rutgers University Press, 2008).

20. Edelman, *No Future*, 30.

21. Shannon Winnubst, "Temporality in Queer Theory and Continental Philosophy," *Philosophy Compass* 5, no. 2 (2010): 138.

22. The only "cure" available for most conditions detected by prenatal testing is selective abortion; there have been recent breakthroughs in fetal surgery, but those are still preliminary and only work for certain conditions. See Pam Belluck, "Success of Spina Bifida Study Opens Fetal Surgery Door," *New York Times*, February 9, 2011, A1.

23. *Buck v. Bell*, 274 U.S. 200, 1927, accessed September 13, 2010, http://laws.findlaw.com/us/274/200.html. See also Paul Lombardo, *Three Generations, No Imbeciles: Eugenics, the Supreme Court, and* Buck v. Bell (Baltimore, MD: The Johns Hopkins University Press, 2008).

24. For histories of eugenics in the United States, see, among others, Susan Burch and Hannah Joyner, *Unspeakable: The Story of Junius Wilson* (Chapel Hill: University of North Carolina Press, 2007); Wendy Kline, *Building a Better Race: Gender, Sexuality, and Eugenics from the Turn of the Century to the Baby Boom* (Berkeley: University of California Press, 2001); Nancy Ordover, *American Eugenics: Race, Queer Anatomy, and the Science of Nationalism* (Minneapolis: University of Minnesota Press, 2003); Martin S. Pernick, *The Black Stork: Eugenics and the Death of "Defective" Babies in American Medicine and Motion Pictures since 1915* (New York: Oxford University Press, 1996); Michael A. Rembis, *Defining Deviance: Sex, Science, and Delinquent Girls, 1890–1960* (Champaign: University of Illinois Press, 2011); Johanna Schoen, *Choice and Coercion: Birth Control, Sterilization, and Abortion in Public Health and Welfare* (Chapel Hill: University of North Carolina Press, 2005); Steven Selden, *Inheriting Shame: The Story of Eugenics and Racism in America* (New York: Teachers College Press, 1999); and James Trent, *Inventing the Feeble Mind: A History of Mental Retardation in the United States* (Berkeley: University of California Press, 1994).

25. See, for example, Elena R. Gutiérrez, *Fertile Matters: The Politics of Mexican-Origin Women's Reproduction* (Austin: University of Texas Press, 2008); Jennifer Nelson, *Women of Color and the Reproductive Rights Movement* (New York: New York University Press, 2003); and Dorothy Roberts, *Killing the Black Body: Race, Reproduction, and the Meaning of Liberty* (New York: Vintage, 1999).

26. For more on institutionalization and the need for community-based care, see Laura Hershey, *Just Help* (unpublished manuscript), 271–72; Harriet MacBryde Johnson, "The Disability Gulag," *New York Times Magazine*, November 23, 2003, http://www.nytimes.com/2003/11/23/magazine/the-disability-gulag.html; and Jennifer LaFleur, "Nursing Homes Get Old for Many with Disabilities," *ProPublica*, June 21, 2009, http://www.propublica.org/article/nursing-homes-get-old-for-many-with-disabilities-621.

27. Mary Storer Kostir, "The Family of Sam Sixty," in *White Trash: The Eugenic Family Studies, 1877–1919*, ed. Nicole Hahn Rafter (Boston: Northeastern University Press, 1988), 208, emphasis in original.

28. The full passage reads: "A community can follow one of three courses in dealing with the problem of parenthood among its mentally diseased and mentally deficient members who are not able to control their own fecundity. 1. It may do nothing at all. That is what most communities are now doing. The results are not satisfactory either to the community or to the patients. They are disastrous in their effect in future generations. 2. It may keep such patients under lock and key for the rest of their lives, or at least for the rest of their reproductive lives. Such a policy is too expensive to reach more than a minority, and is therefore impracticable. Even if possible, it would in many cases be an unnecessary hardship or cruelty to the patient. 3. It may use sterilization in selected cases, as an adjunct to a careful system of parole and supervision, which will aid patients to live in the community, to be self-supporting, and at the same time not put a new burden on society or pass on their handicaps to posterity.

Eugenic sterilization is no panacea, but it is one of the many tested and dependable measures that will help reduce the burdens and increase the happiness and prosperity of the population in this and future generations. As such, it is one among many indispensable procedures in any modern program of social welfare." *Human Sterilization* (Pasadena, CA: Human Betterment Foundation, 1933), 6, Cold Spring Harbor Eugenics Archive, accessed September 13, 2010, http://tinyurl.com/8gcrudb.

29. For examples of this critique of Edelman, see Muñoz, *Cruising Utopia*; and Jasbir K. Puar, *Terrorist Assemblages: Homonationalism in Queer Times* (Durham, NC: Duke University Press, 2007). Shannon Winnubst shares with Edelman a suspicion of the future, and both are wary of political talk of utility or social value. But Winnubst departs from Edelman in her recognition that many people have never had the cultural or economic capital to project themselves into the future in the first place; like Muñoz and Puar, she is concerned with the role of whiteness in the reproductive imaginary. Shannon Winnubst, *Queering Freedom* (Bloomington: Indiana University Press, 2006).

30. Edelman, *No Future*, 11, 29.

31. Heather Love, "Wedding Crashers," *GLQ: A Journal of Lesbian and Gay Studies* 13, no. 1 (2007): 131.

32. Muñoz, *Cruising Utopia*, 95.

33. Sarah Horton and Judith C. Barker. "'Stains' on Their Self-Discipline: Public Health, Hygiene, and the Disciplining of Undocumented Immigrant Parents in the Nation's Borderlands," *American Ethnologist* 36, no. 4 (2009): 785.

34. Susan Schweik similarly describes how categories of health and hygiene were used "as a means of white trashing, in which poor whiteness or bad whiteness (filthy, debilitated, dangerous, debris) sets off the nice body of good whiteness." Susan M. Schweik, *The Ugly Laws: Disability in Public* (New York: New York University Press, 2009), 185; and Anna Stubblefield, "Beyond the Pale: Tainted Whiteness, Cognitive Disability, and Eugenic Sterilization," *Hypatia* 22, no. 2 (2007): 162, 163. For more on historical links between whiteness and (racial) hygiene, see, for example, Mel Y. Chen, *Animacies: Biopolitics, Racial Mattering, and Queer Affect* (Durham, NC: Duke University Press, forthcoming); Natalia Molina, "Constructing Mexicans as Deportable Immigrants: Race, Disease, and the Meaning of 'Public Charge,'" *Identities: Global Studies in Culture and Power* 17 (2010): 641–66; Natalia Molina, "Medicalizing the Mexican: Immigration, Race, and Disability in the Early-Twentieth-Century United States," *Radical History Review* 94 (2006): 22–37; and Nayan Shah, *Contagious Divides: Epidemics and Race in San Francisco's Chinatown* (Berkeley: University of California Press, 2001).

35. Horton and Barker, "'Stains' on Their Self-Discipline," 796.

36. Quoted in Cathy Cohen, "Punks, Bulldaggers, and Welfare Queens: The Radical Potential of Queer Politics?" in *Black Queer Studies: A Critical Anthology*, ed. E. Patrick Johnson and Mae G. Henderson (Durham, NC: Duke University Press, 2005), 40. Cohen offers a concise and incisive critique of Moynihan's project; see also Mattie Udora Richardson, "No More Secrets, No More Lies: African-American History and Compulsory Heterosexuality," *Journal of Women's History* 15, no. 3 (2003): 63–76; and Hortense Spillers, "Mama's Baby, Papa's Maybe: An American Grammar Book," *Diacritics* 17, no. 2 (1987): 64–81.

37. Dorothy Roberts, *Fatal Invention: How Science, Politics, and Big Business Re-create Race in the Twenty-first Century* (New York: The New Press, 2011), 94. See also Erevelles, *Disability and Difference in Global Contexts*; and Beth A. Ferri and David O'Connor, *Reading Resistance: Discourses of Exclusion in Desegregation and Exclusion Debates* (New York: Peter Lang, 2006).

38. I read McRuer's entire *Crip Theory* as a sustained argument to this effect; indeed, to do crip theory *is* to recognize and refuse this call to normalization in all its guises.

39. Puar, *Terrorist Assemblages*, 211.

40. Noam Ostrander, "When Identities Collide: Masculinity, Disability, and Race," *Disability and Society* 23, no. 6 (2008): 594.

41. Kevin Sack, "Research Finds Wide Disparities in Health Care by Race and Region," *New York Times*, June 5, 2008, http://www.nytimes.com/2008/06/05/health/research/05disparities.html; see also Roberts, *Fatal Invention*, 102.

42. As Ed Cohen and Julie Livingston explain, "Inequality does not name a natural imbalance; it bespeaks systematic and relentless devaluations. And, as with all instances of (d)evaluation, the hierarchies it inscribes result from *decisions*." Asking these kinds of questions—of incidence and occurrence—reminds us that decisions can be made differently. Ed Cohen and Julie Livingston, "AIDS," *Social Text* 27, no. 3 (2009): 40.

43. Elizabeth Freeman, introduction to "Queer Temporalities," special issue of *GLQ: A Journal of Gay and Lesbian Studies*, 13 nos. 2–3 (2007): 159, emphasis in the original.

44. Ibid., 160.

45. Ellen Samuels makes this argument about Halberstam, tracing her unmarked relationship to disability studies. Ellen Samuels, "Normative Time: How Queerness, Disability, and Parenthood

Impact Academic Labor," paper presented at the Modern Languages Association Annual Meeting, December 2006.

46. Freeman, introduction, 159.

47. Halberstam, *In a Queer Time and Place*, 1.

48. Ibid., 152.

49. Ibid., 153.

50. Ibid., 2.

51. Ibid., 1.

52. Ibid., 2.

53. Ibid., 2.

54. Robert McRuer has long argued for a more robust and critical investment in the relationships among AIDS theory, queer theory, and disability studies. While such links might already be implicit in some disability and AIDS activism and scholarship, McRuer urges us to make them explicit, "continually focusing on a queer/disabled collectivity, surrounding AIDS theorists with a larger disability community and vice versa." Building on his insights, I think part of this work includes remembering that the time of the epidemic is not over. See Robert McRuer, "Critical Investments: AIDS, Christopher Reeve, and Queer/Disability Studies," *Journal of Medical Humanities* 23, nos. 3–4 (2002): 226.

55. Tom Boellstorff, "When Marriage Fails: Queer Coincidences in Straight Time," *GLQ* 13, nos. 2–3 (2007): 228.

56. Eliza Chandler, "Sidewalk Stories: The Troubling Task of Identification," *Disability Studies Quarterly* 30, nos. 3–4 (2010), http://www.dsq-sds.org/article/view/1293/1329.

57. Jain mentions in passing that prognosis time might be a way to rethink disability beyond identity politics—for don't we all live under prognosis to some degree?—a claim that Puar then takes up in her own ruminations on prognosis time. I share their interest in thinking disability beyond disabled bodies; indeed, part of my fascination with crip temporalities is how thinking through time might push us all to consider disability differently. Sarah Lochlann Jain, "Living in Prognosis: Toward an Elegiac Politics," *Representations* 98 (Spring 2007): 80–81; Jasbir K. Puar, "Prognosis Time: Toward a Geopolitics of Affect, Debility and Capacity," *Women and Performance: A Journal of Feminist Theory* 19, no. 2 (2009): 161–72.

58. Laura Hershey, *Just Help*, 168.

59. Jain discusses these kinds of negotiations as a reckoning with both fantasies of the future and counterfactual futures and pasts. Jain, "Living in Prognosis."

60. Cynthia Daniels discusses the difficulties veterans face in persuading the government to acknowledge the effects of Agent Orange and Iraq War Syndrome on men's reproductive health. *Exposing Men: The Science and Politics of Male Reproduction* (New York: Oxford University Press, 2006).

61. Carolyn Dinshaw et al., "Theorizing Queer Temporalities: A Roundtable Discussion," *GLQ: A Journal of Gay and Lesbian Studies* 13, nos. 2–3 (2007): 192.

62. Nealon asks this question in terms of working-class gay men and gay men of color returning again and again to gay bars where they feel—are made to feel—unwelcome. I deploy it here not only to ask these questions of diagnosis/undiagnosis/misdiagnosis but also out of a recognition that these questions are similarly bound up in questions of race and class. How have popular representations of MCS and chronic fatigue as illnesses (or, often, "illnesses") striking the white and upper/middle class made it impossible to see MCS in populations of color? Or, to put it differently, how have populations of color been seen as always already polluted and therefore exceeding diagnoses of MCS? Moving to other diagnostic categories, how have labels of "learning disability" and "behavioral/emotional disability" been attached to different populations differently, with white students more likely to fit the former classification and students of color the latter? Or, more broadly, how are students of color overrepresented in special education classrooms? For more on these questions, see Chen, *Animacies*;

Nirmala Erevelles and Andrea Minear, "Unspeakable Offenses: Untangling Race and Disability in Discourses of Intersectionality," *Journal of Literary and Cultural Disability Studies* 4, no. 2 (2010): 127–45; and Ferri and O'Connor, *Reading Resistance*.

63. Rhonda Zwillinger, *The Dispossessed: Living with Multiple Chemical Sensitivities* (Paulden, AZ: The Dispossessed Outreach Project, 1999), 61. See also Stacy Alaimo, *Bodily Natures: Science, Environment, and the Material Self* (Bloomington: Indiana University Press, 2010).

64. Mel Y. Chen, "Toxic Animacies, Inanimate Affections," *GLQ: A Journal of Lesbian and Gay Studies* 17, nos. 2–3 (2011): 274.

65. Chen, "Toxic Animacies," 277.

66. Ibid., 274–78. Peggy Munson similarly describes feeling alienated, or even violated, by the bodies of those around her. She reads erotic possibility into going scent-free, describing it as a kind of radical femme surrender. Peggy Munson, "Fringe Dweller: Toward an Ecofeminist Politic of Femme," in *Visible: A Femmethology*, vol. 2., ed. Jennifer Clarke Burke (Ypsilanti, MI: Homofactus Press, 2009), 28–36.

67. Anna Mollow suggests that this "unknowingness" is limited. We may not know, understand, or believe that our use of fragrance- or chemical-laden products makes others ill, but we do expect—and want—our use of fragrances to be apparent to others. As she explains, "the phrase 'personal care products' is something of a misnomer: the fragrances these products contain are designed to affect many others besides those who choose to apply them. People don't pay forty-five dollars for a bottle of Calvin Klein's Eternity so that they can sit alone in their living rooms and inhale its forty-one chemical ingredients (several of which the EPA and other governmental agencies list as toxic). Rather, they expect that these ingredients will permeate the air and enter the bodies of everyone who comes in contact with them." Anna Mollow, "No Safe Place," *WSQ: Women's Studies Quarterly* 39, nos. 1–2 (2011): 194–95.

68. Johnson, "Disability Gulag."

69. For a personal description of such accounting, see Christine Miserandino, "The Spoon Theory," 2003, http://www.butyoudontlooksick.com.

70. Halberstam's book was written before the economic downturn, when "unemployed" was more likely to refer to those considered "unemployable" or those unemployed by choice rather than the massive groups of unemployed people now. Halberstam, *In a Queer Time and Place*, 10.

71. Samuels, "Normative Time," 5.

72. Catherine Kudlick notes that much of the language we use in the academy to evaluate ourselves and our colleagues—measuring up, pulling our own weight—bear the marks of industrial capitalism's focus on fitness and punctuality. Catherine Kudlick, "A History Profession for Every Body," *Journal of Women's History* 18, no. 1 (2006): 163–64. See also Price, *Mad at School*.

73. Halberstam, *In a Queer Time and Place*, 4.

74. Ibid., 4, 152.

75. Ibid., 2.

76. McRuer, *Crip Theory*, 183.

77. Halberstam, *In a Queer Time and Place*, 4.

78. Ibid., 3.

79. Ibid., 3.

80. Winnubst, *Queering Freedom*, 186.

81. Georgina Kleege, *Blind Rage: Letters to Helen Keller* (Washington, DC: Gallaudet University Press, 2006); and Brenda Jo Brueggemann, *Deaf Subjects: Between Identities and Places* (New York: New York University Press, 2009).

82. As Elizabeth Freeman suggests, "[W]riting is a way to speak with the dead, reanimate the past, gamble that there was one at all." Freeman, introduction, 168.

83. Muñoz, *Cruising Utopia*, 37.

84. Le'a Kent, "Fighting Abjection: Representing Fat Women," in *Bodies Out of Bounds: Fatness and Transgression*, ed. Jana Evans Braziel and Kathleen LeBesco (Berkeley: University of California Press, 2001), 135.

85. Elena Levy-Navarro, "Fattening Queer History: Where Does Fat History Go from Here?" in *The Fat Studies Reader*, ed. Esther Rothblum and Sondra Solovay (New York: New York University Press, 2009), 18.

86. Some writers are interested in a cure, some are not, and many are ambivalent, but all feel the need to address the issue in one form or another. See, among others, Eli Clare, *Exile and Pride: Disability, Queerness, and Liberation* (Boston: South End Press, 1999); Nancy Mairs, *Waist-High in the World: A Life among the Nondisabled* (Boston: Beacon Press, 1996); Susan Wendell, *The Rejected Body: Feminist Philosophical Reflections on Disability* (New York: Routledge, 1996); and Susan Wendell, "Unhealthy Disabled: Treating Chronic Illnesses as Disabilities," *Hypatia: A Journal of Feminist Philosophy* 16, no. 4 (2001): 17–33.

87. Wendell, *Rejected Body*, 83.

88. Clare, *Exile and Pride*, 106.

89. Catherine Scott, "Time Out of Joint: The Narcotic Effect of Prolepsis in Christopher Reeve's *Still Me*," *Biography* 29, no. 2 (2006): 309.

90. Halberstam, *In a Queer Time and Place*, 3.

91. Liat Ben-Moshe, Jean Stewart, and Marta Russell have argued for a disability rights movement that recognizes the overlaps between disability and the prison-industrial complex. Liat Ben-Moshe, "Disabling Incarceration: Connecting Disability to Divergent Confinements in the USA," *Critical Sociology* (2011): 1–19; and Jean Stewart and Marta Russell, "Disablement, Prison, and Historical Segregation," *Monthly Review* 53, no. 3 (2001): 61–75.

92. For a powerful reflection and analysis of one example of such effects, see Hiram Perez, "You Can Have My Brown Body and Eat It, Too!" *Social Text* 84–85, vol. 23, nos. 3–4 (2005): 171–91.

93. For the concept of the "lust of recognition," see Mia Mingus, Leah Lakshmi Piepzna-Samarasinha, and Ellery Russian, "Crip Sex, Crip Lust, and the Lust of Recognition," *Leaving Evidence*, May 25, 2010, http://leavingevidence.wordpress.com/2010/05/25/video-crip-sex-crip-lust-and-the-lust-of-recognition/.

94. Robert McRuer and Abby Wilkerson coedited an issue of *GLQ* around this question of "desiring disability." They explain, "[W]e both present this special issue and offer it as part of the project of producing spaces in which desiring disability is not simply tolerated or incorporated into already constituted (able-bodied) spaces (including that of queer theory as it has generally been shaped)." Robert McRuer and Abby L. Wilkerson, introduction to "Desiring Disability: Queer Theory Meets Disability Studies," special issue of *GLQ* 9, nos. 1–2 (2003): 13.

95. Sedgwick, *Tendencies*, 161, emphasis in original. Le'a Kent makes a similar point about fat bodies, particularly fat female bodies. What we need, she argues, is a manual showing that "it might be possible to *live* as a fat woman." Kent, "Fighting Abjection," 132, emphasis in original.

96. Sedgwick, *Tendencies*, 184.

97. Love, *Feeling Backward*, 26.

98. Judith Butler, *Undoing Gender* (New York: Routledge, 2004), 29.

99. Stacey Milbern (Cripchick) urges queer and disability communities to think through how conceptions of "coming out," "out," and "visibility" are marked by privilege. Too often, she laments, coming out requires leaving one's community. Ellen Samuels raises additional questions about the logic of visibility and its presumed relationship to pride. Cripchick, "Thoughts on National Coming Out Day," October 11, 2010, http://blog.cripchick.com/archives/8359; Ellen Samuels, "Bodies in Trouble," in *Restricted Access: Lesbians on Disability*, ed. Victoria A. Brownworth (Seattle: Seal Press, 1999), 192–200.

100. Chandra Talpede Mohanty and Biddy Martin offer insight into the trope of "home" in feminist theory, and in so doing they craft a lineage including both Minnie Bruce Pratt and Bernice Johnson Reagon. Chandra Talpede Mohanty and Biddy Martin, "What's Home Got to Do with It?" in *Feminism Without Borders: Decolonizing Theory, Practicing Solidarity* (Durham, NC: Duke University Press, 2003), 86–105; see also Minnie Bruce Pratt, *Rebellion: Essays, 1980–1991* (Ann Arbor, MI: Firebrand, 1991); and Bernice Johnson Reagon, "Coalition Politics: Turning the Century," in *Home Girls: A Black Feminist Anthology*, ed. Barbara Smith (New York: Kitchen Table Press, 1983), 356–68.

Chapter 2

1. D. F. Gunther and D. S. Diekema, "Attenuating Growth in Children with Profound Developmental Disability: A New Approach to an Old Dilemma," *Archives of Pediatrics and Adolescent Medicine* 160, no. 10 (2006): 1014.

2. Ibid., 1014.

3. Ibid.

4. Following Laura Hershey, I capitalize "treatment" to distinguish between the specific set of surgical and medical interventions used on Ashley (what her parents term "the Ashley Treatment") and the more abstract, general notion of "treatment" as any set of practices that attempt to solve a problem. As Hershey explains, referring to the interventions as a "treatment" accepts and perpetuates the notion that Ashley's body was sick or wrong and in need of a cure. Laura Hershey, "Stunting Ashley," *off our backs* 37, no. 1 (2007): 8.

5. Gunther and Diekema, "Attenuating Growth in Children," 1014.

6. Although bloggers, journalists, and disability rights activists have tended to examine the Treatment as a whole—addressing growth attenuation, breast bud removal, and hysterectomy all at once—some of the medical and bioethics texts have separated these procedures, focusing on either the growth attenuation or the sterilization. See, for example, John Lantos, "It's Not the Growth Attenuation, It's the Sterilization!" *American Journal of Bioethics* 10, no. 1 (2010): 45–46; and Benjamin S. Wilfond, Paul Steven Miller, Carolyn Korfatis, Douglas S. Diekema, Denise M. Dudzinski, Sara Goering, and the Seattle Growth Attenuation and Ethics Working Group, "Navigating Growth Attenuation in Children with Profound Disabilities: Children's Interests, Family Decision-Making, and Community Concerns," *Hastings Center Report* 40, no. 6 (2010): 27–40.

7. Lennard Davis describes disability as "a disruption in the visual, auditory, or perceptual field as it relates to the power of the gaze." As we will see, one of the lines of defense for the Treatment was that it would make it easier for people to see and interact with Ashley; the Treatment would alleviate the alleged visual asynchrony of Ashley's mind and body. Lennard J. Davis, *Enforcing Normalcy: Disability, Deafness, and the Body* (New York: Verso, 1995), 129.

8. Gunther was Ashley's endocrinologist; along with Dr. Douglas Diekema, he is one of the doctors most closely identified with the Ashley Treatment. Gunther committed suicide in September 2007, several months after an investigative report determined that the hospital had acted improperly in sterilizing Ashley. In the years since Gunther's death, Diekema has continued to write about the case, often with Dr. Norman Fost.

9. Gunther and Diekema, "Attenuating Growth in Children," 1013.

10. Ashley's Mom and Dad, *The "Ashley Treatment": Towards a Better Quality of Life for "Pillow Angels,"* March 25, 2007 http://pillowangel.org/Ashley%20Treatment%20v7.pdf; Wilfond et al., "Navigating Growth Attenuation in Children," 27.

11. The effect of the Treatment on Ashley's growth, however, is a matter of some debate. Gunther and Diekema explain that the Treatment had to be started quickly because Ashley had already begun to show signs of a growth spurt; what they do not mention is how much of her final height she had

already achieved by the time the estrogen regimen began. As Rebecca Clarren reports, there is a possibility that Ashley was already approaching her maximum size; perhaps the Treatment had only a small effect. Rebecca Clarren, "Behind the Pillow Angel," *Salon,* February 9, 2007, http://www.salon. com/news/feature/2007/02/09/pillow_angel/index.html.

12. As described in the investigative report, "The Washington Protection and Advocacy System (WPAS) is the federally mandated protection and advocacy (P&A) agency for the state of Washington. The P&As, which exist in every state and territory, are 'watchdog' agencies with legal authority under federal statutes to investigate allegations of abuse and neglect of persons with disabilities and to advocate for their legal and human rights." WPAS changed its name to Disability Rights Washington in 2007 and is part of the National Disability Rights Network. Washington Protection and Advocacy System, "Executive Summary—Investigative Report Regarding the 'Ashley Treatment,'" *Disability Rights Washington,* 1, last modified October 1, 2010, http://www.disabilityrightswa.org/home/Executive_Summary_InvestigativeReportRegardingtheAshleyTreatment.pdf/view?searchterm=ashley. See also http://www.disabilityrightswa.org/.

13. Washington Protection and Advocacy System, "Executive Summary," 1.

14. The committee did, however, sign off on the other two pieces of the Ashley Treatment, the mastectomy and the growth attenuation regimen: "[I]t was the consensus of the Committee members that the potential long term benefit to Ashley herself outweighed the risks; and that the procedures/ interventions would improve her quality of life, facilitate home care, and avoid institutionalization in the foreseeable future." As Clarren notes in her coverage of the case, there were deep divisions in the committee and at the hospital; many at Children's felt uncomfortable with the team's decisions. Washington Protection and Advocacy System, Exhibit L, "Special CHRMC Ethics Committee Meeting/Consultation," *Investigative Report Regarding the "Ashley Treatment,"* May 4, 2004, http://www. disabilityrightswa.org/home/Exhibits_K_T_InvestigativeReportRegardingtheAshleyTreatment. pdf, 1; Clarren, "Behind the Pillow Angel."

15. Washington Protection and Advocacy System, Exhibit O, "Letter from Larry Jones," *Investigative Report Regarding the "Ashley Treatment,"* June 10, 2004, http://www.disabilityrightswa.org/ home/Exhibits_K_T_InvestigativeReportRegardingtheAshleyTreatment.pdf, 1.

16. Washington Protection and Advocacy System, "Letter from Larry Jones," 4.

17. Ibid.

18. David Carlson and Deborah Dorfman, "Full Report—Investigative Report Regarding the 'Ashley Treatment,'" Washington Protection and Advocacy System, May 8, 2007, http://www.disabilityrightswa.org/home/Full_Report_InvestigativeReportRegardingtheAshleyTreatment.pdf, 14.

19. Carlson and Dorfman, "Full Report," 14.

20. Washington Protection and Advocacy System, Exhibit T, "Agreement Between Children's Hospital and Regional Medical Center and the Washington Protection and Advocacy System (Disability Rights Washington) Promoting Protection of Individuals with Developmental Disabilities," *Investigative Report Regarding the "Ashley Treatment,"* May 1, 2007, http://www.disabilityrightswa. org/home/Exhibits_K_T_InvestigativeReportRegardingtheAshleyTreatment.pdf, 1–2.

21. Jessica Marshall, "Hysterectomy on Disabled US Girl Was Illegal," *New Scientist,* May 9, 2007, http://www.newscientist.com/article/dn11809–hysterectomy-on-disabled-us-girl-was-illegal. html.

22. Wilfond et al., "Navigating Growth Attenuation in Children."

23. The report does not define "communicative" or "ambulatory"; according to *Dorland's Illustrated Medical Dictionary,* "ambulatory" refers to someone "able to walk" (*Dorland's* offers no definition for "communicative"). *Dorland's Illustrated Medical Dictionary* (Philadelphia: W. B. Saunders Company, 1994), 54; Wilfond et al., "Navigating Growth Attenuation in Children," 29, 39.

24. Although he supported the group's decision, Norman Fost asserts that "too much deference has been given to the claims of third parties" in medical decision making. He disagrees with the

working group's conclusions that the perspectives of disabled people and disability advocates should be included in the decision-making progress and that families contemplating such decisions should be given information about disability organizations and experiences. Eva Feder Kittay, on the other hand, insists that growth attenuation is never "ethically or medically appropriate," and that limiting the practice to "children with profound developmental and intellectual impairments" is itself abusive and discriminatory. "If growth attenuation should not be done on children without these impairments," she argues, "then it should not be done on any children. To do otherwise amounts to discrimination." Norman Fost, "Offense to Third Parties?" *Hastings Center Report* 40, no. 6 (2010): 30; Eva Feder Kittay, "Discrimination against Children with Cognitive Impairments?" *Hastings Center Report* 40, no. 6 (2010): 32.

25. Gunther and Diekema, "Attenuating Growth in Children," 1016.

26. Ibid., 1015.

27. Amy Burkholder, "Ethicist in Ashley Case Answers Questions," *CNN.com*, January 11, 2007.

28. Daniel Gunther and Douglas Diekema, letter in reply to Carole Marcus, "Only Half of the Story," *Archives of Pediatrics and Adolescent Medicine* 161 (June 2007): 616.

29. Douglas Diekema and Norman Fost, "Ashley Revisited: A Response to the Critics," *American Journal of Bioethics* 10, no. 1 (2010): 30–44.

30. The parents never refer to the procedure as a mastectomy, only as "breast bud removal," but the hospital billing report clearly lists it as "bilat simple mastectomy." Washington Protection and Advocacy System, Exhibit R, "Hospital Billing Report," *Investigative Report Regarding the "Ashley Treatment*," March 28, 2007, http://www.disabilityrightswa.org/home/Exhibits_K_T_InvestigativeReportRegardingtheAshleyTreatment.pdf, 3.

31. Ashley's Mom and Dad, *"Ashley Treatment."*

32. This interpretation makes the absence of any mention of the mastectomy in the doctors' original piece all the more disturbing.

33. Ashley's Mom and Dad, *"Ashley Treatment."*

34. The photographs on the blog are quite remarkable, but not because of their depiction of Ashley. Seen lying on her bed, or strapped into her wheelchair/stroller, she looks like an average disabled kid. What is jarring are the images of her parents and siblings, each depicted with black boxes covering their eyes and faces. For the viewer familiar with medical images of deviant bodies, it is a phenomenal switch; I am accustomed to seeing black boxes over the faces of disabled people, "freaks," and patients, but not over the faces of the normate. Yet the effect is, surprisingly, the same. The disabled person is still clearly marked as other, as fundamentally unlike the other humans in the frame. She is marked as to-be-seen, while the other bodies are protected from gaze.

35. Ashley's Mom and Dad, *"Ashley Treatment."*

36. Amy Burkholder, "Disabled Girl's Parents Defend Growth-Stunting Treatment," *CNN.com*, March 12, 2008.

37. Burkholder, "Ethicist in Ashley Case."

38. Ashley's Parents, "AT Summary," last modified March 17, 2012, http://pillowangel.org/AT-Summary.pdf.

39. John W. Jordan, "Reshaping the 'Pillow Angel': Plastic Bodies and the Rhetoric of Normal Surgical Solutions," *Quarterly Journal of Speech* 95, no. 1 (February 2009): 25.

40. Burkholder, "Ethicist in Ashley Case Answers Questions."

41. Mark Priestley, *Disability: A Life Course Approach* (Cambridge: Polity Press, 2003), 67.

42. Christopher Reeve, *Nothing Is Impossible: Reflections on a New Life* (New York: Random House, 2002), 6.

43. Licia Carlson, *The Faces of Intellectual Disability* (Bloomington: Indiana University Press, 2010), 30.

44. Gunther and Diekema, "Attenuating Growth in Children," 1016.

45. Mims, "The Pillow Angel Case—Three Bioethicists Weigh In," *Scientific American,* January 5, 2007, http://tinyurl.com/9fycg2u.

46. Ashley's Mom and Dad, *"Ashley Treatment."*

47. Gunther and Diekema, "Attenuating Growth in Children," 1016.

48. Christopher Mims, "The Pillow Angel Case."

49. Mikhail Bakhtin describes the grotesque as a temporal category, casting a senile, pregnant hag as the perfect illustration of the grotesque for her blending of youth and old age. But, as Mary Russo argues, "for the feminist reader, this image of the pregnant hag is more than ambivalent. It is loaded with all of the connotations of fear and loathing around the biological processes of reproduction and of aging." Mikhail Bakhtin, *Rabelais and His World*, trans. Helene Iswolsky (Bloomington: Indiana University Press, 1984), 24–27; Mary Russo, *The Female Grotesque: Risk, Excess, and Modernity* (New York: Routledge, 1994), 63. On "matter out of place," see Mary Douglas, *Purity and Danger: An Analysis of Concepts of Pollution and Taboo* (London: Routledge, 2002); on disability and the grotesque, see Rosemarie Garland-Thomson, *Extraordinary Bodies: Figuring Physical Disability in American Culture and Literature* (New York: Columbia University Press, 1997), 111–15; and Margrit Shildrick, *Embodying the Monster: Encounters with the Vulnerable Self* (London: Sage, 2002).

50. George Dvorsky, "Helping Families Care for the Helpless," Institute for Ethics and Emerging Technologies, November 6, 2006, http://ieet.org/index.php/IEET/more/809/.

51. Ashley's Parents, "AT Summary," emphasis mine. Ashley's parents draw the distinction between breasts and breast buds on their blog, describing reports of Ashley's breasts being removed as a media inaccuracy. They explain that "her almond-sized breast buds (not breasts) were removed." Ashley's Mom and Dad, "Updates on Ashley's Story," January 9, 2007, http://www.pillowangel.org/updates.htm.

52. Ashley's Parents, "AT Summary."

53. Ashley's Mom and Dad, *"Ashley Treatment,"* 9–10.

54. Ashley's Parents, "AT Summary."

55. Gunther and Diekema, "Attenuating Growth in Children," 1015.

56. As Patricia Williams notes, it is hard to imagine parents or doctors choosing to castrate a young boy because of fears that his penis or testicles might cause pain and discomfort. Patricia J. Williams, "Judge Not?" *Nation* (New York), March 26, 2007, 9.

57. If we view the hysterectomy as a key component of the Treatment, however, then their "new approach" isn't really all that new. Indeed, this phrasing is one of several moments in which justifications of the Treatment echo early eugenic arguments. Many eugenicists presented sterilization as a "humane" alternative to institutionalization; through sterilization, communities could be "protected" from the reproduction of the "feeble-minded," and the "feeble-minded" could be "allowed" to return to their home communities.

58. Gunther and Diekema, "Attenuating Growth in Children," 1013. This goal of deinstitutionalization has obviously not been met, and the rampant budget cutting underway on both the state and federal level makes progress seem unlikely. The more recent *Healthy People 2020* plan stakes out a similar goal but, like the earlier report, does not include a detailed plan for its achievement. See *Healthy People 2020*, accessed July 8, 2011, http://www.healthypeople.gov/2020/topicsobjectives2020/overview.aspx?topicid=9.

59. Gunther and Diekema, "Attenuating Growth in Children," 1014.

60. Indeed, they criticize media reports for depicting their blog as a defense of the Treatment; on the contrary, they assert, the blog was always intended as a way to share the Treatment with other families. Ashley's Mom and Dad, "Updates on Ashley's Story," January 9, 2007.

61. Ashley's Mom and Dad, *"Ashley Treatment."*

62. Ashley's Mom and Dad, "Third Anniversary Update," January 13, 2010, http://www.pillowangel.org/updates.htm. For the story of one family who, with assistance from Ashley's parents,

successfully acquired the Treatment for their daughter, see Karen McVeigh, "The 'Ashley Treatment': Erica's Story," *Guardian* (UK), March 16, 2012, http://www.guardian.co.uk/society/2012/mar/16/ashley-treatment-ericas-story.

63. Ibid.

64. Indeed, according to a recent article in the *Guardian*, the Treatment is "on the rise." Ed Pilkington and Karen McVeigh, "'Ashley Treatment' On the Rise amid Concerns from Disability Rights Groups," *Guardian* (UK), March 15, 2012, http://www.guardian.co.uk/society/2012/mar/15/ashley-treatment-rise-amid-concerns.

65. Cited in Wilfond et al., "Navigating Growth Attenuation in Children," 27.

66. David Allen, Michael Kappy, Douglas Diekema, and Norman Fost, "Growth-Attenuation Therapy: Principles for Practice," *Pediatrics* 123, no. 6 (2009): 1556–61; Gunther and Diekema, "Attenuating Growth in Children"; and Wilfond et al., "Navigating Growth Attenuation in Children."

67. "Testimonies from Families and Caregivers with Direct Experience,"*"Ashley Treatment,"* accessed March 2, 2012, http://www.pillowangel.org/testimonies.htm.

68. Ashley's Mom and Dad, "Updates on Ashley's Story," May 8, 2007, http://www.pillowangel.org/updates.htm.

69. Haraway distinguishes this traditional understanding of objectivity from the embodied feminist objectivity of partial perspectives and situated knowledges. Donna J. Haraway, *Simians, Cyborgs, and Women: The Reinvention of Nature* (New York: Routledge, 1991), 189.

70. Carol M. Ostrom, "Child's Hysterectomy Illegal, Hospital Agrees," *Seattle Times,* May 9, 2007, http://community.seattletimes.nwsource.com/archive/?date=20070509&slug=childrens09m.

71. Ashley's Mom and Dad, *"Ashley Treatment."*

72. Sarah E. Shannon and Teresa A. Savage, "The Ashley Treatment: Two Viewpoints," *Pediatric Nursing* 32, no. 2 (2007): 177.

73. Adrienne Asch and Anna Stubblefield, "Growth Attenuation: Good Intentions, Bad Decision," *American Journal of Bioethics* 10, no. 1 (2010): 46–48.

74. Harriet McBryde Johnson, "The Disability Gulag," *New York Times Magazine,* November 23, 2003, http://www.nytimes.com/2003/11/23/magazine/the-disability-gulag.html.

75. Laura Hershey, *Just Help,* 207–35. See also Eileen Boris and Rhacel Salazar Parreñas, eds., *Intimate Labors: Cultures, Technologies, and the Politics of Care* (Stanford, CA: Stanford University Press, 2010); and Evelyn Nakano Glenn, *Forced to Care: Coercion and Caregiving in America* (Cambridge, MA: Harvard University Press, 2010).

76. Reed Cooley, "Disabling Spectacles: Representations of Trig Palin and Cognitive Disability," *Journal of Literary and Cultural Disability Studies* 5, no. 3 (2011): 309.

77. For an insightful discussion of "the problem of projection" in determinations of another's quality of life, and especially of the prominence of "suffering" in such determinations, see Carlson, *Faces of Intellectual Disability.*

78. Moreover, as Susan Wendell explains, "function" is also determined by one's cultural and historical context. Susan Wendell, *The Rejected Body: Feminist Philosophical Reflections on Disability* (New York: Routledge, 1996).

79. Adrienne Asch and Anna Stubblefield, "Growth Attenuation: Good Intentions, Bad Decision," *American Journal of Bioethics* 10, no. 1 (2010): 47.

80. Sara Goering, "Revisiting the Relevance of the Social Model of Disability," *American Journal of Bioethics* 10, no. 1 (2010): 55. For one account of such shifts, see Eva Kittay and Jeffrey Kittay, "Whose Convenience? Whose Truth?" *Hastings Center Bioethics Forum,* February 28, 2007, http://www.thehastingscenter.org/Bioethicsforum/Post.aspx?id=350&blogid=140.

81. Anne McDonald describes herself as a former pillow angel; she spent most of her childhood in an institution where she was assumed to be fully, and permanently, noncommunicative. Anne McDonald, "The Other Story from a 'Pillow Angel,'" *Seattle Post-Intelligencer,* June 16, 2007,

http://www.seattlepi.com/opinion/319702_noangel17.html. See also Jeremy L. Brunson and Mitchell E. Loeb, eds., "Mediated Communication," special issue of *DSQ: Disability Studies Quarterly* 31, no. 4 (2011); and Nirmala Erevelles, "Signs of Reason: Rivière, Facilitated Communication, and the Crisis of the Subject," in *Foucault and the Government of Disability*, ed. Shelley Tremain (Ann Arbor: University of Michigan Press, 2005): 45–64.

82. Kittay, "Discrimination against Children with Cognitive Impairments?" 32.

83. Asch and Stubblefield make a similar point, stressing that neither the supporters nor the critics of the Treatment can know for certain how the interventions have affected Ashley or what her experiences of them were. They explain, "Ashley's parents and doctors decided to proceed with her growth attenuation with good intentions in circumstances of uncertainty about how Ashley experiences herself and the world. Our objection to performing growth attenuation procedures on children like Ashley is also based on good intentions in identical circumstances of uncertainty. So the acceptability of this intervention cannot be decided based on which side has better intentions or on which side has more certain knowledge of what life is like for Ashley." Asch and Stubblefield, "Growth Attenuation," 46–47.

84. Ashley's Parents, "AT Summary."

85. For more on violence against people with disabilities, see, for example, Mark Sherry, *Disability Hate Crimes: Does Anyone Really Hate Disabled People?* (Burlington, VT: Ashgate, 2010); and Dick Sobsey, D. Wells, R. Lucardie, and S. Mansell, eds., *Violence and Disability: An Annotated Bibliography* (Baltimore, MD: Paul H. Brookes Publishing Company, 1995).

86. I refer here only to the kind of sensations I mentioned above: the binding and release of her seat belts; the feel of her clothes rubbing across her skin; warm bathwater. To be clear, I am not in any way condoning or encouraging sexual acts with someone unable to consent. Urging for a recognition that Ashley might feel pleasure in her body, through her skin, is significantly different from encouraging others to take pleasure (or power, or control) in her body.

87. Ashley is not the only child to have had her body medically and surgically altered through interventions that were cast as necessary to her quality of life. Children born intersexed or with "ambiguous" genitalia have faced all kinds of surgical interventions intended to normalize them without regard to their pain, sense of self, or relation to their bodies. Other children have endured limb-lengthening or limb-straightening procedures or have been made to wear braces and splints that often led to chronic pain and no real increase in function.

88. Williams, "Judge Not?" 9.

89. Anita J. Tarzian notes that a similar phenomenon and critique happened with the Terri Schiavo case: disability rights activists, organizations, and scholars treated the case as a disability issue (even as they disagreed about the proper course of action), while critics disputed the relevance of the case to disability rights. Anita J. Tarzian, "Disability and Slippery Slopes," *Hastings Center Report* 37, no. 5 (2007): c3.

90. Ashley's Parents, "AT Summary."

91. Tarzian, "Disability and Slippery Slopes," c3.

Chapter 3

1. A wide range of feminist studies and disability studies scholars have addressed the issue of prenatal testing and selective abortion, analyzing the impact these practices have on women and disabled people and deconstructing the assumptions about gender, pregnancy, and disability that underlie them. For examples of this work, see, among others, Adrienne Asch, "A Disability Equality Critique of Routine Testing and Embryo or Fetus Elimination Based on Disabling Traits," *Political Environments* 11 (2007): 43–47, 78; Dena S. Davis, *Genetic Dilemmas: Reproductive Technology, Parental Choices, and Children's Futures* (New York: Routledge, 2001); Anne Finger, *Past Due: A*

Story of Disability, Pregnancy, and Birth (Seattle: Seal Press, 1990); Erik Parens and Adrienne Asch, eds., *Prenatal Testing and Disability Rights* (Washington, DC: Georgetown University Press, 2000); Rayna Rapp, *Testing Women, Testing the Fetus: The Social Impact of Amniocentesis in America* (New York: Routledge, 1999); Janelle Taylor, *The Public Life of the Fetal Sonogram: Technology, Consumption, and the Politics of Reproduction* (New Brunswick, NJ: Rutgers University Press, 2008); Karen H. Rothenberg and Elizabeth J. Thomson, eds., *Women and Prenatal Testing: Facing the Challenges of Genetic Technology* (Columbus: Ohio State University Press, 1994); Marsha Saxton, "Disability Rights and Selective Abortion," in *Abortion Wars: A Half-Century of Struggle: 1950–2000*, ed. Rickie Solinger (Berkeley: University of California Press, 1998), 374–93; and Tom Shakespeare, "Arguing about Genetics and Disability," *Interaction* 13, no. 3 (2000): 11–14. See also Generations Ahead, *Bridging the Divide: Disability Rights and Reproductive Rights and Justice Advocates Discussing Genetic Technologies*, July 2009; and Generations Ahead, *A Disability Rights Analysis of Genetic Technologies: Report on a Convening of Disability Rights Leaders*, March 2010, http://www.generations-ahead.org/resources.

2. Timothy J. Dailey, "Homosexual Parenting: Placing Children at Risk," *Insight* no. 238, accessed November 8, 2006, www.frc.org. See also Caryle Murphy, "Gay Parents Find More Acceptance," *Washington Post*, June 14, 1999, A1.

3. Susan Merrill Squier makes a case for literature, specifically science fiction, in analyses of biomedicine and reproductive technology. Fascinated by representations of reproductive technology in feminist fiction, she urges cultural critics to attend to the "ideological construction . . . being carried out through the production and dissemination" of these texts. Susan Merrill Squier, *Babies in Bottles: Visions of Reproductive Technology* (New Brunswick, NJ: Rutgers University Press, 1994), 19; Susan Merrill Squier, *Liminal Lives: Imagining the Human at the Frontiers of Biomedicine* (Durham, NC: Duke University Press, 2004).

4. Piercy's utopian village shares its name with a small town in southeastern Massachusetts that was incorporated in 1857. According to the town website, the town's "name is said to come from an old Indian word meaning 'a place of resting.'" "Mattapoisett," accessed November 7, 2011, http://www.mattapoisett.net/Pages/index. Piercy does not specify the year of the dystopic New York, suggesting only that it is another possible future, an alternative to the one found in Mattapoisett.

5. Marge Piercy, *Woman on the Edge of Time* (New York: Fawcett Crest, 1976), 96.

6. WMST-L, a women's studies teaching and research listserve, has featured several discussions over the years about teaching the book to undergraduate women's studies students. Searching Google for "syllabus" and "Woman on the Edge of Time" produces multiple links to individual courses and women's and gender studies departments/programs that include the novel in their curricula. For a (dated) collection of such courses, see "Women's Studies Syllabi," University of Maryland, last modified July 24, 2002, http://www.mith2.umd.edu/WomensStudies/Syllabi.

7. José van Dijck, *Imagenation: Popular Images of Genetics* (New York: New York University Press, 1998), 86, 87; Josephine Carubia Glorie, "Feminist Utopian Fiction and the Possibility of Social Critique," in *Political Science Fiction*, ed. Donald M. Hassler and Clyde Wilcox (Columbia: University of South Carolina Press, 1997), 156; Cathleen McGuire and Colleen McGuire, "Grassroots Ecofeminism: Activating Utopia," in *Ecofeminist Literary Criticism: Theory, Interpretation, Pedagogy*, ed. Greta Gaard and Patrick D. Murphy (Urbana: University of Illinois Press, 1998). See also, for example, Patricia Huckle, "Women in Utopias," in *The Utopian Vision: Seven Essays on the Quincentennial of Sir Thomas More*, ed. E. D. S. Sullivan (San Diego: San Diego State University Press, 1983), 115–36; and Kathy Davis, "'My Body is My Art': Cosmetic Surgery as Feminist Utopia?" in *Embodied Practices: Feminist Perspectives on the Body*, ed. Kathy Davis (Thousand Oaks, CA: Sage, 1997), 168–81. Even feminist theorists who take a more critical stance toward Piercy's vision of utopia, finding fault with its use of violence or its reliance on small communities, praise Mattapoisett's system of participatory democracy, particularly its embodiment in the Shaper/Mixer

debates. See, for example, Erin McKenna, *The Task of Utopia* (Lanham, MD: Rowman and Little-field, 2001).

8. For discussion of these issues, see, among others, Lori B. Andrews, *Future Perfect: Confronting Decisions about Genetics* (New York: Columbia University Press, 2001); Glenn McGee, *The Perfect Baby: Parenthood in the New World of Cloning and Genetics* (Lanham, MD: Rowman and Little-field, 2000); and Dena S. Davis, *Genetic Dilemmas: Reproductive Technology, Parental Choices, and Children's Futures* (New York: Routledge, 2001). Some entrepreneurs have hoped to profit from this desire to breed "the perfect baby," establishing sperm banks that accept sperm only from "successful" men. Perhaps the most notorious of these projects was Robert K. Graham's Repository for Germinal Choice, formed with the intent of collecting sperm from Nobel Prize winners and other high achievers in order to increase the number of intelligent and creative people in the population. Because of Graham's racist and explicitly eugenicist views, the company was widely reviled in the media and had difficulty attracting donors of the desired caliber. It eventually closed in 1999, after almost twenty years in existence (and after creating over two hundred children). Although the Repository for Germinal Choice is the most well-known "genius sperm bank," other companies share its mission to collect sperm from successful, healthy, and intelligent men. Heredity Choice, based in Nevada and run by former Graham employee Paul Smith, is one such example. David Plotz, "The 'Genius Babies' and How They Grew," *Slate*, February 8, 2001, http://www.slate.com.

9. The use of "Deaf," with a capital "D," emerged in the late twentieth century as a way to signal pride in one's identity and in the cultural practices and historical traditions of deaf people. Deaf with a capital letter is thus a way to draw attention to a cultural deaf identity, whereas Deaf with a small "d" simply connotes being unable to hear or hard-of-hearing. This use is not universally accepted, however, with some deaf people and deaf studies scholars moving away from the "big D/little d" convention. For a recent reflection on this question, and on larger questions of deaf identity, see Brenda Jo Brueggemann, *Deaf Subjects: Between Identities and Places* (New York: New York University Press, 2009); for discussion about the limitations of American discourses of deaf identity, see Susan Burch and Alison Kafer, eds., *Deaf and Disability Studies: Interdisciplinary Perspectives* (Washington, DC: Gallaudet University Press, 2010).

10. Carol Padden and Tom Humphries, *Deaf in America: Voices from a Culture* (Cambridge, MA: Harvard University Press, 1988); John Vickrey Van Cleve and Barry Crouch, *A Place of Their Own: Creating the Deaf Community in America* (Washington, DC: Gallaudet University Press, 1989).

11. Harlan Lane, "Constructions of Deafness," in *The Disability Studies Reader*, ed. Lennard J. Davis (New York: Routledge, 1997), 161. Lane acknowledges that there are differences between Deaf people and other linguistic minorities. He notes, "Deaf people cannot learn English as a second language as easily as other minorities. Second and third generation Deaf children find learning English no easier than their forbears, but second and third generation immigrants to the United States frequently learn English before entering school. . . . Normally, Deaf people are not proficient in this native language [sign language] until they reach school age. Deaf people are more scattered geographically than many linguistic minorities. The availability of interpreters is even more vital for Deaf people than for many other linguistic minorities because there are so few Deaf lawyers, doctors, and accountants, etc." Lane, "Constructions of Deafness," 163–64.

12. Nora Ellen Groce, *Everyone Here Spoke Sign Language: Hereditary Deafness on Martha's Vineyard* (Cambridge, MA: Harvard University Press, 1985). For a more recent discussion of deafness on Martha's Vineyard, see Annelies Kusters, "Deaf Utopias? Reviewing the Sociocultural Literature on the World's 'Martha's Vineyard Situations,'" *Journal of Deaf Studies and Deaf Education* 15, no. 1 (2010): 3–16.

13. Unfortunately, there is an extensive history of requiring Deaf people to do precisely that: to learn to lip-read, speak orally, and abandon signing, and to undergo painful surgeries and medical treatments in order to "correct" their hearing loss. Scholars of Deaf studies have documented

histories of Deaf people being punished, often brutally, for engaging in sign language, and of the campaigns waged against residential schools and Deaf communities. In spite of such treatment, the Deaf community continued to use and fight for sign language. Robert M. Buchanan, *Illusions of Equality: Deaf Americans in School and Factory, 1850–1950* (Washington, DC: Gallaudet University Press, 1999); Susan Burch, *Signs of Resistance: American Deaf Cultural History, 1900 to World War II* (New York: New York University Press, 2002).

14. For one example of these kinds of coalitions, see Corbett Joan O'Toole, "Dale Dahl and Judy Heumann: Deaf Man, Disabled Woman—Allies in 1970s Berkeley," in *Deaf and Disability Studies: Interdisciplinary Perspectives*, ed. Susan Burch and Alison Kafer (Washington, DC: Gallaudet University Press, 2010): 162–87. For a recent discussion on whether deaf equals disability, see H-Dirksen Bauman, ed., *Open Your Eyes: Deaf Studies Talking* (Minneapolis: University of Minnesota Press, 2008). For some Deaf studies scholars, deaf/disability coalition requires not seeing deaf as disability; Lane stresses that recognizing the "great common cause" between culturally Deaf people and people with disabilities means respecting the "self-construction of culturally Deaf people" as not disabled. Lane, "Constructions of Deafness," 165.

15. Deafness is not the only trait screened out of the gene pool. Sperm banks exclude male donors who have family histories of cystic fibrosis, Tay-Sachs, alcoholism, and other conditions deemed problematic or undesirable. Under guidelines established by the FDA, most sperm banks forbid gay men and men who have had sex with men in the last five years from donating. For discussion of the politics of sperm banks and sperm donation, see Cynthia Daniels, *Exposing Men: The Science and Politics of Male Reproduction* (New York: Oxford University Press, 2006); and Laura Mamo, *Queering Reproduction: Achieving Pregnancy in the Age of Technoscience* (Durham, NC: Duke University Press, 2007).

16. Indeed, Gauvin's deafness was not a given. There are many different genetic combinations that result in deafness, but the trait is recessive; two congenitally deaf parents will not automatically or necessarily produce deaf children.

17. Liza Mundy, "A World of their Own," *Washington Post Magazine*, March 31, 2002, www.washingtonpost.com. Sadly, Gauvin died suddenly and unexpectedly from an inherited condition (unrelated to his deafness). In sharp contrast to his birth, his passing was met with very little news coverage or public reaction.

18. Mundy, "A World of Their Own."

19. MJ Bienvenu makes a similar point, although she more optimistically attributes the lack of focus on their lesbianism to the "strides made by the L/G community." "Queer as Deaf: Intersections," in *Open Your Eyes: Deaf Studies Talking*, ed. H-Dirksen Bauman (Minneapolis: University of Minnesota Press, 2008), 270.

20. Family Research Council, "*Washington Post* Profiles Lesbian Couple Seeking to Manufacture a Deaf Child," PR Newswire Association, April 1, 2002. There are strong parallels here between Connor's warning and the eugenic tracts in wide circulation in the late nineteenth and early twentieth centuries. Alexander Graham Bell, for example, worried about the development of deaf culture and any related rise in deaf populations. See his "Memoir Upon the Formation of a Deaf Variety of the Human Race" for one iteration of these fears. I thank Susan Burch for pointing me in the direction of this text.

21. In tying together the women's sexuality with their deafness, and presenting both as if they could, and should, be eliminated, Connor seems to be yearning for (his understanding of) a better world; his preference for households that do not bear the burden of disability or queerness supports Robert McRuer's contention that the "dream of an able-bodied future is . . . thoroughly intertwined with the heterosexist fantasy of a world without queers." Robert McRuer, "Critical Investments: AIDS, Christopher Reeve, and Queer/Disability Studies," in *Thinking the Limits of the Body*, ed. Jeffrey Jerome Cohen and Gail Weiss (Albany: State University of New York Press, 2003), 154–55.

22. Jeanette Winterson, "How Would We Feel If Blind Women Claimed the Right to a Blind Baby?" *Guardian* (UK), April 9, 2002.

23. For feminist and queer deconstructions of nature rhetoric, particularly uses of "nature" to proscribe gender and sexuality identities and practices, see, for example, Catriona Mortimer-Sandilands and Bruce Erickson, eds. *Queer Ecologies: Sex, Nature, Politics, Desire* (Bloomington: Indiana University Press, 2010); and Noël Sturgeon, *Environmentalism in Popular Culture: Gender, Race, Sexuality, and the Politics of the Natural* (Tucson: University of Arizona Press, 2009).

24. Winterson is not alone in this exaggeration. Although Mundy's original article made it clear that the use of a Deaf sperm donor only increased the women's chances of having a Deaf baby to 50 percent, wire reports and stories in other papers consistently described the women as manipulating nature and technology to "guarantee" a Deaf baby, a misrepresentation of the facts that depicts the women as meddling with the future. Even essays in medical journals followed this pattern, referring to the use of the donor as "guaranteeing" and "ensuring" a Deaf child. (I do not mean to suggest that criticisms of the couple would have been justified if the use of a Deaf donor had increased the odds to more than 50 percent, and I doubt that critics would have left the women alone if the odds had been less than 50 percent.) Critics condemned these women for failing to do everything in their power to prevent disability, a failure that, in the ableist worldview, sentenced their children to a negative, imperfect future. See, for example, a set of essays in the *Journal of Medical Ethics*, both of which determined the women to have acted inappropriately: K. W. Anstey, "Are Attempts to Have Impaired Children Justifiable?" *Journal of Medical Ethics* 28 (2002): 286–89; and N. Levy, "Deafness, Culture, and Choice," *Journal of Medical Ethics* 28 (2002): 284–85.

25. Winterson refers to McCullough and Duchesneau's decision as "a bad joke," a sign of "psychosis," "paranoid," and a form of "genetic imperialism."

26. For an essay on a blind woman reflecting on her desire for a blind child, see Deborah Kent, "Somewhere a Mockingbird," in *Prenatal Testing and Disability Rights*, ed. Erik Parens and Adrienne Asch (Washington, DC: Georgetown University Press, 2000). Kent movingly describes her internal struggles in realizing that her parents and her husband, all sighted, do not share her understanding of blindness as a "neutral trait" and are concerned about the possible blindness of her future children.

27. Mundy, "A World of Their Own."

28. These comments were not left unaddressed by other members on the listserv, however. Participants questioned the assumptions about the "burdens" caused by disability and about the inappropriateness of Deaf women choosing a donor that reflected their own lives, a choice nondisabled couples make regularly. They also challenged the contention that Deaf children pose a financial strain on the state, arguing that economic arguments about the "strain" caused by people with disabilities have often been used to justify coerced and forced sterilization, institutionalization, and coerced abortion.

29. Sarah Franklin, "Essentialism, Which Essentialism? Some Implications of Reproductive and Genetic Technoscience," in *If You Seduce a Straight Person, Can You Make Them Gay? Issues in Biological Essentialism versus Social Constructionism in Gay and Lesbian Identities*, ed. John P. DeCecco and John P. Elia (Binghamton, NY: Harrington Park, 1993); 30; italics in original.

30. Patrick Steptoe, known as the "father of in vitro fertilization," remarked that "it would be unthinkable to willingly create a child to be born into an unnatural situation such as a gay or lesbian relationship." Quoted in Franklin, "Essentialism, Which Essentialism?" 31.

31. Mamo, *Queering Reproduction*, 72.

32. Ibid., 134.

33. Dorothy Roberts, *Killing the Black Body: Race, Reproduction, and the Meaning of Liberty* (New York: Vintage, 1998); Elizabeth Weil, "Breeder Reaction," *Mother Jones* 31, no. 4 (2006): 33–37.

34. Franklin, "Essentialism, Which Essentialism?" 29.

35. Roberts, *Killing the Black Body,* 254. In her more recent work, Roberts notes that fertility clinics are increasingly including *elite* women of color in their campaigns; even as these technologies become available to a wider range of women, their availability mirrors the unequal distribution of health care in this country. See, for example, Dorothy Roberts, "Race, Gender, and Genetic Technologies: A New Reproductive Dystopia?" *Signs: Journal of Women in Culture and Society* 34, no. 4 (2009): 783–804.

36. This trend is only the latest in a long history of marginalization, discrimination, and abuse; disabled, African American, Latina, and Native American women have undergone forced and coerced sterilization, medical experimentation, and coerced abortion at the hands of medical professionals and government employees who deemed them unfit. See, for example, Elena R. Gutiérrez, *Fertile Matters: The Politics of Mexican-Origin Women's Reproduction* (Austin: University of Texas Press, 2008); Jennifer Nelson, *Women of Color and the Reproductive Rights Movement* (New York: New York University Press, 2003); Nancy Ordover, *American Eugenics: Race, Queer Anatomy, and the Science of Nationalism* (Minneapolis: University of Minnesota Press, 2003); and Roberts, *Killing the Black Body.*

37. Jo Litwinowicz, "In my Mind's Eye: I," in *Bigger than the Sky: Disabled Women on Parenting,* ed. Michele Wates and Rowen Jade (London: Women's Press, 1999).

38. Jim Hughes, "Blind Woman Sues Fertility Clinic: Englewood Facility Halted Treatments after Questions about Her Fitness as a Parent," *Denver Post,* November 7, 2003.

39. In her influential study of amniocentesis in the United States, Rayna Rapp notes that "selfishness" is a key lens through which white middle-class couples, and especially white women, understand their reproductive decisions. Rapp, *Testing Women,* 136–42.

40. Laura Hershey, "Disabled Woman's Lawsuit Exposes Prejudices," *The Ragged Edge,* accessed December 2003, http://www.raggededgemagazine.com/extra/hersheychamberstrial.html.

41. The Colorado Cross-Disability Coalition filed suit in Chambers's behalf. Hershey, "Disabled Woman's Lawsuit."

42. Quoted in David Teather, "Lesbian Couple Have Deaf Baby by Choice," *Guardian* (UK), April 8, 2002, http://www.guardian.co.uk/world/2002/apr/08/davidteather.

43. Glenn Stanton from Focus on the Family scolds, "[A] wise and compassionate society always comes to the aid of children in motherless or fatherless families, but a wise and compassionate society never intentionally subjects children to such families. But every single same-sex home would do exactly that, for no other reason than that a small handful of adults desire such kinds of families." Same-sex households are to be discouraged, in other words, because they "subject" children to situations in which they will need "aid" and rescue. Quoted in McCreery, "Save Our Children/Let Us Marry," 196.

44. Michael Warner, *The Trouble with Normal: Sex, Politics, and the Ethics of Queer Life* (New York: Free Press, 1999), 183. Ellen Samuels examines the limits of substitution, rightly noting that there is often an imprecision in meaning and an effacement of specificity when "disability" is used in place of "sexuality" (or "porn," in my example). In this case, however, my substitution points to important parallels between disability and queerness: both queerness and disability have been cast as entities to be avoided and as drains on a child's quality of life; moreover, as I have argued here, their *combination* has proved especially threatening. Ellen Samuels, "Critical Divides: Judith Butler's Body Theory and the Question of Disability," *NWSA Journal* 14, no. 3 (2002): 58–76.

45. Susan Wendell, "Unhealthy Disabled: Treating Chronic Illnesses as Disabilities," *Hypatia: A Journal of Feminist Philosophy* 16, no. 4 (2001); 31, emphasis in original.

46. Wendell, *Rejected Body,* 69.

47. H-Dirksen L. Bauman, "Designing Deaf Babies and the Question of Disability," *Journal of Deaf Studies and Deaf Education* 10, no. 3 (2005): 313.

48. Lennard J. Davis, "Postdeafness," in *Open Your Eyes: Deaf Studies Talking,* ed. H-Dirksen Bauman (Minneapolis: University of Minnesota Press, 2008), 319.

49. For an analysis of sex selection and "family balancing," see Rajani Bhatia, "Constructing Gender from the Inside Out: Sex Selection Practices in the United States," *Feminist Studies* 36, no. 2 (2010): 260–91.

Chapter 4

1. The Foundation for a Better Life, February 7, 2010, http://www.values.com/.

2. All of the billboards can be viewed on the foundation's website, which also features "inspirational stories," "good news stories," and short vignettes about specific values. See the Foundation for a Better Life, February 7, 2010, http://www.values.com.

3. The image of the Tiananmen Square protestor has been removed from the organization's website, but I am unsure as to when it disappeared. It was still on the site in 2007, but by 2010 it was gone, and there is no mention of it on the organization's website.

4. Of course, as any disability studies scholar (or social services gatekeeper) will note, determining who is and who is not disabled is easier said than done. For the purposes of this discussion, I have focused only on those figures who are widely recognized as disabled, who have publicly identified as disabled, and/or whose illnesses and disabilities are highlighted in the campaign itself.

5. The italicized words are the values highlighted in each billboard; on the billboard, the value is in white bold capitals, inside a red text box. The phrases in quotation marks are the captions on the billboards.

6. The Foundation for a Better Life, "About FBL," June 30, 2004, http://www.forbetterlife.org/main.asp?section=about&language=eng.

7. Amy Vidali offers a useful analysis of the relationship between vision and knowledge, critically examining the assumption that "knowing is seeing." Amy Vidali, "Seeing What We Know: Disability and Theories of Metaphor," *Journal of Literary and Cultural Disability Studies* 4, no. 1 (2010): 33–54. See also Georgina Kleege, *Sight Unseen* (New Haven: Yale University Press, 1999). Both the FBL billboards ("VISION") and the stylistic conventions of footnotes (e.g., "see Kleege") rely on this history of representation and this epistemology.

8. It is useful here to read the FBL's representation of Muhammad Ali in light of Anna Mollow's discussion of overcoming. Mollow rightly notes that a story of overcoming illness or disability does not have to be "a denial of political realities" but can instead be "an assertion of personal strength amid overwhelming social oppression." In the case of the FBL, however, their overcoming narratives do not highlight "individuals' power in relation to oppressive political and economic structures"— Mollow's criteria for understanding overcoming narratives differently—but rather deny that such oppression exists at all. Anna Mollow, "'When *Black* Women Start Going on Prozac': Race, Gender, and Mental Illness in Meri Nana-Ama Danquah's *Willow Weep for Me*," *MELUS* 31, no. 3 (2006): 89, 68.

9. Foundation for a Better Life, "Our Mission Statement," accessed February 7, 2010, http://www.values.com/about-us/mission-statement.

10. The FBL's Internet domain name is registered to the Anschutz Exploration Corporation, an oil and gas exploration company owned by Anschutz. See Nathan Callahan, "Corporate Vulture: Philip Anschutz Tries to Thread His Way into Heaven," *OC Weekly* 8, no. 35 (2003), accessed September 18, 2004, http://www.ocweekly.com/ink/03/35/news-callahan.php; Stuart Elliott, "A Campaign Promotes Noble Behavior," *New York Times*, November 9, 2001; Colleen Kenney, "Lincoln Receives Several Messages of Hope from Up Above" *Lincoln Journal Star*, February 5, 2004; Jeremy David Stolen, "Foundation for a Better Life," Portland Independent Media Center, accessed July 4, 2004, http://portlandindymedia.org/2002/02/7617.shtml; and Jeremy David Stolen, "Big Money behind 'Inspirational' Billboard Campaign," accessed April 15, 2006, http://www.theportlandalliance.org/2002/april/billboard.html. See also Sandra Thompson, "Billboards Marketing Virtues We Can Use Now,"

St. Petersburg Times, February 2, 2002, http://saintpetersburgtimes.com/2002/02/02/Columns/Billboards_marketing_.shtml.

11. These kinds of responses likely feel familiar to many of us with visible disabilities. I have more than once been stopped by a stranger who wanted to tell me that seeing me made their day. As one woman put it, "I was feeling so sorry for myself today, but then I saw you and realized how lucky I am."

12. David M. Halperin, *Saint Foucault: Toward a Gay Hagiography* (New York: Oxford University Press, 1995), 67.

13. There has been some attention to the campaign in the blogosphere, and I address those responses below. Thus far scholars have largely ignored the billboards, and most news coverage has been positive.

14. Graham Bowley, "Goal! He Spends It on Beckham," *New York Times,* April 22, 2007, http://www.nytimes.com/2007/04/22/business/yourmoney/22phil.html?pagewanted=1&_r=1&ref=media&adxnnlx=1313886061–H/sYx4pZH4V3t39yunqx3A.

15. The billboards are not dated on the FBL website, making it difficult to determine when each billboard debuted nationwide. The Shirley billboard was not one of the original images.

16. The Iraq and Afghanistan Veterans of America organization (IAVA) includes official casualty statistics from the Department of Defense on its website, but it also encourages visitors to research the statistics provided by private organizations and individual researchers. Available at http://iava.org, accessed August 10, 2011. For additional statistics, see, for example, the website http://icasualties.org, accessed August 10, 2011.

17. For example, *Newsweek*'s editors chose an image of an amputee to illustrate their cover story, "Failing Our Wounded," March 5, 2007, on newly disabled veterans and their troubles with Veterans Affairs.

18. Lee Edelman, *No Future: Queer Theory and the Death Drive* (Durham, NC: Duke University Press, 2004), 2. In focusing on the figure of the child in American politics, Edelman draws on the work of Lauren Berlant's *The Queen of America Goes to Washington City: Essays on Sex and Citizenship* (Durham, NC: Duke University Press, 1997). Berlant traces the ways in which the ideal American citizen is imagined through the figure of the child.

19. Katie, August 29, 2005, http://majikthise.typepad.com/majikthise_/2004/11/what_is_the_fou/comments/page/2/#comments, last accessed July 29, 2010. The "majikthise" blog is no longer active and this link now leads to a blank page. (I first saw the entry in April 2006.)

20. Niles eventually decides that the ads make her too uncomfortable, but that discomfort seems to stem from her distrust of Anschutz rather than the content or rhetoric of the billboards themselves. Maria Niles, "Am I Too Cynical for a Better Life?" *BlogHer*, June 7, 2008, http://www.blogher.com/am-i-too-cynical-better-life.

21. Justin Berrier, "Fox Hides Anti-Gay, Right-Wing Background of Foundation for a Better Life," *MediaMatters*, December 16, 2010, http://mediamatters.org/blog/201012160022.

22. *Observer*, May 4, 2002, http://portland.indymedia.org/en/2002/02/7617.shtml; JYPD, May 1, 2002, http://portland.indymedia.org/en/2002/02/7617.shtml.

23. Robert McRuer offers necessary caution about disability rhetorics and frameworks, noting that they can and are being used in ways counter to radical crip politics. See, for example, Robert McRuer, "Taking It to the Bank: Independence and Inclusion on the World Market," *Journal of Literary Disability* 1, no. 2 (2007): 5–14.

24. Noël Sturgeon, *Environmentalism in Popular Culture: Gender, Race, Sexuality, and the Politics of the Natural* (Tucson: University of Arizona Press, 2009), 28.

25. Rosemarie Garland-Thomson, "Seeing the Disabled: Visual Rhetorics of Disability in Popular Photography," in *The New Disability History: American Perspectives*, ed. Paul K. Longmore and Lauri Umansky (New York: New York University Press, 2001), 338.

26. Iris Marion Young, *Justice and the Politics of Difference* (Princeton, NJ: Princeton University Press, 1990), 227–34; Betty Sasaki, "Toward a Pedagogy of Coalition," *Twenty-First-Century Feminist Classrooms: Pedagogies of Identity and Difference*, ed. Amie A. MacDonald and Susan Sánchez-Casal (New York: Palgrave, 2002), 33.

27. Judith Butler, *Gender Trouble: Feminism and the Subversion of Identity*, 10th anniversary ed. (New York: Routledge, 1999), viii. See also Judith Butler, "Contingent Foundations," in *Feminist Contentions: A Philosophical Exchange,* ed. Seyla Benhabib, Judith Butler, Drucilla Cornell, and Nancy Fraser (New York: Routledge, 1995), 50–51; and Chantal Mouffe, *The Return of the Political* (London: Verso, 1993), 8.

28. Susan Stewart, of the Kiss and Tell Collective, notes, "Some of us have been reading across the grain for so long that our eyes have splinters." Kiss and Tell, *Her Tongue on my Theory* (Vancouver: Press Gang, 1994), 51.

29. Rosemarie Garland-Thomson, "The Politics of Staring: Visual Rhetorics of Disability in Popular Photography," *Disability Studies: Enabling the Humanities*, ed. Sharon L. Snyder, Brenda Jo Brueggemann, and Rosemarie Garland-Thomson (New York: Modern Language Association, 2002), 63.

30. Photographs of these altered billboards are available on the Portland Independent Media Center's website, accessed July 4, 2004, http://portland.indymedia.org/en/2002/02/7617.shtml

31. Edelman, *No Future*, 2.

32. I am influenced here by Heather Love and her insistence that we attend to negative affect. Heather Love, *Feeling Backward: Loss and the Politics of Queer History* (Cambridge, MA: Harvard University Press, 2007).

33. Nomy Lamm, "Private Dancer: Evolution of a Freak," *Restricted Access: Lesbians on Disability*, ed. Victoria A. Brownworth and Susan Raffo (Seattle: Seal Press, 1999), 152–61. For an incisive critique of the inspiring disabled person, see John B. Kelly, "Inspiration," *Ragged Edge Online* (January/February 2003), accessed February 7, 2010, http://www.raggededgemagazine.com/0103/0103ft1.html.

34. The disability rights organization ADAPT was a key player in transportation struggles in the 1980s; ADAPT originally stood for American Disabled for Accessible Public Transit. For more information on ADAPT, see http://www.adapt.org. For a more extensive history of disability rights activism, including transit battles, see, for example, Sharon N. Barnartt and Richard K. Scotch, *Disability Protests: Contentious Politics, 1970–1999* (Washington, DC: Gallaudet University Press, 2001); Doris Zames Fleischer and Frieda Zames, *The Disability Rights Movement: From Charity to Confrontation* (Philadelphia: Temple University Press, 2001); and Joseph Shapiro, *No Pity: People with Disabilities Forging a New Civil Rights Movement* (New York: Three Rivers Press, 1994).

35. See, for example, Jasbir Puar's analysis of homonationalism. Jasbir Puar, *Terrorist Assemblages: Homonationalism in Queer Times* (Durham, NC: Duke University Press, 2007). See also McRuer, "Taking It to the Bank."

36. As Robert McRuer shows in his analysis of disability imagery, it is not enough to frame some images of disability as "positive" and others as "negative." McRuer, *Crip Theory*, 171–98.

Chapter 5

1. Donna Haraway, "Cyborgs, Coyotes, and Dogs: A Kinship of Feminist Figurations: An Interview with Nina Lykke, Randi Markussen, and Finn Olesen," in *The Haraway Reader*, ed. Donna Haraway (New York: Routledge, 2004), 323–24.

2. Donna J. Haraway, "A Manifesto for Cyborgs: Science, Technology, and Socialist Feminism in the 1980s," *Socialist Review*, no. 80 (1985): 65–108. Unless otherwise noted, all references to the manifesto are taken from the revised version, published as "A Cyborg Manifesto: Science, Technology, and Socialist-Feminism in the Late Twentieth Century" in Donna J. Haraway, *Simians, Cyborgs, and Women: The Reinvention of Nature* (New York: Routledge, 1991), 149–81.

3. Haraway, *Simians, Cyborgs, and Women*, 151–53.

4. Donna Haraway, "Introduction: A Kinship of Feminist Figurations," in *The Haraway Reader*, ed. Donna Haraway (New York: Routledge, 2004), 1; Haraway, *Simians, Cyborgs, and Women*, 154.

5. Haraway, *Simians, Cyborgs, and Women*, 181.

6. Ibid.

7. Ibid., 154.

8. Ibid.

9. Haraway, "Introduction," 3; Haraway, *Simians, Cyborgs, and Women*, 149.

10. Haraway, "Cyborgs, Coyotes, and Dogs," 326; Haraway, *Simians, Cyborgs, and Women*, 181.

11. Haraway, *Simians, Cyborgs, and Women*, 154.

12. Ibid., 1.

13. Ibid., 156.

14. Ibid., 156. For more on the manifesto's debt to the work of women of color, see Chela Sandoval, "New Sciences: Cyborg Feminism and the Methodology of the Oppressed," in *The Cyborg Handbook*, ed. Chris Hables Gray, Steven Mentor, and Heidi J. Figueroa-Sarriera (New York: Routledge, 1995), 407–21.

15. Haraway, *Simians, Cyborgs, and Women*, 180.

16. Haraway, "Cyborgs, Coyotes, and Dogs," 324.

17. "[W]e are all chimeras, theorized and fabricated hybrids of machine and organism; in short, we are cyborgs." Haraway, *Simians, Cyborgs, and Women*, 150.

18. For an excellent overview of the uses of the cyborg manifesto, see Zoë Sofoulis, "Cyberquake: Haraway's Manifesto," in *Prefiguring Cyberculture: An Intellectual History*, ed. Darren Tofts, Annemarie Jonson, and Allesio Cavallaro (Cambridge, MA: MIT Press, 2002), 84–103.

19. Several essays in the anthology *The Prosthetic Impulse*, for example, suggest that the cyborg needs to be replaced with a newer theoretical framework, such as the prosthetic. Marquard Smith and Joanne Morra, eds., *The Prosthetic Impulse: From a Posthuman Present to a Biocultural Future* (Cambridge, MA: MIT Press, 2006).

20. Haraway, *Simians, Cyborgs, and Women*, 178.

21. See, for example, the introduction to and framing of *The Cyborg Handbook*, edited by Chris Hables Gray, Heidi J. Figueroa-Sarriera, and Steven Mentor.

22. For an overview of the cyborg's appearance in disability studies, see Alison Kafer, "Cyborg," in *Encyclopedia of U.S. Disability History*, ed. Susan Burch (New York: Facts on File, 2009), 223–24. For examples of scholars in disability studies who take up the figure, see Sharon Betcher, "Putting my Foot (Prosthesis, Crutches, Phantom) Down: Considering Technology as Transcendence in the Writings of Donna Haraway," *Women's Studies Quarterly* 29, nos. 3–4 (2001): 35–53; Fiona Kumari Campbell, *Contours of Ableism: The Production of Disability and Abledness* (New York: Palgrave Macmillan, 2009); Nirmala Erevelles, "In Search of the Disabled Subject," in *Embodied Rhetorics: Disability in Language and Culture*, ed. James C. Wilson and Cynthia Lewiecki-Wilson (Carbondale: Southern Illinois University Press, 2001), 92–111; David Mitchell and Sharon Snyder, "Introduction: Disability Studies and the Double Bind of Representation," in *The Body and Physical Difference: Discourses of Disability*, ed. David Mitchell and Sharon Snyder (Ann Arbor: University of Michigan Press, 1999), 1–31; Katherine Ott, "The Sum of Its Parts: An Introduction to Modern Histories of Prosthetics," in *Artificial Parts, Practical Lives: Modern Histories of Prosthetics*, ed. Katherine Ott, David Serlin, and Stephen Mihm (New York: New York University Press, 2002), 1–42; Donna Reeve, "Cyborgs and Cripples: What Can Haraway Offer Disability Studies?" in *Disability and Social Theory: New Developments and Directions*, ed. Dan Goodley, Bill Hughes, and Lennard Davis (New York: Palgrave Macmillan, forthcoming); Alexa Schriempf, "Hearing Deafness: Subjectness, Articulateness, and Communicability," *Subjectivity* 28 (2009): 279–96; and Tobin Siebers, "Disability in Theory: From Social Constructionism to the New Social Realism of the Body," *American Literary History* (2001): 737–54.

23. James L. Cherney, "Deaf Culture and the Cochlear Implant Debate: Cyborg Politics and the Identity of People with Disabilities," *Argumentation and Advocacy* 36 (Summer 1999): 22–34; and Margaret Quinlan and Benjamin Bates, "*Bionic Woman* (2007): Gender, Disability, and Cyborgs," *Journal of Research in Special Educational Needs* 9, no. 1 (2009): 48–58. For scholars who take up the figure of the cyborg in terms of disability in film and performance more generally, see, for example, Petra Kuppers, "Addenda, Phenomenology, Embodiment: Cyborgs and Disability Performance," in *Performance and Technology: Practices of Virtual Embodiment and Interactivity,* ed. Susan Broadhurst and Josephine Machon (New York: Palgrave Macmillan, 2006): 169–80; and Helen Meekosha, "Superchicks, Clones, Cyborgs, and Cripples: Cinema and Messages of Bodily Transformations," *Social Alternatives* 18, no. 1 (1999): 24–28.

24. A few notable exceptions would be the works of Rosemarie Garland-Thomson, Diane Price Herndl, Robert McRuer, and Margrit Shildrick, each of whom (briefly) examines the cyborg in the context of feminist theory and feminist disability studies. Although Garland-Thomson initially approaches the figure enthusiastically, in later work she expresses more misgivings about the figure; Herndl and Shildrick are more optimistic, linking the cyborg to their respective articulations of the posthuman and the monstrous. McRuer does not explicitly take up the cyborg figure itself, but he casts crip theory as "allied" with cyborg theory in its critical, and feminist, approach to identity. Rosemarie Garland-Thomson, *Extraordinary Bodies: Figuring Physical Disability in American Culture and Literature* (New York: Columbia University Press, 1997); Rosemarie Garland-Thomson, "Integrating Disability, Transforming Feminist Theory," in *Gendering Disability,* ed. Bonnie G. Smith and Beth Hutchison (New Brunswick, NJ: Rutgers University Press, 2004): 73–103; Diane Price Herndl, "Reconstructing the Posthuman Body Twenty Years after Audre Lorde's *Cancer Journals,*" in *Disability Studies: Enabling the Humanities,* ed. Sharon L. Snyder, Brenda Jo Brueggemann, and Rosemarie Garland-Thomson (New York: Modern Language Association, 2002), 144–55; Margrit Shildrick, *Embodying the Monster: Encounters with the Vulnerable Self* (London: Sage, 2002); and Robert McRuer, *Crip Theory: Cultural Signs of Queerness and Disability* (New York: New York University Press, 2006), 226n37.

25. Haraway, *Simians, Cyborgs, and Women,* 180.

26. Ibid., 150, 177.

27. Haraway uses the slogan "cyborgs for earthly survival!" several times in *Simians, Cyborgs, and Women,* explaining that it is the phrase on her "favorite political button" (244n1).

28. For feminist critiques of the hypermasculinity of contemporary cyborgs, see Anne Balsamo, *Technologies of the Gendered Body: Reading Cyborg Women* (Durham, NC: Duke University Press, 1996); Gill Kirkup, Linda Janes, Kath Woodward, and Fiona Hovenden, eds., *The Gendered Cyborg: A Reader* (London: Routledge, 2000); Cristina Masters, "Bodies of Technology: Cyborg Soldiers and Militarized Masculinities," *International Feminist Journal of Politics* 7, no. 1 (2005): 112–32; and Claudia Springer, "The Pleasure of the Interface," in *Sex/Machine: Readings in Culture, Gender, and Technology,* ed. Patrick D. Hopkins (Bloomington: Indiana University Press, 1998), 484–500.

29. See, for example, Cherney, "Deaf Culture and the Cochlear Implant Debate"; Johnson Cheu, "De-gene-erates, Replicants, and Other Aliens: (Re)Defining Disability in Futuristic Film," in *Disability/Postmodernity: Embodying Disability Theory,* ed. Mairian Corker and Tom Shakespeare (New York: Continuum, 2002), 199–212; and Meekosha, "Superchicks, Clones, Cyborgs, and Cripples."

30. Jennifer Gonzalez, "Envisioning Cyborg Bodies: Notes from Current Research," in *The Gendered Cyborg: A Reader,* ed. Gill Kirkup, Linda Janes, Kath Woodward, and Fiona Hovenden (London: Routledge, 2000), 64.

31. Sherry Baker, "The Rise of the Cyborgs," *Discover,* October 2008, http://discovermagazine.com/2008/oct/26-rise-of-the-cyborgs; Tim Kelly, "Rise of the Cyborg," *Forbes,* October 4, 2006, http://www.forbes.com/forbes/2006/0904/090.html; and Tim Kelly, "Cyborg Waiting List," *Forbes,* September 3, 2007,http://www.forbes.com/forbes/2007/0903/038.html.

32. In 2009, only 16.8 percent of disabled people were employed. S. von Schrader, W. A. Erickson, and C. G. Lee, *Disability Statistics from the Current Population Survey* (Ithaca, NY: Cornell University Rehabilitation Research and Training Center on Disability Demographics and Statistics, 2010), www.disabilitystatistics.org.

33. Lewis Page, "Cyborg-Style 'iLimb' Hand a Big Hit with Iraq Veterans," *Register* (UK), July 18, 2007, http://www.theregister.co.uk/2007/07/18/robo_hand_gets_big_hand.

34. For more on economic disparity and cyborgization, see Erevelles, "In Search of the Disabled Subject"; Gonzalez, "Envisioning Cyborg Bodies"; and Mitchell and Snyder, "Introduction."

35. Siebers, "Disability in Theory," 745.

36. Baker, "Rise of the Cyborgs."

37. Baker's language of immediacy is a bit of an overstatement when it comes to disability as well. Many of the advanced technologies heralded in her article remain in the experimental phase; other cybertechnology remains financially out of reach for most disabled people, as does more "mundane"—and less celebrated—technology like lightweight wheelchairs.

38. Leslie Swartz and Brian Watermeyer, "Cyborg Anxiety: Oscar Pistorius and the Boundaries of What It Means to be Human," *Disability and Society* 23, no. 2 (2008): 187–90.

39. Anna Salleh, "Cyborg Rights 'Need Debating Now,'" *ABC Science Online,* June 5, 2010, http://www.abc.net.au/news/stories/2010/06/05/2918723.htm.

40. Swartz and Watermeyer, "Cyborg Anxiety," 188. Hari Kunzru takes the description still further, arguing that elite athletes' high-performance clothing and scientifically tested diet and exercise regimens qualify them for cyborg status. Hari Kunzru, "You Are Cyborg," *Wired* 5, no. 2 (1997), accessed September 22, 2004, http://www.wired.com/wired/archive/5.02/ffharaway_pr.html.

41. Gonzalez offers a compelling critique of this conceptualization of the cyborg in terms of hybridity and racial purity. She cautions against using the language of miscegenation or unlawful coupling in describing the cyborg's boundary-crossing; such terms cannot be stripped of their violent past to function solely as metaphor. This presumption of the cyborg as the blending of two previously pure entities is similarly complicit in racist notions of purity and miscegenation. Gonzalez, "Envisioning the Cyborg."

42. Chris Hables Gray, *Cyborg Citizen: Politics in the Posthuman Age* (New York: Routledge, 2001), 1.

43. This choice seems significant given that several pages later he introduces a group of students at MIT who explicitly and proudly identify themselves as cyborgs. Gray, *Cyborg Citizen*, 9.

44. Ibid., 1.

45. Chris Hables Gray and Steven Mentor, "The Cyborg Body Politic and the New World Order," in *Prosthetic Territories: Politics and Hypertechnologies*, ed. Gabriel Brahm, Jr., and Mark Driscoll (Boulder, CO: Westview, 1995), 223.

46. Gray, *Cyborg Citizen*, 1.

47. For more on medicalized language and the construction of disability as a master identity, see Linton, *Claiming Disability.*

48. Gray, *Cyborg Citizen*, 1.

49. In a footnote to his text, Gray acknowledges that some disability activists find Reeve's cure work troubling, but only because they felt he "encouraged false hopes among the crippled." Gray makes no mention of those who oppose the whole cure narrative, suggesting everyone would have supported Reeve's work if only his timetable for success had been more reasonable. This acknowledgement, however, never appeared in the book itself, but only on the publisher's website; Routledge has since closed that site, but Gray has moved its content to his personal website. Chris Hables Gray, "Cyborg Citizen," first accessed July 16, 2002, http://www.routledge-ny.com/CyborgCitizen/chappgs/introduction.html (site discontinued); now available at http://www.chrishablesgray.org/CyborgCitizen.

50. Annie Potts, "Cyborg Masculinity in the Viagra Era," *Sexualities, Evolution, and Gender* 7, no. 1 (2005): 4.

51. See, for example, "Scientists Test First Human Cyborg," *CNN.com,* March 22, 2002, http://archives.cnn.com/2002/TECH/science/03/22/human.cyborg/.

52. I refer to the "imagined figure of the quadriplegic" to stress the cultural construction of this figure. Not all quadriplegics need ventilators, and some use manual rather than power wheelchairs. Spinal cord injuries vary widely, and although we tend to assume that paraplegics can move their arms and quadriplegics cannot, the reality is much more complicated.

53. Indeed, Haraway is quick to admit as much: "I have a perverse love of words, which have always seemed like tart physical beings to me." Haraway, "Introduction: A Kinship," 2.

54. Haraway, *Simians, Cyborgs, and Women,* 245n4.

55. Ibid., 178.

56. Ibid., 178.

57. Linton, *Claiming Disability,* 13.

58. Corinne Kirchner and Liat Ben-Moshe, "Language and Terminology," in *Encyclopedia of U.S. Disability History,* ed. Susan Burch (New York: Facts on File, 2009), 546–50.

59. Haraway, *Simians, Cyborgs, and Women,* 247–48n28.

60. For an exploration of how to reimagine these associations with "severe," see McRuer, *Crip Theory,* 30–31.

61. Haraway, *Simians, Cyborgs, and Women,* 178.

62. Malini Johar Schueller argues that this split implies a hard boundary between the two groups, as if all science fiction writers were white. She finds the split all the more mystifying given Haraway's inclusion of Octavia Butler, a black science fiction writer (Butler appears in the science fiction section, not the women of color section). Haraway does describe the two groups of texts as "overlapping," but Schueller sees the framing as indicative of Haraway's treatment of all women of color as the same. Malini Johar Schueller, "Analogy and (White) Feminist Theory: Thinking Race and the Color of the Cyborg Body," *Signs* 31, no. 1 (Autumn 2005): 79.

63. Haraway, *Simians, Cyborgs, and Women,* 174.

64. Compare this description to those of *The Female Man* by Joanna Russ or *Wild Seed* and *Xenogenesis* by Octavia Butler. Haraway, *Simians, Cyborgs, and Women,* 178–79.

65. Ibid., 180.

66. Ibid., 154.

67. Later in the essay, Haraway gets slightly more specific, but more in terms of the production line than the women working it. She offers as one example of "real-life cyborgs" "the Southeast Asian village women workers in Japanese and US electronics firms." Haraway, *Simians, Cyborgs, and Women,* 177.

68. Schueller, "Analogy and (White) Feminist Theory," 81.

69. Scott, "Cyborgian Socialists?" 216–17. For yet another critique of this passage, see, for example, Carol A. Stabile, *Feminism and the Technological Fix* (Manchester: Manchester University Press, 1994).

70. Constance Penley and Andrew Ross, Cyborgs at Large: An Interview with Donna Haraway," in *Technoculture,* ed. Constance Penley and Andrew Ross (Minneapolis: University of Minnesota Press, 1991), 12–13. Even in the manifesto, Haraway raises concerns about naming. "[W]ho counts as 'us' in my own rhetoric?" she queries. Haraway, *Simians, Cyborgs, and Women,* 155.

71. See, for example, Carol Mason, "Terminating Bodies: Toward a Cyborg History of Abortion," in *Posthuman Bodies,* ed. Judith Halberstam and Ira Livingston (Bloomington: Indiana University Press, 1995), 225–43; Penley and Ross, "Cyborgs at Large: An Interview with Donna Haraway"; Scott, "Cyborgian Socialists?"; and Stabile, *Feminism and the Technological Fix.*

72. Alexander G. Weheliye stresses that "the literal and virtual whiteness of cybertheory" is directly related to the kinds of texts and technologies recognized as "cyborg." He argues for greater attention to aural technologies in general and black popular music in particular. Alexander G. Weheliye, "'Feenin':

Posthuman Voices in Contemporary Black Popular Music," *Social Text 71* vol. 20, no. 2 (2002): 21–47; Beth E. Kolko, Lisa Nakamura, and Gilbert B. Rodman, introduction to *Race in Cyberspace*, ed. Beth E. Kolko, Lisa Nakamura, and Gilbert B. Rodman (New York: Routledge, 2000), 8.

73. Vivian Sobchack, "A Leg to Stand On: Prosthetics, Metaphor, and Materiality," in *The Prosthetic Impulse: From a Posthuman Present to a Biocultural Future*, ed. Marquard Smith and Joanne Morra (Cambridge, MA: MIT Press, 2006), 19.

74. Haraway, *Companion Species Manifesto*, 4. See also Haraway, *When Species Meet*.

75. On vampires, see Ingrid Bartsch, Carolyn DiPalma, and Laura Sells, "Witnessing the Postmodern Jeremiad: (Mis)Understanding Donna Haraway's Method of Inquiry," *Configurations* 9, no. 1 (Winter 2001): 127–64; and Shannon Winnubst, "Vampires, Anxieties, and Dreams: Race and Sex in the Contemporary United States," *Hypatia* 18, no. 3 (2003): 1–20. On the cyborg and the grotesque, see Sara Cohen Shabot, "Grotesque Bodies: A Response to Disembodied Cyborgs," *Journal of Gender Studies* 15, no. 3 (2006): 223–35. On the grotesque, the monstrous, and disability, see Garland-Thomson, *Extraordinary Bodies*; Garland-Thomson, "Integrating Disability"; and Shildrick, *Embodying the Monster*.

76. According to the American Kennel Club (AKC), "Dogs disfigured as the result of accident or injury but otherwise qualified shall·be eligible provided that the disfigurement does not interfere with functional movement. Dogs should be physically sound. Dogs that are blind or deaf shall not be eligible. Blind means without useful vision, and deaf means without useful hearing. No dog shall compete if it is taped or bandaged or in any way has anything attached to it for medical purposes." The North American Dog Agility Council similarly excludes lame, blind, or deformed dogs, but it specifies that such exclusions are to preserve the "health and welfare" of the dogs; unlike the AKC, they admit deaf (and mixed breed) dogs. I appreciate the desire to protect dog athletes from injury, and I want to be clear that I am not advocating for the elimination of such guidelines; I do not know enough about dogs or dog agility to make such demands. My concern is more with using *agility* as a way to think through feminist relationality. I am not sure disability politics is well-served by a figure so invested in "useful," "sound" bodies. American Kennel Club, *Regulations for Agility Trials,* 2010, accessed July 30, 2010, http://www.akc.org/pdfs/rulebooks/REAGIL.pdf; North American Dog Agility Council, *Exhibitor's Handbook: Rules for NADAC Trials,* 2010, accessed July 30, 2010, http://www. nadac.com/Rules_for_NADAC_trials.htm#_Eligibility_For_Entry.

There is at least one organization for disabled people involved in agility, and it describes itself as open to anyone who identifies as disabled: the Disabled Handlers Annual Agility League. For more information, see their website http://agilitynet.co.uk/reference/disabledhandlersleague_rulesandregs2006.html.

77. Christina Crosby, "Allies and Enemies," in *Coming to Terms: Feminism, Theory, Politics*, ed. Elizabeth Weed (New York: Routledge, 1989), 206. See also Mason, "Terminating Bodies," 226; and Penley and Ross, "Cyborgs at Large."

78. Sofoulis, "Cyberquake."

79. The quotation comes from the editors' blurb introducing Haraway's essay. Susan Stryker and Stephen Whittle, eds., *The Transgender Studies Reader* (New York: Routledge, 2006), 103.

80. Attending to such erasures—to what Gloria Wekker calls "the politics of citation" in her discussion of the work of Gloria Anzaldúa—should be an integral part of cyborg theory, given its attention to troubling single origins. See Chela Sandoval, "New Sciences: Cyborg Feminism and the Methodology of the Oppressed," in *The Cyborg Handbook*, ed. Chris Hables Gray, Steven Mentor, and Heidi J. Figueroa-Sarriera (New York: Routledge, 1995), 413; and Gloria Wekker, "The Arena of Disciplines: Gloria Anzaldúa and Interdisciplinarity," in *Doing Gender in Media, Art, and Culture*, ed. Rosemarie Buikema and Iris van der Tuin (New York: Routledge, 2007), 56.

81. Mariana Ortega, "Being Lovingly, Knowingly Ignorant: White Feminism and Women of Color," *Hypatia* 21, no. 3 (Summer 2006): 56–74; and Schueller, "Analogy and (White) Feminist Theory," 81.

82. Wilkerson identifies this question at the heart of the manifesto: "How are those who experience some form of social privilege to address work articulating the experiences of corresponding forms of oppression?" Abby Wilkerson, "Ending at the Skin: Sexuality and Race in Feminist Theorizing," *Hypatia* 12, no. 3 (1997): 165.

83. Haraway, *Simians, Cyborgs, and Women*, 150; emphasis in original.

84. Donna J. Haraway, *How Like a Leaf: An Interview with Thyrza Nichols Goodeve* (New York: Routledge, 2000), 136.

85. Brenda Brueggemann raises this question about pagers, Blackberries, and other instant communication devices in terms of deaf and hearing people, and Katherine Ott questions the very concept of assistive technology. Brueggemann, *Deaf Subjects*, 17; and Ott, "The Sum of Its Parts," 21.

86. Erevelles, "In Search of the Disabled Subject." See also Mitchell and Snyder, "Introduction: Disability Studies."

87. Kirkup, *Gendered Cyborg*, 5. Stabile shares Kirkup's assessment, but she links this gap to the cyborg's inability to address "the increasingly insurmountable walls that divide classes." Stabile, *Feminism and the Technological Fix*, 152–55.

88. Stacy Alaimo notes, "Even though Haraway underscores the fact that the cyborg transgresses the boundaries between human and nature as well as between human and machine, it is telling that the cyborg has become much more popular as a creature of technology, rather than as a creature of nature." Stacy Alaimo, *Undomesticated Ground: Recasting Nature as Feminist Space* (Ithaca: Cornell University Press, 2000),186; see also Alaimo, *Bodily Natures*, 6–7.

89. Rod Michalko, *The Two in One: Walking with Smokie, Walking with Blindness* (Philadelphia: Temple University Press, 1999).

90. Cary Wolfe, "Learning from Temple Grandin, or, Animal Studies, Disability Studies, and Who Comes after the Subject," *New Formations* 64 (2008): 110–23.

91. Loree Erickson, "Revealing Femmegimp: A Sex Positive Reflection on Sites of Shame as Sites of Resistance for People with Disabilities," *Atlantis* 31, no. 2 (2007): 42–52; Hershey, *Just Help*.

92. Erickson's description of their activities reads "helping me prepare food, helping me get dressed, take a shower, change the batteries in my vibrator, get into bed and out again, use the toilet, and the list goes on." Notice the shift in syntax, with the "helping me" dropping away. Erickson, "Revealing Femmegimp," 45. Barbara E. Gibson addresses attendants' experiences of this relation; see "Disability, Connectivity, and Transgressing the Autonomous Body," *Journal of Medical Humanities* 27 (2006): 187–96.

93. Garland-Thomson, *Extraordinary Bodies*, 114.

94. Steven L. Kurzman, "Presence and Prosthesis: A Response to Nelson and Wright," *Cultural Anthropology* 16, no. 3 (2001): 382.

95. Berkeley Bionics, "Introducing eLEGS," posted October 6, 2010, http://www.youtube.com/watch?v=WcMoruq28dc; Berkeley Bionics, "Human Universal Load Carrier (HULC), TM," posted April 30, 2010, http://www.youtube.com/watch?v=jPB6uwc7aWs.

96. For an extended analysis of the militarized cyborg, see Masters, "Bodies of Technology."

97. Judy Rohrer, "Toward a Full-Inclusion Feminism: A Feminist Deployment of Disability Analysis," *Feminist Studies* 31, no. 1 (Spring 2005): 43–44.

98. Haraway, *Simians, Cyborgs, and Women*, 181.

99. Corbett Joan O'Toole, "The View from Below: Developing a Knowledge Base about an Unknown Population," *Sexuality and Disability* 18, no. 3 (2000): 220. See also Siebers, *Disability Theory*, 151.

100. Laura Hershey, "Crip Commentary," accessed September 5, 2004, http://www.cripcommentary.com/LewisVsDisabilityRights.html. See also Laura Hershey, "From Poster Child to Protestor," *Spectacle* (Spring/Summer 1997), The Independent Living Institute, accessed September 5, 2004, http://www.independentliving.org/docs4/hershey93.html.

101. Mike Ervin, another former poster child turned telethon protestor, has long worked with Hershey to critique Lewis's rhetoric and assumptions about disability. For more on the Oscar protests, see his essay, "Jerry Lewis Doesn't Deserve a Humanitarian Award at the Oscars," *Progressive* (Madison, WI), February 19, 2009, http://tinyurl.com/awlyn5.

102. Haraway, *Simians, Cyborgs, and Women*, 181.

103. McRuer, *Crip Theory*, 31.

104. Panzarino died in 2001 at the age of fifty-three; Hershey died in 2010 at the age of forty-eight. I write about them in the present tense partly out of academic convention (Panzarino's protest sign, for example, lives on in the present as a text), but more out of an awareness that their work continues to impact queer crip communities, particularly disabled lesbian communities. For more on Panzarino's advocacy, see the obituary from Justice For All, accessed May 24, 2010, http://tinyurl.com/2fcpby6; for more on Hershey, see http://www.laurahershey.com.

105. Bradley Lewis, *Moving Beyond Prozac, DSM, and the New Psychiatry: The Birth of Postpsychiatry* (Ann Arbor: University of Michigan Press, 2006), 133, emphasis in original.

106. Lewis, *Moving Beyond Prozac*, 142. Elizabeth A. Wilson's analysis of Prozac suggests another way the cyborg can facilitate an understanding of psychopharmacology. She explains that, as a manufactured psychopharmaceutical, Prozac illustrates the difficulty of definitively distinguishing between nature and culture, between one's body and one's culture. Where does the body stop and the drug begin? Although Wilson does not take up the figure of the cyborg, her framing of the drug makes possible a reading of the drug through the lens of cyborgian boundary blurring. Elizabeth A. Wilson, "Organic Empathy: Feminism, Psychopharmaceuticals, and the Embodiment of Depression," in *Material Feminisms*, ed. Stacy Alaimo and Susan Hekman (Bloomington: Indiana University Press, 2008), 373–99.

107. Michelle O'Brien, "Tracing This Body: Transsexuality, Pharmaceuticals, and Capitalism," *deadletters: scattered notes toward the remembering of a misplaced present* (Summer 2003): 1–14, accessed June 22, 2010, http://www.deadletters.biz/body.html (site discontinued).

108. Ibid., 3.

109. Ibid., 11–12.

110. Ibid., 13.

111. Dean Spade, "Resisting Medicine, Re/modeling Gender," *Berkeley Women's Law Journal* 18 (2003): 15–37. See also Anna Kirkland, "When Transgendered People Sue and Win: Feminist Reflections on Strategy, Activism, and the Legal Process," in *The Fire This Time: Young Activists and the New Feminism*, ed. Vivien Labaton and Dawn Lundy Martin (New York: Anchor, 2004), 181–219; and Cayden Mak, "Cyborg Theory, Cyborg Practice," May 11, 2010, http://tinyurl.com/2wm7vag.

112. Spade, "Resisting Medicine," 35.

113. Ibid., 35.

114. The original essay is included in the anthology *The Cyborg Handbook*, and Haraway credits editor Chris Hables Gray with uncovering this lost history. Manfred E. Clynes and Nathan S. Kline, "Cyborgs and Space," in *The Cyborg Handbook*, ed. Chris Hables Gray, Steven Mentor, and Heidi J. Figueroa-Sarriera (New York: Routledge, 1995), 29–33.

115. According to Clynes, Kline was invited to write something about psychopharmacology, and he invited Clynes to coauthor. Chris Hables Gray, "An Interview with Manfred Clynes," in *The Cyborg Handbook*, ed. Chris Hables Gray, Heidi J. Figueroa-Sarriera, and Steven Mentor (New York: Routledge, 1995), 47.

116. Clynes and Kline, "Cyborgs and Space," 30.

117. Ibid., 30.

118. Ibid., 33.

119. Some of this drug research is described in a biography of Kline on the Nathan Kline Institute's web page "The Man Behind the Institute," accessed May 26, 2010, http://www.rfmh.org/nki/welcome/kline.cfm.

120. Quoted in Jackie Orr, *Panic Diaries: A Genealogy of Panic Disorder* (Durham, NC: Duke University Press, 2006), 312n159. Orr briefly discusses Kline's research in her analysis of postwar psychiatry and the rise of psychopharmacology. Haraway also mentions this psychiatric research in passing, noting that she discovered descriptions of experiments with "neural-chemical implants and telemetric monitoring" at Rockland when reading through old grant proposals from the National Science Foundation and the National Institutes of Mental Health. Donna J. Haraway, "Cyborgs and Symbionts: Living Together in the New World Order," in *The Cyborg Handbook*, ed. Chris Hables Gray, Steven Mentor, and Heidi J. Figueroa-Sarriera (New York: Routledge, 1995), xvi.

121. For discussion of Rockland during the 1940s and 1950s, see "Herded Like Cattle," *Time*, December 20, 1948, http://tinyurl.com/8b6wmv7; and Donna Cornachio, "Changes in Mental Care," *New York Times*, January 3, 1999. For examples of such accusations, see Pranay Gupte, "Tranquilizing Held a Factor in Deaths of Mental Patients," *New York Times*, July 17, 1978; Ronald Sullivan, "Panel Rejects Charges that Tranquilizer Use Led to Patient Deaths," *New York Times*, March 27, 1979; "Psychiatric Aide Accused of Rape," *New York Times*, November 26, 1979; and Cecilia Cummings, "Rockland Psychiatric Center Faulted in a Death," *New York Times*, July 17, 1988. Decades later, state institutions continue to come under scrutiny for negligence and abuse. See, for example, Danny Hakim, "At State-Run Homes, Abuse and Impunity," *New York Times*, March 12, 2011.

122. Hiram Perez, "You Can Have My Brown Body and Eat It, Too!" *Social Text* 84–85, vol. 23, nos. 3–4 (2005): 190n17.

123. Haraway, "Introduction: A Kinship," 3.

124. Haraway, *Simians, Cyborgs, and Women*, 153.

125. Ibid., 177.

Chapter 6

1. Tom Shakespeare, *Disability Rights and Wrongs* (New York: Routledge, 2006), 45.

2. Shakespeare, *Disability Rights and Wrongs*, 46.

3. Catriona Mortimer-Sandilands and Bruce Erickson discuss Joe Hermer's work on campgrounds in their thorough examination of queer ecologies. Catriona Mortimer-Sandilands and Bruce Erickson, "Introduction: A Genealogy of Queer Ecologies," in *Queer Ecologies: Sex, Nature, Politics, Desire*, ed. Catriona Mortimer-Sandilands and Bruce Erickson (Bloomington: Indiana University Press, 2010), 19.

4. William Cronon, "Introduction: In Search of Nature," in *Uncommon Ground: Toward Reinventing Nature*, ed. by William Cronon (New York: W. W. Norton, 1995), 23–56; and William Cronon, "The Trouble with Wilderness; or, Getting Back to the Wrong Nature," in *Uncommon Ground: Toward Reinventing Nature*, ed. William Cronon (New York: W. W. Norton, 1995), 69–90. See also Chaia Heller, "For the Love of Nature: Ecology and the Cult of the Romantic," in *Ecofeminism: Women, Animals, Nature*, ed. Greta Gaard (Philadelphia: Temple University Press, 1993), 219–42; and Lauret Savoy, "The Future of Environmental Essay: A Discourse," *Terrain* (Summer/Fall 2008), terrain.org.

5. Evelyn C. White, "Black Women and the Wilderness," in *The Stories That Shape Us: Contemporary Women Write about the West*, ed. Teresa Jordan and James Hepworth (New York: W. W. Norton, 1995): 376–83; on Carolyn Finney's work, see Barry Bergman, "Black, White, and Shades of Green," *Berkeleyan*, November 28, 2007, http://berkeley.edu/news/berkeleyan/2007/11/28_finney.shtml. Surveys of parkgoers support these claims, revealing that visitors to wilderness parks such as Yosemite or Yellowstone tend to be overwhelmingly white. A survey conducted at Yosemite in 2009 found white people constituted 77 percent of park visitors; 11 percent were Latino, 11 percent were Asian, and only 1 percent were black. Mireya Navarro, "National Parks Reach Out to Blacks Who Aren't Visiting," *New York Times*, November 2, 2010, http://www.nytimes.com/2010/11/03/science/earth/03parks.html?scp=2&sq=race+national+parks&st=nyt. See also Jason Byrne and Jennifer

Wolch, "Nature, Race, and Parks: Past Research and Future Directions for Geographic Research," *Progress in Human Geography* 33, no. 6 (2009): 743–65; and John Grossmann, "Expanding the Palette," *National Parks,* Summer 2010, accessed July 15, 2011, http://www.npca.org/magazine/2010/summer/expanding-the-palette.html.

6. Mei Mei Evans, "'Nature' and Environmental Justice," in *The Environmental Justice Reader: Politics, Poetics, and Pedagogy,* ed. Joni Adamson, Mei Mei Evans, and Rachel Stein (Tucson: University of Arizona Press, 2002), 191–92.

7. Evans, "'Nature' and Environmental Justice," 191, 192.

8. Cronon, "Introduction: In Search of Nature," 25.

9. I am excited by the rethinking of materiality taking place in feminist theory and environmental studies; I agree we need, in Stacy Alaimo's framing, "investigations that account for the ways in which nature, the environment, and the material world itself signify, act upon, or otherwise affect human bodies, knowledges, and practices." Although I focus more here on discursive constructions of nature, I see my project as a necessary complement to that work, as we have yet to reckon closely with relationships between dis/ability and "nature." Stacy Alaimo, *Bodily Natures: Science, Environment, and the Material Self* (Bloomington: Indiana University Press, 2010), 7–8.

10. Linda Vance, "Ecofeminism and Wilderness," *NWSA Journal* 9, no. 3 (Fall 1997): 71.

11. According to blurbs on the book's cover, the *New Yorker* called the book "an American masterpiece," while the *New York Times Book Review* praised it for its "power and beauty." This is not to say that Abbey is without critics; on the contrary, Abbey has long been challenged for his views on women and immigration. He himself describes *Desert Solitaire* as "coarse, rude, bad-tempered, violently prejudiced, unconstructive" and likely to draw criticism from "[s]erious critics, serious librarians, serious associate professors." Edward Abbey, *Desert Solitaire: A Season in the Wilderness* (New York: Touchstone, 1990), xii. I thank Cathy Kudlick for pushing me to engage with this text.

12. Abbey, *Desert Solitaire,* 49, 51, 233.

13. Sarah Jaquette Ray, "Risking Bodies in the Wild: The 'Corporeal Unconscious' of American Adventure Culture," *Journal of Sport and Social Issues* 33, no. 3 (2009): 271.

14. Ibid., 272.

15. Abbey, *Desert Solitaire,* 233.

16. Ibid., 49.

17. The whole genre of nature writing relies heavily on the epistemological assumption that walking brings knowledge. As both George Hart and Sarah Jaquette Ray note in their discussion of nature writing, walking is the privileged method of attaining a sense of unity and wholeness with nature. George Hart, "'Enough Defined': Disability, Ecopoetics, and Larry Eigner," *Contemporary Literature* 51, no. 1 (2010): 152–79; and Ray, "Risking Bodies in the Wild."

18. Ray, "Risking Bodies in the Wild," 260. Abbey was himself influenced by Thoreau and other writers who came before him.

19. For a discussion of such exclusions, see Giovanna Di Chiro, "Nature as Community: The Convergence of Environment and Social Justice," in *Uncommon Ground: Toward Reinventing Nature,* ed. William Cronon (New York: W. W. Norton, 1995), 298–319; Evans, "'Nature' and Environmental Justice"; Gaard, "Ecofeminism and Wilderness"; Linda Vance, "Ecofeminism and the Politics of Reality"; and Richard T. Twine, "Ma(r)king Essence: Ecofeminism and Embodiment," *Ethics and the Environment* 6, no. 2 (2001): 31–57.

20. It issued its first apology on October 24, 2000, wherein the company expressed regret for the offensive nature of the ad and stressed its own connection to the disability community, a connection embodied by the fact that a former Nike executive was "confined to a wheelchair." The company tried again a day later, stating that disabilities "are no laughing matter" and that disabled people "demonstrate more courage in a day than most of us will in a lifetime." Striking some activists as

condescending for its assumption that any attempt to live with disability is worthy of praise, that apology was followed shortly thereafter with a more straightforward one. Taken together, the group of apologies maps out the overlapping models of disability available to Nike: disability as tragedy; disabled people as inspiration to others; disability as the site of pity. The apologies were all posted on Nike's website, although disability activists argued that Nike should print its apologies in the same publications in which the ad originally appeared; only then could Nike begin to rectify the damage of the original ad. The ad and the apologies have since been removed from the company's website.

My understanding of the Nike controversy comes from the following: Bruce Steele, "Faculty Member Encourages Boycott over Ad," *University Times* (University of Pittsburgh), November 22, 2000; "Crip Community Outraged at Nike Ad," *Ragged Edge Online Extra,* 2000, accessed March 12, 2003, http://www.ragged-edge-mag.com/extra/nikead.htm; and "Nike Issues Formal Apology, " *Ragged Edge Online Extra,* 2000, accessed March 12, 2003, http://www.ragged-edge-mag.com/extra/ nikead.htm. On the use of disability and disabled people in advertising, see Rosemarie Garland-Thomson, "Seeing the Disabled: Visual Rhetorics of Disability in Popular Photography," in *The New Disability History: American Perspectives,* ed. Paul K. Longmore and Lauri Umansky (New York: New York University Press, 2001), 335–74.

21. Nike has long had a reputation for running edgy advertisements, and they very well may have suspected that the ad would generate some controversy (and thereby garner some free publicity). But even that strategy would rely on the assumption that they could offend or anger disability communities without alienating their consumers or affecting their bottom line.

22. Although the freak show did not disappear in the 1940s, it was no longer as acceptable or as widespread as it had been in the previous decades. For accounts of this history, see, for example, Leslie Fiedler, *Freaks: Myths and Images of the Secret Self* (New York: Simon and Schuster, 1978); Robert Bogdan, *Freak Show: Presenting Human Oddities for Amusement and Profit* (Chicago: University of Chicago Press, 1988); Rosemarie Garland-Thomson, ed., *Freakery: Cultural Spectacles of the Extraordinary Body* (New York: New York University Press, 1996); Rosemarie Garland-Thomson, *Extraordinary Bodies: Figuring Physical Disability in American Culture and Literature* (New York: Columbia University Press, 1997); Leonard Cassuto, *The Inhuman Race: The Racial Grotesque in American Literature and Culture* (New York: Columbia University Press, 1997); and Rachel Adams, *Sideshow U.S.A.: Freaks and the American Cultural Imagination* (Chicago: University of Chicago Press, 2001).

23. Rosemarie Garland-Thomson, *Extraordinary Bodies,* 41.

24. Ray, "Risking Bodies in the Wild," 263.

25. Linda Vance, "Ecofeminism and the Politics of Reality," in *Ecofeminism: Women, Animals, and Nature,* ed. Greta Gaard (Philadelphia: Temple University Press, 1993), 133.

26. See, for example, Linda Vance, "Ecofeminism and Wilderness," *NWSA Journal* 9 no. 3 (Fall 1997): 60–76.

27. According to a survey of people with learning disabilities and cognitive impairments, a lack of materials in alternative formats is one of the more alienating dimensions of public parks. The survey covered only urban parks, but it seems likely that the same would be true of wilderness parks. A. R. Mathers, "Hidden Voices: The Participation of People with Learning Disabilities in the Experience of Public Open Space," *Local Environment* 13, no. 6 (2008): 515–29.

28. Rob Imrie and Huw Thomas, "The Interrelationships between Environment and Disability," *Local Environment* 13, no. 6 (2008): 477.

29. For a discussion of the access battles at Maine's Allagash Waterway, see A. J. Higgins, "Canoe Launch Divides Environmentalists, Disabled," *Boston Globe,* June 4, 2000, C1; and Joe Huber, "Accessibility vs. Wilderness Preservation—Maine's Allagash Wilderness Waterway," *Palaestra: Forum of Sport, Physical Education, and Recreation for Those with Disabilities* 16, no. 4 (2000), accessed December 16, 2002, http://www.palaestra.com/allagash.html. (Huber's article has since been removed from the Palaestra site). For a more general discussion of accessibility, wilderness, and

the law, see Jennie Bricker, "Wheelchair Accessibility in Wilderness Areas: The Nexus Between the ADA and the Wilderness Act," *Environmental Law* 25, no. 4 (1995): 1243–70.

30. Bruce was responding to a front-page article in the *Times* about the modifications to the hut at Galehead and the integrated hiking team. Carey Goldberg, "For These Trailblazers, Wheelchairs Matter," *New York Times,* August 17, 2000; Dan Bruce, "Letters to the Editor," *New York Times,* August 21, 2000, available at http://www.nytimes.com/2000/08/21/opinion/l-destructive-hiking-748404.html.

31. Quoted in "Trailblazing in a Wheelchair: An Oxymoron?" *Palaestra: Forum of Sport, Physical Education, and Recreation for Those with Disabilities* 17, no. 4 (2001): 52.

32. Gravink was the director of the Northeast Passage program at the University of New Hampshire, the organization sponsoring the hike. Quoted in Goldberg, "For These Trailblazers."

33. Whole Access was founded in 1983 by Phyllis Cangemi; although the group often served as a clearinghouse for individuals interested in accessible trails, its primary goal was to educate park managers and planners about accessibility. Cangemi, who served as the executive director of the organization, died in 2005, and Whole Access closed not long after.

34. Steep trails (which hinder the use of wheelchairs) tend to collect water and create erosion channels, eventually damaging the trail and surrounding terrain. Phyllis Cangemi, "Trail Design: Balancing Accessibility and Nature," *Universal Design Newsletter,* July 1999, 4.

35. "Accessibility Guidelines for Trails," *Universal Design Newsletter,* July 1999, 5.

36. Ann Sieck, "On a Roll: A Wheelchair Hiker Gets Back on the Trail," *Bay Nature,* October 2006, accessed April 28, 2007, http://baynature.org/articles/on-a-roll. See also Claire Tregaskis, "Applying the Social Model in Practice: Some Lessons from Countryside Recreation," *Disability and Society* 19, no. 6 (2004): 601–11.

37. Hershey includes the excised section of the essay on her website, as well as a brief description of her exchange with the editor. Laura Hershey, "Along Asphalt Trails (The Rest of the Story)," September 18, 2008, http://www.laurahershey.com/?p=4; Laura Hershey, "Along Asphalt Trails," *National Parks,* Fall 2008, accessed June 8, 2011, http://www.npca.org/magazine/2008/fall/along-asphalt-trails.html.

38. Sieck, "On a Roll."

39. Erik Weihenmayer, *Touch the Top of the World: A Blind Man's Journey to Climb Farther than the Eye Can See* (New York: Plume, 2002), 5–7.

40. Petra Kuppers, "Outsides: Disability Culture Nature Poetry," *Journal of Literary Disability* 1, no. 1 (2007): 1.

41. Catriona Sandilands, "Unnatural Passions? Toward a Queer Ecology," *Invisible Culture,* no. 9 (2005), accessed June 10, 2010, http://www.rochester.edu/in_visible_culture/Issue_9/title9.html.

42. Eli Clare, *Exile and Pride: Disability, Queerness, and Liberation* (Boston: South End, 1999), 4.

43. Ibid., 5.

44. Ibid., 8–9.

45. Ibid., 8.

46. Ray, "Risking Bodies in the Wild," 265.

47. Kuppers, "Outsides," 2.

48. Samuel Lurie, "Loving You Loving Me," in *Queer Crips: Disabled Gay Men and their Stories,* ed. Bob Guter and John R. Killacky (New York: Harrington Park Press, 2004), 85.

49. A. M. Baggs, "In My Language," uploaded January 14, 2007, http://www.youtube.com/watch?v=JnylM1hI2jc.

50. Eli Clare, "Stolen Bodies, Reclaimed Bodies: Disability and Queerness," *Public Culture* 13, no. 3 (2001): 362.

51. Indeed, the relationship between disability rights and animal rights movements, not to mention the overlaps and gaps between the categories of disability and animality, is a rich site for analysis.

Philosopher Peter Singer's use of cognitive disability to make arguments for animal rights has long been criticized by disability studies scholars and activists (and with good reason), and the representation of disabled people as animals has a deep and troubling history that is thoroughly entwined with scientific racism and eugenics. At the same time, there are exciting possibilities for political and theoretical collaboration between disability studies and animal studies. Several sessions of the Society for Disability Studies conference in recent years have addressed the potential for animal rights/disability rights alliances, and there are scholars, activists, and artists working to deconstruct and reimagine the relationship between animality and disability. See, for example, Licia Carlson, *The Faces of Intellectual Disability* (Bloomington: Indiana University Press, 2010); Mel Y. Chen, *Animacies: Biopolitics, Racial Mattering, and Queer Affect* (Durham, NC: Duke University Press, forthcoming); Nora Ellen Groce and Jonathan Marks, "The Great Ape Project and Disability Rights: Ominous Undercurrents of Eugenics in Action," *American Anthropologist* 102, no. 4 (2001): 818–22; Sunaura Taylor, "Beasts of Burden: Disability Studies and Animal Rights," *Qui Parle: Critical Humanities and Social Sciences* 19, no. 2 (2011): 191–222; and Cary Wolfe, "Learning from Temple Grandin, or, Animal Studies, Disability Studies, and Who Comes After the Subject," *New Formations* 64 (2008): 110–23. See also the artwork of painter Sunaura Taylor, whose recent *Animal* exhibition tracked the overlapping visual iconography of freak shows, medical textbooks, and butcher-shop diagrams: Sunaura Taylor, *Animal*, Rowan Morrison Gallery, Oakland, California, October 2009. Images from the show, as well as my gallery essay about the show, "Seeing Animals," are available through Taylor's website, http://www.sunaurataylor.org/portfolio/animal/.

Chapter 7

1. Douglas C. Baynton, "Disability and the Justification of Inequality in American History," in *The New Disability History: American Perspectives*, ed. Paul K. Longmore and Lauri Umansky (New York: New York University Press, 2001), 52.

2. Ranu Samantrai, *AlterNatives: Black Feminism in the Postimperial Nation* (Stanford, CA: Stanford University Press, 2002), 1, 25.

3. Ibid., 132. Audre Lorde makes a similar point, urging, "Do not let the differences pull you apart. Use them, examine them, go through them, grow from them." Jennifer Abod, *The Edge of Each Other's Battles: The Vision of Audre Lorde* (Long Beach, CA: Profile Productions, 2002), VHS.

4. Chantal Mouffe, "Feminism, Citizenship, and Radical Democratic Politics," in *Feminists Theorize the Political*, ed. Judith Butler and Joan W. Scott (New York: Routledge, 1992), 380; Samantrai, *AlterNatives*, 132.

5. Bernice Johnson Reagon, "Coalition Politics: Turning the Century," in *Home Girls: A Black Feminist Anthology*, ed. Barbara Smith (New York: Kitchen Table, 1983): 356–68. I thank Sue Schweik for encouraging me to focus on this text.

6. These struggles were part of the 1981 festival itself. For brief descriptions of what transpired, see Barbara Gagliardi, "West Coast Women's Music Festival," *Big Mama Rag* 9, no. 10 (1981): 3, 22; and Loraine Hutchins, "Trouble and Mediation at Yosemite," *off our backs* 11, no. 10 (1981): 12–13, 25. For an analysis of Reagon's presentation in the context of the festival and the women's movement more broadly, see Becky Thompson, *A Promise and a Way of Life: White Antiracist Activism* (Minneapolis: University of Minnesota, 2001), 201–04.

7. Reagon, "Coalition Politics," 356.

8. Ibid., 356.

9. Stacy Alaimo makes a similar move in her reading of Audre Lorde's *Cancer Journals*. She argues against reading the memoir "as an abstraction disentangled from the context of Lorde's breast cancer," seeing it only "as a generalized call to refuse to be silenced." Divorcing the text from Lorde's physical, embodied experience dilutes the political thrust of the text, suggests Alaimo. Stacy Alaimo,

Bodily Natures: Science, Environment, and the Material Self (Bloomington: Indiana University Press, 2010), 85–86.

10. Reagon, "Coalition Politics," 356.

11. Reagon mentions disability in her discussion of how women find themselves identified with, or identify themselves with, other groups; gender is not always primary: "You are Black or you are Chicana or you are Disabled or you are Racist or you are White." Ibid., 349.

12. I take the first part of my title from the title of an article I cowrote with fellow members of PISSAR (People In Search of Safe and Accessible Restrooms). This section, as well as my understandings of coalition politics and queer activism, has benefited tremendously from my time with them; I remain grateful for our intellectual and political work together. Simone Chess, Alison Kafer, Jessi Quizar, and Mattie Udora Richardson, "Calling All Restroom Revolutionaries," in *That's Revolting: Queer Strategies for Resisting Assimilation*, ed., Mattilda (aka Matt Bernstein Sycamore) (Brooklyn: Soft Skull Press, 2004), 189–206.

13. Plaskow lists "the civil rights movement, feminism, disability rights, and rights for transgendered persons." Judith Plaskow, "Embodiment, Elimination, and the Role of Toilets in Struggles for Social Justice," *Cross Currents* (Spring 2008): 52.

14. For an early articulation of the argument that public toilets are a necessary site for feminist theorizing and activism, see Taunya Lovell Banks, "Toilets as a Feminist Issue: A True Story," *Berkeley Women's Law Journal* (1990): 263–89. See also Mary Anne Case, "Changing Room? A Quick Tour of Men's and Women's Rooms in U.S. Law over the Last Decade, from the U.S. Constitution to Local Ordinances," *Public Culture* 13, no. 2 (2001): 333–36; and Patricia Cooper and Ruth Oldenziel, "Cherished Classifications: Bathrooms and the Construction of Gender/Race on the Pennsylvania Railroad during World War II," *Feminist Studies* 25, no. 1 (1999): 7–41.

15. Judith Plaskow offers one example from her personal history, describing a feminist takeover of a campus bathroom during her career as a graduate student. The library at Yale's divinity school had no toilet for women, so she and her comrades put flowers in the men's room urinal and declared the space unisex. Plaskow, "Embodiment, Elimination, and the Role of Toilets," 55.

16. Elizabeth Abel, "Bathroom Doors and Drinking Fountains: Jim Crow's Racial Symbolic," *Critical Inquiry* 25 (Spring 1999): 439. See also Cooper and Oldenziel, "Cherished Classifications."

17. Laura Norén reveals the difficulty that New York cabdrivers and other officeless workers (e.g., bike messengers and street vendors) have in finding a toilet that they can safely and reliably use. Restaurant and other business owners often refuse to let them use their facilities ("for customers and employees only"), and the city has closed a significant number of its public toilets. Laura Norén, "Only Dogs Are Free to Pee: New York Cabbies' Search for Civility," in *Toilet: Public Restrooms and the Politics of Sharing*, ed. Harvey Molotch and Laura Norén (New York: New York University Press, 2010): 93–114.

18. See, for example, Sheila L. Cavanagh, *Queering Bathrooms: Gender, Sexuality, and the Hygienic Imagination* (Toronto: University of Toronto Press, 2010); Olga Gershenson and Barbara Penner, eds., *Ladies and Gents: Public Toilets and Gender* (Philadelphia: Temple University Press, 2009); Molotch and Norén, *Toilet: Public Restrooms and the Politics of Sharing*; and Christine Overall, "Public Toilets: Sex Segregation Revisited," *Ethics and the Environment* 12, no. 2 (2007): 71–91.

19. In the past decade or so, activists have become increasingly vocal about the importance of accessible restrooms for genderqueer and trans-identified people. San Francisco–based PISSR (People In Search of Safe Restrooms); *Toilet Training*, Dean Spade's documentary film and teaching kit; and student groups on college campuses across the country, from Harvard to the University of Washington—all make the case for expanding access to include the needs of genderqueer people, casting the presence of gender-neutral restrooms as necessary for a space to be considered accessible. A number of activist and academic conferences have re-signed the doors on (at least some of) the public toilets in their meeting places, rendering them temporarily unisex; my first exposure to

such activism was at the 2002 Queer Disability Conference in San Francisco. For an overview of an early site of toilet activism, the University of Massachusetts, see Olga Gershenson, "The Restroom Revolution: Unisex Toilets and Campus Politics," in Molotch and Norén, *Toilet*, 191–207. For a comprehensive overview of toilet activism in general, see Dean Spade, *Toilet Training: Companion Guide for Activists and Educators*, Sylvia Rivera Law Project (New York: Urban Justice Center, 2004).

This kind of activism is necessary, explains Leslie Feinberg, because having to decide over and over again which bathroom to use takes a toll on one's humanity. Yet the decision keeps repeating because gender-segregated public toilets place genderqueer people at risk: "If I go into the women's bathroom, am I prepared for the shouting and shaming? Will someone call security or the cops? If I use the men's room, am I willing to fight my way out? Am I really ready for the violence that could ensue?" Leslie Feinberg, *Trans Liberation: Beyond Pink or Blue* (Boston: Beacon, 1998), 68–69.

20. History provides other examples of moments when gender was not the primary organizing principle at work in public toilets, or, rather, when the toilet served as a way to un-gender some bodies but not others. During the era of Jim Crow, "white" bathrooms were strictly segregated by gender, while many "colored" restrooms were not. The imperative to protect women's purity and safety, or to preserve strict distinctions between male and female, applied only to whites; black women were not seen as needing such protections, and unisex bathrooms served as yet another way to deny the manhood of black men. See Abel, "Bathroom Doors and Drinking Fountains," 440–41n5. As Cooper and Oldenzeil note, both race and gender were "cherished classifications" when it came to public spaces. Cooper and Oldenzeil, "Cherished Classifications."

21. While large, single-stall restrooms with diaper-changing tables and room for small children are necessary, labeling them "family," with a male icon and a female icon surrounding an icon of an infant, simply creates a different kind of (hetero)sex-segregation.

22. Sally Munt notes that "the disabled toilet provides isolated privacy and secrecy for the marked body," but we can also see it as offering privacy *from* the marked body. Cultural fears of disability intertwine with shame about elimination and taboos of contamination; although Sheila Cavanagh's interviewees document intense curiosity about what disabled people do in the bathroom, it is a curiosity that prefers a "safe" distance from the disabled body. Sally R. Munt, "The Butch Body," in *Contested Bodies*, ed. Ruth Holliday and John Hassard (London: Routledge, 2001), 102; Cavanagh, *Queering Bathrooms*, 101–03.

23. Munt, "The Butch Body," 102.

24. Ibid., 103.

25. Reading disability narratives alongside trans or genderqueer narratives makes this shared inaccessibility readily apparent. For example, Connie Panzarino, a wheelchair user unable to transfer independently in and out of her chair, explains that as a child she was allowed to attend public schools only if she could refrain from using the restroom while on campus. For years, she restricted her fluid intake and controlled her bladder in order to get an education. Respondents to a survey about gender-segregated toilets describe disciplining their bodies much like Panzarino, restricting their liquid intake or altering their plans in order to avoid having to use gender-specific restrooms. Banks traces a historical parallel in the experiences of African Americans living under Jim Crow who tried to anticipate their toilet needs before leaving home. Banks, "Toilets as a Feminist Issue," 287; Connie Panzarino, *The Me in the Mirror* (Seattle: Seal Press, 1994); and the Transgender Law Center, accessed May 4, 2007, http://www.transgenderlawcenter.org/. See also Kath Browne, "Genderism and the Bathroom Problem: (Re)Materialising Sexed Sites, (Re)Creating Sexed Bodies," *Gender, Place, and Culture* 11, no. 3 (2004): 331–46.

26. Munt, "The Butch Body," 102.

27. PISSAR was inspired in part by materials created for the 2002 Queer Disability Conference. Participants at the conference were given a "Statement on Bathrooms and Gender" that was also posted on bathroom doors throughout the conference center (see Appendix B). The "Statement"

explicitly framed the issue of gender-neutral restrooms as an access issue: "Part of making this conference accessible is recognizing that sex segregated bathrooms are limiting for people who do not fit easily into Men's or Women's Rooms." Queer Disability Conference Organizers, "Statement on Bathrooms and Gender," Queer Disability Conference, San Francisco, California, June 2002. For more on PISSAR, see Chess et al., "Calling All Restroom Revolutionaries!"

28. TransBrandeis, "Mapping Brandeis Bathrooms," accessed July 24, 2011, http://people.brandeis.edu/~trisk/brms/concept.html.

29. Contrast TransBrandeis, for example, with the Harvard Trans Task Force, accessed July 24, 2011, http://www.hcs.harvard.edu/queer/ttf/activism.html.

30. Tobin Seibers makes a similar point about "color-blind" and "race-blind," arguing that they need "to be interrogated from a disability perspective alert to the metaphor of blindness." Tobin Siebers, *Disability Theory* (Ann Arbor: University of Michigan, 2008), 206n4.

31. See, for example, two studies about the inaccessibility of public toilets that make no mention of gender segregation or trans and genderqueer exclusion: Rob Kitchin and Robin Law, "The Socio-spatial Construction of (In)accessible Public Toilets," *Urban Studies* 38, no. 2 (2001): 287–98; and Tanya Titchkosky, "'To Pee or Not to Pee?': Ordinary Talk about Extraordinary Exclusions in a University Environment," *Canadian Journal of Sociology/Cahiers Canadiens de Sociologie* 33, no. 1 (2008): 37–60. For an overview of potential connections between the two fields, see Ashley Mog and Amanda Lock Swarr, "Threads of Commonality in Transgender and Disability Studies," *Disability Studies Quarterly* 28, no. 4 (2008), www.dsq-sds.org.

32. Harvey Molotch, "Learning from the Loo," introduction to *Toilet: Public Restrooms and the Politics of Sharing*, ed. Harvey Molotch and Laura Norén (New York: New York University Press, 2010), 17.

33. Jennifer Levi and Bennett Klein, "Pursuing Protection for Transgender People through Disability Laws," in *Transgender Rights*, ed. Paisley Currah, Richard M. Juang, and Shannon Price Minter (Minneapolis: University of Minnesota, 2006), 77. For more on the relationship between trans and disability in terms of legal protections, see Anna Kirkland, "When Transgendered People Sue and Win: Feminist Reflections on Strategy, Activism, and the Legal Process," in *The Fire This Time: Young Activists and the New Feminism*, ed. Vivien Labaton and Dawn Lundy Martin (New York: Anchor, 2004): 181–219; and Dean Spade, "Resisting Medicine, Re/modeling Gender," *Berkeley Women's Law Journal* 18 (2003): 15–37.

34. Titchkosky, "'To Pee or Not to Pee?'" 39.

35. Carrie Sandahl, "Anarcha Anti-Archive: Depends®," *Liminalities: A Journal of Performance Studies* 4, no. 2 (2008), accessed July 24, 2011, http://liminalities.net/4-2/anarcha. John B. Kelly notes how often discussion of assisted suicide and euthanasia turns to, and turns on, discussion of incontinence. Reading through news coverage of Dr. Jack Kevorkian, he explains, makes clear how profoundly afraid our culture is of those who cannot toilet themselves, so much so that death begins to look better than diapers. John B. Kelly, "Incontinence," *Ragged Edge*, no. 1 (2002), accessed July 24, 2011, http://www.ragged-edge-mag.com/0102/0102ft3.htm.

36. Sandahl, "Depends®."

37. For more on teratology, see Rosemarie Garland-Thomson, ed., *Freakery: Cultural Spectacles of the Extraordinary Body* (New York: New York University Press, 1996).

38. As a wheelchair user, I can easily tell when I have rolled into a poor, undervalued neighborhood: The sidewalk becomes cracked and curb cuts get increasingly precarious or disappear altogether. In his poem "Two Cities Separated Identities," Leroy Moore contrasts Berkeley with Oakland by making reference to the cities' sidewalks: "The most accessible city shares roads/leading to potholes, crack sidewalks and mountain curbs of Oaktown." Anne Finger makes a similar observation about race, class, and infrastructure in her rumination on disability and Hurricane Katrina, noting that the sidewalks of New Orleans were in trouble long before the storm hit. Anne Finger,

"Hurricane Katrina, Race, Class, Tragedy, and Charity," *DSQ: Disability Studies Quarterly* 25, no. 4 (2005), accessed May 9, 2011, http://www.dsq-sds.org/article/view/630/807.

39. Johnson focuses on the persistence of "food deserts," or areas without affordable and reliable access to safe, fresh, and healthy foods, as an issue linking both disability and environmental justice. Andrew Charles and Huw Thomas similarly call environmental justice movements to task, but their focus is more on encouraging those movements to support local improvements to disability access; they urge greater recognition that the built environment of cities is part of the environment. I share their concerns, but my interest is more with encouraging disability studies scholars and activists to engage more fully with environmental justice movements. Valerie Ann Johnson, "Bringing Together Feminist Disability Studies and Environmental Justice," Barbara Faye Waxman Fiduccia Papers on Women and Girls with Disabilities, Center for Women Policy Studies, February 2011, 3, http://www.centerwomenpolicy.org/programs/waxmanfiduccia/BFWFP_BringingTogetherFeministDisabilityStudiesandEnvironmentalJustice_ValerieAnnJohnso.pdf; and Andrew Charles and Huw Thomas, "Deafness and Disability—Forgotten Components of Environmental Justice: Illustrated by the Case of Local Agenda 21 in South Wales," *Local Environment* 12, no. 3 (June 2007): 209–21.

40. Alaimo, *Bodily Natures*, 12.

41. Giovanna Di Chiro, "Polluted Politics? Confronting Toxic Discourse, Sex Panic, and Eco-Normativity," in *Queer Ecologies: Sex, Nature, Politics, Desire*, ed. Catriona Mortimer-Sandilands and Bruce Erickson (Bloomington: Indiana University Press, 2010), 202.

42. Ibid., 202; see also 218–19.

43. And, as Di Chiro's analysis suggests, queer fear and disability fear are hard to untangle. LGBT people and intersexed people appear as "disabled" within this literature, their bodies and orientations "unjustly harmed" by their environments. Acknowledging that link, I still think it is useful to focus on the disability fear in addition to, and separately from, fears about sexual abnormalities. The imperative to eliminate disability—"defects" in environmental discourses—is firmly entrenched in environmental movements and discourses.

44. Ted Schettler, "Developmental Disabilities—Impairment of Children's Brain Development and Function: The Role of Environmental Factors," The Collaborative on Health and the Environment, February 8, 2003, http://healthandenvironment.org/learning_behavior/peer_reviewed.

45. Alaimo, *Bodily Natures*, 86.

46. Ibid., 86–87.

47. Breast Cancer Action, "Our Priorities," accessed July 24, 2011, http://bcaction.org/about/priorities/. Stacy Alaimo and Giovanna Di Chiro extend this critique, arguing that attending exclusively to genetic factors opens the door to conceptualizing individual people or "genomic subsets of the population" as particularly susceptible to toxic exposures; the problem to "solve" then becomes those people's susceptibility rather than the release or use of those toxins. Di Chiro refers to this scenario as creating "Roundup Ready®" or "Beryllium Ready" communities. See Alaimo, *Bodily Natures*, 127–28; and Giovanna Di Chiro, "Producing 'Roundup Ready®' Communities? Human Genome Research and Environmental Justice Policy," in *New Perspectives on Environmental Justice: Gender, Sexuality, and Activism*, ed. Rachel Stein (New Brunswick, NJ: Rutgers University Press, 2004), 146, 149.

48. Disability Rights Education and Defense Fund, "Environmental Justice," accessed July 15, 2011, http://www.dredf.org/envirojustice/index.shtml.

49. Queer Disability Conference Organizers, "How and Why to Be Scent-Free," Queer Disability Conference, San Francisco, California, June 2002. For a more recent example of a conference responding to, and struggling with, scent-free/low-scent spaces, see nolose (a conference for folks "dedicated to ending the oppression of fat people and creating vibrant fat queer culture"), accessed May 9, 2011, http://www.nolose.org/10/access.php.

50. See, for example, Mel Y. Chen, "Toxic Animacies, Inanimate Affections," *GLQ: A Journal of Lesbian and Gay Studies* 17, nos. 2–3 (2011): 265–86; Anna Mollow, "No Safe Place," *WSQ: Women's*

Studies Quarterly 39, nos. 1–2 (2011): 188–99; Peggy Munson, "Fringe Dweller: Toward an Ecofeminist Politic of Femme," in *Visible: A Femmethology*, vol. 2., ed. Jennifer Clarke Burke (Ypsilanti, MI: Homofactus Press, 2009), 28–36; and Rhonda Zwillinger, *The Dispossessed: Living with Multiple Chemical Sensitivities* (Paulden, AZ: The Dispossessed Outreach Project, 1999).

51. Chen, "Toxic Animacies, Inanimate Affections," 274.

52. Although their influence on this project is not limited to this section, I am deeply grateful to my colleagues in Generations Ahead (GA) for the ideas and actions discussed here, as well as to the disability and reproductive rights and justice activists who participated in the GA roundtables and convenings on disability. Thanks especially to Patty Berne, Julia Epstein, Anne Finger, Emily Galpern, Sujatha Jesudason, Jessica Lehman, Mia Mingus, Dorothy Roberts, Marsha Saxton, Tracy Weitz, and Silvia Yee.

53. Andrea Smith, "Beyond Pro-Choice versus Pro-Life: Women of Color and Reproductive Justice," *NWSA Journal* 17, no. 1 (2005): 120.

54. See, among others, Jennifer Nelson, *Women of Color and the Reproductive Rights Movement* (New York: New York University Press, 2003); Dorothy Roberts, *Killing the Black Body: Race, Reproduction, and the Meaning of Liberty* (New York: Vintage, 1999); Jael Silliman, Marlene Gerber Fried, Loretta Ross, and Elena R. Gutiérrez, *Undivided Rights: Women of Color Organize for Reproductive Justice* (Boston: South End Press, 2004); Rickie Solinger, *Beggars and Choosers: How the Politics of Choice Shapes Adoption, Abortion, and Welfare in the United States* (New York: Hill and Wang, 2001); and Rickie Solinger, *Pregnancy and Power: A Short History of Reproductive Politics in America* (New York: New York University Press, 2005).

55. Silliman et al., *Undivided Rights*, 4.

56. We saw how this limitation played out in the case of a Deaf lesbian couple in chapter 3. Marsha Saxton, "Disability Rights and Selective Abortion," in *Abortion Wars: A Half-Century of Struggle: 1950–2000*, ed. Rickie Solinger (Berkeley: University of California Press, 1998), 375. See also Laura Hershey, "Choosing Disability," *Ms.* (July/August 1994): 26–32; and Ruth Hubbard, "Abortion and Disability: Who Should and Who Should Not Inhabit the World?" in *The Disability Studies Reader*, ed. Lennard J. Davis (New York: Routledge, 2006): 93–103.

57. Shelley Tremain, "Reproductive Freedom, Self-Regulation, and the Government of Impairment in Utero," *Hypatia* 21, no. 1 (2006): 37.

58. Silliman et al., *Undivided Rights*, 22n36.

59. Smith makes this argument from the position of indigenous feminism and the need to challenge those pro-choice activists who have allied with population control groups; she singles out Planned Parenthood. Smith, "Beyond Pro-Choice versus Pro-Life," 132–33.

60. The organization Asian Communities for Reproductive Justice offers a particularly compelling definition of reproductive justice, one that easily encompasses attention to disability: "We believe Reproductive Justice exists when all people have the social, political and economic power and resources to make healthy decisions about our gender, bodies, sexuality and families for ourselves and our communities. Reproductive Justice aims to transform power inequities and create long-term systemic change, and therefore relies on the leadership of communities most impacted by reproductive oppression. The reproductive justice framework recognizes that all individuals are part of families and communities and that our strategies must lift up entire communities in order to support individuals." Asian Communities for Reproductive Justice, accessed December 14, 2010, http://reproductivejustice.org/what-is-reproductive-justice.

61. Examples would include attempts to ban race- and sex-selective abortions and billboards describing black children as "endangered species." Organizations such as SisterSong and Generations Ahead have posted responses to these kinds of campaigns on their websites.

62. For a feminist analysis of FFL and pro-life feminism, see Laury Oaks, "What Are Pro-Life Feminists Doing on Campus?" *NWSA Journal* 21, no. 1 (2009): 178–203.

63. See, for example, Generations Ahead, "Bridging the Divide: Disability Rights and Reproductive Rights and Justice Advocates Discussing Genetic Technologies," (2009), accessed March 8, 2010, http://www.generations-ahead.org/resources; and Saxton, "Disability Rights and Selective Abortion." Of course, even as they agreed with the poster's critical stance toward selective abortion, many disability activists and scholars would challenge the poster's positioning of disability as an adversity to be overcome.

64. Brian Skotko has conducted several studies asking women about the kind of information they received about disability, particularly Down syndrome, in conjunction with prenatal testing and genetic counseling. They report widespread dissatisfaction with both the content and the tone of the information they were given by their doctors. Brian Skotko, "Prenatally Diagnosed Down Syndrome: Mothers Who Continued Their Pregnancies Evaluate Their Health Care Providers," *American Journal of Obstetrics and Gynecology*192 (2005): 670–77.

65. For a description of Generation Ahead's work on the bill, see "Dodging Old Traps: Aligning, Affirming, and Addressing Disability Rights and Reproductive Autonomy," accessed August 19, 2011, http://www.generations-ahead.org/files-for-download/success-stories/K_Brownback_2011.pdf.

66. Edwards made this statement during his comments to the 1999 meetings of the European Society of Reproduction and Embryology. Lois Rogers, "Having Disabled Babies Will Be Sin, Says Scientist," *Sunday Times* (London), July 4, 1999.

67. For examples of pro-life/antiabortion criticisms that condemn Edwards's statements on disability, see Jenna Lyle, "Vatican Official Objects to IVF Scientist's Nobel Prize Win," *Christian Post*, October 5, 2010, http://www.christianpost.com/news/vatican-official-objects-to-ivf-scientists-nobel-prize-win-47083/; and "Pro-Life Group Objects to Nobel Honors for IVF Co-inventor," *Catholic News Agency*, October 5, 2010, http://www.catholicnewsagency.com/news/pro-life-group-objects-to-nobel-honors-for-ivf-co-inventor/.

68. Vanessa Allen, "Outrage as Agony Aunt Tells TV Audience 'I Would Suffocate a Child to End Its Suffering," *Daily Mail*, October 5, 2010, http://www.dailymail.co.uk/news/article-1317400/Virginia-Ironside-sparks-BBC-outrage-Id-suffocate-child-end-suffering.html.

69. During the television program, disability activist Clair Lewis called in to the show to challenge Ironside's comments, and she describes the encounter and her position in a blog post. See Clair Lewis, "Why I Called Virginia Ironside a Eugenicist on Live TV," *Heresy Corner*, October 5, 2010, http://heresycorner.blogspot.com/2010/10/why-i-called-virginia-ironside.html. In her column in the *Guardian*, Zoe Williams agreed with those condemning Ironside for her comments on euthanasia, but she defended Ironside's position on abortion and disability. See Zoe Williams, "Abortion and Euthanasia: Was Virginia Ironside Right?" *Guardian*, October 5, 2010, http://www.guardian.co.uk/world/2010/oct/04/virginia-ironside-tv-euthanasia-abortion.

70. Julia Epstein, Laura Hershey, Sujatha Jesudason, Dorothy Roberts, Silvia Yee, and I wrote the text collaboratively over email and the telephone. The statement remains active, and new signatories are still being added. "Robert Edwards, Virginia Ironside, and the Unnecessary Opposition of Rights," accessed October 15, 2010, http://www.generations-ahead.org/resources/the-unnecessary-opposition-of-rights.

71. We knew that such a clear statement was necessary because of the long history of disability being used not only to justify specific abortions but to make abortion in general more acceptable. Leslie Reagan describes the process by which middle-class, married, heterosexual white women talking publicly about their own desire for abortion in the wake of the german measles/rubella epidemic "made abortion respectable"; through their stories, abortion came to be seen as a potentially "ethical and responsible" decision. As mentioned in previous chapters, this dynamic is not new; Licia Carlson, among others, details how early twentieth-century feminists deployed eugenic rhetoric about the dangers of "feebleminded offspring" in their battle for women's reproductive rights. Carlson, *Faces of Intellectual Disability*, 175–76; Reagan, *Dangerous Pregnancies*, 104.

72. One of the motivations of this chapter is to honor and name that work. When someone at a feminist studies conference recently lamented to me that "no one is talking about the relationship between disability and abortion," I understood and shared her frustration; I had given a paper making that very point a few years earlier. Certainly on one level we were right—much more open and difficult dialogue is necessary, both within disability studies and beyond it. On another level, though, our concerns reveal an erasure of activist and intellectual histories. We need to gather the stories of those people, primarily but not exclusively disabled women, who pioneered this work.

73. See, for example, Adrienne Asch and Michelle Fine, "Shared Dreams: A Left Perspective on Disability Rights and Reproductive Rights," in *Women with Disabilities: Essays in Psychology, Culture, and Politics*, ed. Michelle Fine and Adrienne Asch (Philadelphia: Temple University Press, 1988): 297–305; Anne Finger, *Past Due: A Story of Disability, Pregnancy, and Birth* (Seattle: Seal Press, 1990); Dorothy Roberts, *Killing the Black Body: Race, Reproduction, and the Meaning of Liberty* (New York: Vintage, 1999); and Saxton, "Disability Rights and Selective Abortion."

74. Hubbard, "Abortion and Disability," 99, 101, 102.

75. Ibid., 102.

76. Asch and Fine, "Shared Dreams," 297.

77. Ibid., 298.

78. Adrienne Asch, "A Disability Equality Critique of Routine Testing and Embryo or Fetus Elimination Based on Disabling Traits," *Political Environments* 11 (2007): 43–47, 78.

79. Silliman et al., *Undivided Rights*, 22n36.

80. Jesudason is the founder and executive director of Generations Ahead. Sujatha Anbuselvi Jesudason, "In the Hot Tub: The Praxis of Building New Alliances for Reprogenetics," *Signs: Journal of Women in Culture and Society* 34, no. 4 (2009): 901–24.

81. Roberts, *Fatal Invention*, 301.

82. Roberts, *Fatal Invention*, 302–6. See also Eli Clare, preface to the 2009 South End Press Classics edition of *Exile and Pride: Disability, Queerness, and Liberation* (Boston: South End Press, 2009), xi.

83. Liat Ben-Moshe, "Disabling Incarceration: Connecting Disability to Divergent Confinements in the USA," *Critical Sociology* (2011): 1–19.

84. Robert McRuer, *Crip Theory: Cultural Signs of Queerness and Disability* (New York: New York University Press, 2006), 36, 57.

85. McRuer makes this point during his reading of Grace Chang's *Disposable Domestics*. Chang writes about immigrant women of color who populate domestic service jobs, such as home health workers, and McRuer urges disability studies scholars to recognize their stories as disability stories. As he explains, "[A] system that wants 'young and strong workers' is always haunted by disability, and the need for surplus profit ensures that a system that generates disability must immediately conjure it away when it appears." McRuer, *Crip Theory*, 204; see also 199–208.

86. For one description of the gaps between these two movements, and of the possibilities for bridging them, see Bob Kafka, "Disability Rights vs. Workers Rights: A Different Perspective," *Znet*, November 14, 2003, http://www.zcommunications.org/disability-rights-vs-workers-rights-a-different-perspective -by-bob-kafka.

Bibliography

Abbey, Edward. *Desert Solitaire: A Season in the Wilderness*. New York: Touchstone, 1990.

Abel, Elizabeth. "Bathroom Doors and Drinking Fountains: Jim Crow's Racial Symbolic." *Critical Inquiry* 25 (Spring 1999): 435–81.

Abod, Jennifer. *The Edge of Each Other's Battles: The Vision of Audre Lorde*. Long Beach, CA: Profile Productions, 2002. VHS.

Adams, Rachel. *Sideshow U.S.A.: Freaks and the American Cultural Imagination*. Chicago: University of Chicago Press, 2001.

Alaimo, Stacy. *Bodily Natures: Science, Environment, and the Material Self*. Bloomington: Indiana University Press, 2010.

———. "MCS Matters: Material Agency in the Science and Practices of Environmental Illness." *Topia: Canadian Journal of Cultural Studies* 21 (March 2009): 9–27.

———. *Undomesticated Ground: Recasting Nature as Feminist Space*. Ithaca: Cornell University Press, 2000.

Allen, David, Michael Kappy, Douglas Diekema, and Norman Fost. "Growth-Attenuation Therapy: Principles for Practice." *Pediatrics* 123, no. 6 (2009): 1556–61.

Allen, Vanessa. "Outrage as Agony Aunt Tells TV Audience 'I Would Suffocate a Child to End Its Suffering." *Daily Mail*. October 5, 2010. http://www.dailymail.co.uk/news/article-1317400/Virginia-Ironside-sparks-BBC-outrage-Id-suffocate-child-end-suffering.html.

Andrews, Lori B. *Future Perfect: Confronting Decisions about Genetics*. New York: Columbia University Press, 2001.

Anstey, K. W. "Are Attempts to Have Impaired Children Justifiable?" *Journal of Medical Ethics* 28 (2002): 286–89.

Anzaldúa, Gloria. "Disability and Identity." In *The Gloria Anzaldúa Reader*, ed. AnaLouise Keating, 298–302. Durham, NC: Duke University Press, 2009.

Asch, Adrienne. "Critical Race Theory, Feminism, and Disability: Reflections on Social Justice and Personal Identity." In *Gendering Disability*, ed. Bonnie G. Smith and Beth Hutchison, 9–44. New Brunswick, NJ: Rutgers University Press, 2004.

———. "A Disability Equality Critique of Routine Testing and Embryo or Fetus Elimination Based on Disabling Traits." *Political Environments* 11 (2007): 43–47, 78.

Asch, Adrienne, and Michelle Fine. "Shared Dreams: A Left Perspective on Disability Rights and Reproductive Rights." In *Women with Disabilities: Essays in Psychology, Culture, and Politics*, ed. Michelle Fine and Adrienne Asch, 297–305. Philadelphia: Temple University Press, 1988.

Asch, Adrienne, and Gail Geller. "Feminism, Bioethics, and Genetics." In *Feminism and Bioethics: Beyond Reproduction*, ed. Susan M. Wolf, 318–50. New York: Oxford University Press, 1996.

Asch, Adrienne, and Anna Stubblefield. "Growth Attenuation: Good Intentions, Bad Decision." *American Journal of Bioethics* 10, no. 1 (2010): 46–48.

Ashley's Mom and Dad. *The "Ashley Treatment": Towards a Better Quality of Life for "Pillow Angels."* March 25, 2007. Accessed from http://pillowangel.org/Ashley%20Treatment%20v7.pdf.

———. "Third Anniversary Update." January 13, 2010. Accessed from http://www.pillowangel. org/updates.htm.

———. "Updates on Ashley's Story." January 9, 2007. Accessed from http://www.pillowangel. org/updates.htm.

Ashley's Parents. "AT Summary." Last modified March 17, 2012. Accessed from http://pillowangel.org/AT-Summary.pdf.

Baker, Sherry. "The Rise of the Cyborgs." *Discover.* October 2008. http://discovermagazine. com/2008/oct/26-rise-of-the-cyborgs.

Bakhtin, Mikhail. *Rabelais and His World.* Trans. Helene Iswolsky. Bloomington, IN: Indiana University Press, 1984.

Balsamo, Anne. *Technologies of the Gendered Body: Reading Cyborg Women.* Durham, NC: Duke University Press, 1996.

Banks, Taunya Lovell. "Toilets as a Feminist Issue: A True Story." *Berkeley Women's Law Journal* (1990): 263–89.

Barnartt, Sharon N., and Richard K. Scotch. *Disability Protests: Contentious Politics, 1970–1999.* Washington, DC: Gallaudet University Press, 2001.

Bartsch, Ingrid, Carolyn DiPalma, and Laura Sells. "Witnessing the Postmodern Jeremiad: (Mis)Understanding Donna Haraway's Method of Inquiry." *Configurations* 9, no. 1 (Winter 2001): 127–64.

Bastian, Michelle. "Haraway's Lost Cyborg and the Possibilities of Transversalism." *Signs* 31, no. 4 (2006): 1027–49.

Bauman, H-Dirksen L. "Designing Deaf Babies and the Question of Disability." *Journal of Deaf Studies and Deaf Education* 10, no. 3 (2005): 311–15.

———., ed. *Open Your Eyes: Deaf Studies Talking.* Minneapolis: University of Minnesota Press, 2008.

Baynton, Douglas C. "Disability and the Justification of Inequality in American History." In *The New Disability History: American Perspectives*, ed. Paul K. Longmore and Lauri Umansky, 33–57. New York: New York University Press, 2001.

Bell, Chris. "Introducing White Disability Studies: A Modest Proposal." In *The Disability Studies Reader,* 2nd ed. 275–82. New York: Routledge, 2006.

Belluck, Pam. "Success of Spina Bifida Study Opens Fetal Surgery Door." *New York Times.* February 9, 2011.

Ben-Moshe, Liat. "Disabling Incarceration: Connecting Disability to Divergent Confinements in the USA." *Critical Sociology* (2011): 1–19.

———. "New Resistance to Old Power? Disablement and Global Anti-Incarceration Movements." Paper presented at the Society for Disability Studies Annual Meeting, Philadelphia, PA. June 4, 2010.

Ben-Moshe, Liat, and Justin Powell. "Sign of Our Times: Revis(it)ing the International Symbol of Access." *Disability and Society* 22, no. 5 (2007): 489–505.

Bergman, Barry. "Black, White, and Shades of Green." *Berkeleyan.* November 28, 2007. http:// berkeley.edu/news/berkeleyan/2007/11/28_finney.shtml.

Berlant, Lauren. *The Queen of America Goes to Washington City: Essays on Sex and Citizenship.* Durham, NC: Duke University Press, 1997.

Berrier, Justin. "Fox Hides Anti-Gay, Right-Wing Background of Foundation for a Better Life," *Media Matters,* December 16, 2010. http://mediamatters.org/blog/201012160022.

Bérubé, Michael. "Afterword: If I Should Live So Long." In *Disability Studies: Enabling the Humanities*, ed. Sharon Snyder, Brenda Brueggemann, and Rosemarie

Garland-Thomson, 337–43. New York: The Modern Language Association of America, 2002.

———. "Term Paper." *Profession* (2010): 112–16.

Betcher, Sharon. "Putting my Foot (Prosthesis, Crutches, Phantom) Down: Considering Technology as Transcendence in the Writings of Donna Haraway." *Women's Studies Quarterly* 29, nos. 3–4 (2001): 35–53.

Bhatia, Rajani. "Constructing Gender from the Inside Out: Sex Selection Practices in the United States." *Feminist Studies* 36, no. 2 (2010): 260–91.

Bhavnani, Kum-Kum, and Donna Haraway. "Shifting the Subject: A Conversation between Kum-Kum Bhavnani and Donna Haraway, 12 April 1993, Santa Cruz, California." *Feminism and Psychology* 4, no. 1 (1994): 19–39.

Bienvenu, MJ. "Queer as Deaf: Intersections." In *Open Your Eyes: Deaf Studies Talking*, ed. H-Dirksen Bauman, 264–73. Minneapolis: University of Minnesota Press, 2008.

Blaser, Art. "Awareness Days: Some Alternatives to Simulation Exercises." *Ragged Edge Online*, September/October 2003. Accessed from http://www.raggededgemagazine.com/0903/0903ft1.html.

Blumberg, Lisa. "Public Stripping." In *The Ragged Edge: The Disability Experience from the Pages of the First Fifteen Years of the Disability Rag*, ed. Barrett Shaw, 77–81. Louisville, KY: Advocado Press, 1994.

Boellstorff, Tom. "When Marriage Fails: Queer Coincidences in Straight Time." *GLQ* 13, nos. 2–3 (2007): 227–48.

Bogdan, Robert. *Freak Show: Presenting Human Oddities for Amusement and Profit*. Chicago: University of Chicago Press, 1988.

Boggan, Steve, and Glenda Cooper. "Nobel Winner May Sue over Gay Baby Abortion Claim." *Independent* (UK). February 17, 1997. http://www.independent.co.uk/news/nobel-winner-may-sue-over-gay-baby-abortion-claim-1279127.html.

Boris, Eileen, and Rhacel Salazar Parreñas, eds. *Intimate Labors: Cultures, Technologies, and the Politics of Care*. Stanford, CA: Stanford University Press, 2010.

Bornstein, Kate. *Gender Outlaw: On Men, Women, and the Rest of Us*. New York: Vintage, 1995.

Bowley, Graham. "Goal! He Spends It on Beckham." *New York Times*. April 22, 2007.

Brahm, Gabriel, Jr. Introduction to *Prosthetic Territories: Politics and Hypertechnologies*, ed. Gabriel Brahm, Jr., and Mark Driscoll, 1–2. Boulder: Westview, 1995.

Bricker, Jennie. "Wheelchair Accessibility in Wilderness Areas: The Nexus Between the ADA and the Wilderness Act." *Environmental Law* 25, no. 4 (1995): 1243–70.

Browne, Kath. "Genderism and the Bathroom Problem: (Re)Materialising Sexed Sites, (Re)Creating Sexed Bodies." *Gender, Place and Culture* 11, no. 3 (2004): 331–46.

Brueggemann, Brenda. *Deaf Subjects: Between Identities and Places*. New York: New York University Press, 2009.

———. *Lend Me Your Ear: Rhetorical Constructions of Deafness*. Washington, DC: Gallaudet University Press, 1999.

Brunson, Jeremy L., and Mitchell E. Loeb, eds. "Mediated Communication." Special issue. *DSQ: Disability Studies Quarterly* 31, no. 4 (2011).

Buchanan, Robert M. *Illusions of Equality: Deaf Americans in School and Factory, 1850–1950*. Washington, DC: Gallaudet University Press, 1999.

Burch, Susan. *Signs of Resistance: American Deaf Cultural History, 1900 to World War II*. New York: New York University Press, 2002.

Burch, Susan, and Hannah Joyner. *Unspeakable: The Story of Junius Wilson*. Chapel Hill: University of North Carolina Press, 2007.

Burch, Susan, and Alison Kafer, eds. *Deaf and Disability Studies: Interdisciplinary Perspectives*. Washington, DC: Gallaudet University Press, 2010.

Burkholder, Amy. "Disabled Girl's Parents Defend Growth-Stunting Treatment." *CNN.com*. March 12, 2008.

———. "Ethicist in Ashley Case Answers Questions." *CNN.com*. January 11, 2007.

Butler, Judith. *Bodies That Matter: On the Discursive Limits of "Sex."* New York: Routledge, 1993.

———. "Contingent Foundations." In *Feminist Contentions: A Philosophical Exchange*, ed. Seyla Benhabib, Judith Butler, Drucilla Cornell, and Nancy Fraser, 35–57. New York: Routledge, 1995.

———. *Gender Trouble: Feminism and the Subversion of Identity*. 10th anniversary ed. New York: Routledge, 1999.

———. *Undoing Gender*. New York: Routledge, 2004.

Byrne, Jason, and Jennifer Wolch. "Nature, Race, and Parks: Past Research and Future Directions for Geographic Research." *Progress in Human Geography* 33, no. 6 (2009): 743–65.

Callahan, Nathan. "Corporate Vulture: Philip Anschutz Tries to Thread His Way into Heaven." *OC Weekly* 8, no. 35 (2003). http://www.ocweekly.com/ink/03/35/news-callahan.php.

Campbell, Fiona Kumari. *Contours of Ableism: The Production of Disability and Abledness*. New York: Palgrave Macmillan, 2009.

Cangemi, Phyllis. "Trail Design: Balancing Accessibility and Nature." *Universal Design Newsletter*. July 1999.

Carlson, David, and Deborah Dorfman. "Full Report—Investigative Report Regarding the 'Ashley Treatment.'" Washington Protection and Advocacy System. May 8, 2007. Accessed from http://www.disabilityrightswa.org/home/Full_Report_InvestigativeReportRegardingtheAshleyTreatment.pdf.

Carlson, Licia. "Cognitive Ableism and Disability Studies: Feminist Reflections on the History of Mental Retardation." *Hypatia* 16, no. 4 (2001): 128–33.

———. *The Faces of Intellectual Disability*. Bloomington: Indiana University Press, 2010.

Case, Mary Anne. "Changing Room? A Quick Tour of Men's and Women's Rooms in U.S. Law over the Last Decade, from the U.S. Constitution to Local Ordinances." *Public Culture* 13, no. 2 (2001): 333–36.

Casper, Monica J. "Fetal Cyborgs and Technomoms on the Reproductive Frontier: Which Way to the Carnival?" In *The Cyborg Handbook*, ed. Chris Hables Gray, Steven Mentor, and Heidi J. Figueroa-Sarriera, 183–202. New York: Routledge, 1995.

Casper, Monica J., and Lisa Jean Moore. *Missing Bodies: The Politics of Visibility*. New York: New York University Press, 2009.

Cassuto, Leonard. *The Inhuman Race: The Racial Grotesque in American Literature and Culture*. New York: Columbia University Press, 1997.

Cavanagh, Sheila L. *Queering Bathrooms: Gender, Sexuality, and the Hygienic Imagination*. Toronto: University of Toronto Press, 2010.

Chandler, Eliza. "Sidewalk Stories: The Troubling Task of Identification." *Disability Studies Quarterly* 30, nos. 3–4 (2010). Accessed from http://www.dsq-sds.org/article/view/1293/1329.

Charles, Andrew, and Huw Thomas. "Deafness and Disability—Forgotten Components of Environmental Justice: Illustrated by the Case of Local Agenda 21 in South Wales." *Local Environment* 12, no. 3 (June 2007): 209–21.

Charo, R. Alta, and Karen H. Rothenberg, "'The Good Mother': The Limits of Reproductive Accountability and Genetic Choice." In *Women and Prenatal Testing: Facing the Challenges of Genetic Technology*, ed. Karen H. Rothenberg and Elizabeth J. Thomson, 105–30. Columbus: Ohio State University Press, 1994.

Chen, Mel Y. *Animacies*. Durham, NC: Duke University Press, forthcoming.

———. "Racialized Toxins and Sovereign Fantasies." *Discourse* 29, nos. 2–3 (2007): 367–83.

———. "Toxic Animacies, Inanimate Affections." *GLQ: A Journal of Lesbian and Gay Studies* 17, nos. 2–3 (2011): 265–86.

Cherney, James L. "Deaf Culture and the Cochlear Implant Debate: Cyborg Politics and the Identity of People with Disabilities." *Argumentation and Advocacy* 36 (Summer 1999): 22–34.

Chess, Simone, Alison Kafer, Jessi Quizar, and Mattie Udora Richardson. "Calling All Restroom Revolutionaries!" In *That's Revolting! Queer Strategies for Resisting Assimilation*, ed. Matt Bernstein Sycamore, 189–206. New York: Soft Skull, 2004.

Cheu, Johnson. "De-gene-erates, Replicants, and Other Aliens: (Re)Defining Disability in Futuristic Film." In *Disability/Postmodernity: Embodying Disability Theory*, ed. Mairian Corker and Tom Shakespeare, 199–212. New York: Continuum, 2002.

Chorost, Michael. *Rebuilt: My Journey Back to the Hearing World*. Boston: Mariner, 2005.

Clare, Eli. *Exile and Pride: Disability, Queerness, and Liberation*. Boston: South End Press, 1999.

———. "Stolen Bodies, Reclaimed Bodies: Disability and Queerness." *Public Culture* 13, no. 3 (2001): 359–65.

Clark, David L., and Catherine Myser. "Being Humaned: Medical Documentaries and the Hyperrealization of Conjoined Twins." In *Freakery: Cultural Spectacles of the Extraordinary Body*, ed. Rosemarie Garland-Thomson, 338–55. New York: New York University Press, 1996.

Clarren, Rebecca. "Behind the Pillow Angel." *Salon*. February 9, 2007. Accessed from http://www.salon.com/news/feature/2007/02/09/pillow_angel/index.html.

Clynes, Manfred E., and Nathan S. Kline. "Cyborgs and Space." In *The Cyborg Handbook*, ed. Chris Hables Gray, Steven Mentor, and Heidi J. Figueroa-Sarriera, 29–33. New York: Routledge, 1995.

Cohen, Cathy. "Punks, Bulldaggers, and Welfare Queens: The Radical Potential of Queer Politics?" In *Black Queer Studies: A Critical* Anthology, ed. E Patrick Johnson and Mae G. Henderson, 21–51. Durham, NC: Duke University Press, 2005.

Cohen, Ed, and Julie Livingston. "AIDS." *Social Text* 27, no. 3 (2009): 39–42.

Cooley, Reed. "Disabling Spectacles: Representations of Trig Palin and Cognitive Disability." *Journal of Literary and Cultural Disability Studies* 5, no. 3 (2011): 303–20.

Cooper, Patricia, and Ruth Oldenziel. "Cherished Classifications: Bathrooms and the Construction of Gender/Race on the Pennsylvania Railroad during World War II." *Feminist Studies* 25, no. 1 (1999): 7–41.

Cornachio, Donna. "Changes in Mental Care." *New York Times*. January 3, 1999.

Crenshaw, Kimberlé. "Mapping the Margins: Intersectionality, Identity Politics, and Violence against Women of Color." *Stanford Law Review* 43 (July 1991): 1241–65.

Crewe, Jonathan. "Transcoding the World: Haraway's Postmodernism." *Signs* 22, no. 4 (Summer 1997): 891–905.

Cronon, William. "Introduction: In Search of Nature." In *Uncommon Ground: Toward Reinventing Nature*, ed. William Cronon, 23–65. New York: W. W. Norton, 1995.

———. "The Trouble with Wilderness; or, Getting Back to the Wrong Nature." In *Uncommon Ground: Toward Reinventing Nature*, ed. William Cronon, 69–90. New York: W. W. Norton, 1995.

Crosby, Christina. "Allies and Enemies." In *Coming to Terms: Feminism, Theory, Politics*, ed. Elizabeth Weed, 205–8. New York: Routledge, 1989.

Crow, Liz. "Including All of Our Lives: Renewing the Social Model of Disability." In *Encounters with Strangers: Feminism and Disability*, ed. Jenny Morris, 206–26. London: The Women's Press, 1996.

Cuomo, Chris J. *Feminism and Ecological Communities: An Ethics of Flourishing*. New York: Routledge, 1998.

Cummings, Cecilia. "Rockland Psychiatric Center Faulted in a Death." *New York Times*. July 17, 1988.

Cvetkovich, Ann. *An Archive of Feelings: Trauma, Sexuality, and Lesbian Public Cultures*. Durham, NC: Duke University Press, 2003.

Dailey, Timothy J. "Homosexual Parenting: Placing Children at Risk." *Insight* 238, www.frc.org.

Daniels, Cynthia. *Exposing Men: The Science and Politics of Male Reproduction*. New York: Oxford University Press, 2006.

Darnovsky, Marcy. "Overhauling the Meaning Machines: An Interview with Donna Haraway." *Socialist Review* 21, no. 2 (1991): 65–84.

Davis, Alison. "Women with Disabilities: Abortion and Liberation." *Disability, Handicap and Society* 2, no. 3 (September 1987): 275–84.

Davis, Dena S. *Genetic Dilemmas: Reproductive Technology, Parental Choices, and Children's Futures*. New York: Routledge, 2001.

Davis, Kathy. "'My Body Is My Art': Cosmetic Surgery as Feminist Utopia?" In *Embodied Practices: Feminist Perspectives on the Body*, ed. Kathy Davis, 168–81. Thousand Oaks, CA: Sage, 1997.

Davis, Lennard J. *Bending Over Backwards: Disability, Dismodernism, and Other Difficult Positions*. New York: New York University Press, 2002.

———. *Enforcing Normalcy: Disability, Deafness, and the Body*. New York: Verso, 1995.

———. *My Sense of Silence: Memoirs of a Childhood with Deafness*. Champaign: University of Illinois Press, 2000.

———. "Postdeafness." In *Open Your Eyes: Deaf Studies Talking*, ed. H-Dirksen Bauman, 314–25. Minneapolis: University of Minnesota Press, 2008.

Dawkins, Richard. "Letter: Women to Decide on Gay Abortion." *Independent* (UK). February 19, 1997. http://www.independent.co.uk/opinion/letter-women-to-decide-on-gay-abortion-1279433.html.

Dean, Jodi. "Introduction: The Interface of Political Theory and Cultural Studies." In *Cultural Studies and Political Theory*, ed. Jodi Dean, 1–19. Ithaca, NY: Cornell University Press, 2000.

DeKoven, Marianne. "*Jouissance*, Cyborgs, and Companion Species: Feminist Experiment." *PMLA* 121, no. 5 (2006): 1690–96.

Di Chiro, Giovanna. "Living Environmentalisms: Coalition Politics, Social Reproduction, and Environmental Justice." *Environmental Politics* 17, no. 2 (2008): 276–98.

———. "Nature as Community: The Convergence of Environment and Social Justice." In *Uncommon Ground: Toward Reinventing Nature*, ed. William Cronon, 298–319. New York: W. W. Norton, 1995.

———. "Polluted Politics? Confronting Toxic Discourse, Sex Panic, and Eco-Normativity." In *Queer Ecologies: Sex, Nature, Politics, Desire*, ed. Catriona Mortimer-Sandilands and Bruce Erickson, 199–230. Bloomington: Indiana University Press, 2010.

———. "Producing 'Roundup Ready®' Communities? Human Genome Research and Environmental Justice Policy." In *New Perspectives on Environmental Justice: Gender, Sexuality, and Activism*, ed. Rachel Stein, 139–60. New Brunswick, NJ: Rutgers University Press, 2004.

Diekema, Douglas S., and Norman Fost. "Ashley Revisited: A Response to the Critics." *American Journal of Bioethics* 10, no. 1 (2010): 30–44.

Dinshaw, Carolyn, et al. "Theorizing Queer Temporalities: A Roundtable Discussion." *GLQ: A Journal of Gay and Lesbian Studies* 13, nos. 2–3 (2007): 177–95.

Donaldson, Elizabeth J. "Revisiting the Corpus of the Madwoman: Further Notes toward a Feminist Disability Studies Theory of Mental Illness." In *Feminist Disability Studies*, ed. Kim Q. Hall, 91–113. Bloomington: Indiana University Press, 2011.

Dorn, Michael. "Beyond Nomadism: The Travel Narratives of a 'Cripple.'" In *Places Through the Body*, ed. Heidi J. Nast and Steve Pile, 183–206. New York: Routledge, 1998.

Douglas, Mary. *Purity and Danger: An Analysis of Concepts of Pollution and Taboo*. London: Routledge, 2002.

Dugdale, Richard L. "Hereditary Pauperism as Illustrated in the 'Juke' Family." In *White Trash: The Eugenic Family Studies, 1877–1919*, ed. Nicole Hahn Rafter, 33–47. Boston: Northeastern University Press, 1988.

Dutton, Denis. "What Are Editors For." *Philosophy and Literature* 20 (1996): 551–66. Accessed from http://www.denisdutton.com/what_are_editors_for.htm.

Dvorsky, George. "Helping Families Care for the Helpless." Institute for Ethics and Emerging Technologies. November 6, 2006. http://ieet.org/index.php/IEET/more/809/.

Edelman, Lee. *No Future: Queer Theory and the Death Drive*. Durham, NC: Duke University Press, 2004.

Edwards, Julia, and Linda McKie. "Women's Public Toilets: A Serious Issue for the Body Politic." In *Embodied Practices: Feminist Perspectives on the Body*, ed. Kathy Davis, 135–49. London: Sage, 1997.

Elliott, Stuart. "A Campaign Promotes Noble Behavior." *New York Times*. November 9, 2001.

Enke, Anne. *Finding the Movement: Sexuality, Contested Space, and Feminist Activism*. Durham, NC: Duke University Press, 2007.

Erevelles, Nirmala. *Disability and Difference in Global Contexts: Enabling a Transformative Body Politic*. New York: Palgrave Macmillan, 2011.

———. "In Search of the Disabled Subject." In *Embodied Rhetorics: Disability in Language and Culture*, ed. James C. Wilson and Cynthia Lewiecki-Wilson, 92–111. Carbondale: Southern Illinois University Press, 2001.

———. "Signs of Reason: Rivière, Facilitated Communication, and the Crisis of the Subject." In *Foucault and the Government of Disability*, ed. Shelley Tremain, 45–64. Ann Arbor: University of Michigan Press, 2005.

Erevelles, Nirmala, and Andrea Minear. "Unspeakable Offenses: Untangling Race and Disability in Discourses of Intersectionality." *Journal of Literary and Cultural Disability Studies* 4, no. 2 (2010): 127–45.

Erickson, Loree. "Revealing Femmegimp: A Sex Positive Relection on Sites of Shame as Sites of Resistance for People with Disabilities." *Atlantis* 31, no. 2 (2007): 42–52.

———. *Want*. Toronto: Femmegimp Productions, 2006. DVD.

Ervin, Mike. "Jerry Lewis Doesn't Deserve a Humanitarian Award at the Oscars." *Progressive* (Madison, WI). February 19, 2009. http://tinyurl.com/awlyn5.

Evans, Mei Mei. "'Nature' and Environmental Justice." In *The Environmental Justice Reader: Politics, Poetics, and Pedagogy*, ed. Joni Adamson, Mei Mei Evans, and Rachel Stein, 181–93. Tucson: University of Arizona Press, 2002.

Family Research Council. "*Washington Post* Profiles Lesbian Couple Seeking to Manufacture a Deaf Child." PR Newswire Association, Inc. April 1, 2002.

Ferri, Beth A., and David O'Connor. *Reading Resistance: Discourses of Exclusion in Desegregation and Exclusion Debates*. New York: Peter Lang, 2006.

Ferris, Jim, ed. "In (Disability) Time." *DSQ: Disability Studies Quarterly* 30, nos. 3–4 (2010).

Fiedler, Leslie. *Freaks: Myths and Images of the Secret Self*. New York: Simon and Schuster, 1978.

Finger, Anne. "Hurricane Katrina, Race, Class, Tragedy, and Charity." *DSQ: Disability Studies Quarterly* 25, no. 4 (2005). Accessed from http://www.dsq-sds.org/article/view/630/807.

———. *Past Due: A Story of Disability, Pregnancy, and Birth*. Seattle: Seal Press, 1990.

Fleischer, Doris Zames, and Frieda Zames. *The Disability Rights Movement: From Charity to Confrontation*. Philadelphia: Temple University Press, 2001.

Fost, Norman. "Offense to Third Parties?" *Hastings Center Report* 40, no. 6 (2010): 30.

Franklin, Sarah. "Essentialism, Which Essentialism? Some Implications of Reproductive and Genetic Technoscience." In *If You Seduce a Straight Person, Can You Make Them Gay? Issues in Biological Essentialism versus Social Constructionism in Gay and Lesbian Identities*, ed. John P. DeCecco and John P. Elia, 27–40. Binghamton, NY: Harrington Park, 1993.

Freccero, Carla. "Fuck the Future." *GLQ: A Journal of Gay and Lesbian Studies* 12, no. 2 (2006): 332–34.

Freeman, Elizabeth. Introduction to "Queer Temporalities." Special issue. *GLQ: A Journal of Gay and Lesbian Studies*, 13 nos. 2–3 (2007): 159–76.

———. *Time Binds: Queer Temporalities, Queer Histories*. Durham, NC: Duke University Press, 2010.

Fries, Kenny. *The History of My Shoes and the Evolution of Darwin's Theory*. New York: Carroll & Graf, 2007.

"'Frozen Girl' Debate." BBC News. January 4, 2007. http://news.bbc.co.uk/2/hi/6230045.stm;

Gaard, Greta. "Ecofeminism and Wilderness." *Environmental Ethics* 19, no. 1 (1997): 5–24.

———. "Living Interconnections with Animals and Nature." In *Ecofeminism: Women, Animals, Nature*, ed. Greta Gaard, 1–12. Philadelphia: Temple University Press, 1993.

———. "Toward a Queer Ecofeminism." *Hypatia* 12, no. 1 (1997): 114–37.

Gagliardi, Barbara. "West Coast Women's Music Festival." *Big Mama Rag* 9, no. 10 (1981): 3, 22.

Garland-Thomson, Rosemarie. "The Cultural Logic of Euthanasia: 'Sad Fancyings' in Herman Melville's 'Bartleby.'" *American Literature* 76, no. 4 (2004): 777–806.

———. *Extraordinary Bodies: Figuring Physical Disability in American Culture and Literature*. New York: Columbia University Press, 1997.

———, ed. *Freakery: Cultural Spectacles of the Extraordinary Body*. New York: New York University Press, 1996.

———. "Integrating Disability, Transforming Feminist Theory." In *Gendering Disability*, ed. Bonnie G. Smith and Beth Hutchison, 73–103. New Brunswick, NJ: Rutgers University Press, 2004.

———. "The Politics of Staring: Visual Rhetorics of Disability in Popular Photography." In *Disability Studies: Enabling the Humanities*, ed. Sharon L. Snyder, Brenda Jo Brueggemann, and Rosemarie Garland-Thomson, 56–75. New York: Modern Language Association, 2002.

———. "Seeing the Disabled: Visual Rhetorics of Disability in Popular Photography." In *The New Disability History: American Perspectives*, ed. Paul K. Longmore and Lauri Umansky, 335–74. New York: New York University Press, 2001.

———. *Staring: How We Look*. New York: Oxford University Press, 2009.

———. "Welcoming the Unbidden: The Case for Preserving Human Biodiversity." In *What Democracy Looks Like: A New Critical Realism for a Post-Seattle World*, ed. Amy Shrager Lang and Cecelia Tichi, 77–87. New Brunswick, NJ: Rutgers University Press, 2006.

Garver, Kenneth L., and Bettylee Garver. "The Human Genome Project and Eugenic Concerns." *American Journal of Human Genetics* 54 (1994): 148–58.

Generations Ahead. *Bridging the Divide: Disability Rights and Reproductive Rights and Justice Advocates Discussing Genetic Technologies*. 2009. http://www.generations-ahead.org/resources.

———. *A Disability Rights Analysis of Genetic Technologies: Report on a Convening of Disability Rights Leaders*. 2010. http://www.generations-ahead.org/resources.

Gershenson, Olga. "The Restroom Revolution: Unisex Toilets and Campus Politics." In *Toilet: Public Restrooms and the Politics of Sharing*, ed. Harvey Molotch and Laura Norén, 191–207. New York: New York University Press, 2010.

Gershenson, Olga, and Barbara Penner, eds. *Ladies and Gents: Public Toilets and Gender*. Philadelphia: Temple University Press, 2009.

Gerson, Michael. "The Eugenics Temptation." *Washington Post*. October 24, 2007, A19.

Gibson, Barbara E. "Disability, Connectivity, and Transgressing the Autonomous Body." *Journal of Medical Humanities* 27 (2006): 187–96.

Gill, Carol. "Cultivating Common Ground: Women with Disabilities." In *Manmade Medicine: Women's Health, Public Policy, and Reform*, ed. K. L. Moss, 183–93. Durham, NC: Duke University Press, 1996.

———. "A Psychological View of Disability Culture." *DSQ: Disability Studies Quarterly* 15, no. 4 (1995): 16–19.

Gilmore, Stephanie. *Feminist Coalitions: Historical Perspectives on Second-Wave Feminism in the United States*. Urbana: University of Illinois Press, 2008.

Gleeson, B. J. "Disability Studies: A Historical Materialist View" *Disability and Society* 12, no. 2 (1997): 179–202.

Glenn, Evelyn Nakano. *Forced to Care: Coercion and Caregiving in America*. Cambridge, MA: Harvard University Press, 2010.

Glorie, Josephine Carubia. "Feminist Utopian Fiction and the Possibility of Social Critique." In *Political Science Fiction*, ed. Donald M. Hassler and Clyde Wilcox, 148–59. Columbia: University of South Carolina Press, 1997.

Goering, Sara. "Revisiting the Relevance of the Social Model of Disability." *American Journal of Bioethics* 10, no. 1 (2010): 54–55.

Gonzalez, Jennifer. "Envisioning Cyborg Bodies: Notes from Current Research." In *The Gendered Cyborg: A Reader*, ed. Gill Kirkup, Linda Janes, Kath Woodward, and Fiona Hovenden, 58–73. London: Routledge, 2000.

Gopinath, Gayatri. *Impossible Desires: Queer Diasporas and South Asian Public Cultures*. Durham, NC: Duke University Press, 2005.

Gough, Annette. "Body/Mine: A Chaos Narrative of Cyborg Subjectivities and Liminal Experiences." *Women's Studies* 34, nos. 3–4 (2005): 249–64.

Gray, Chris Hables. *Cyborg Citizen: Politics in the Posthuman Age.* New York: Routledge, 2001.
———. "An Interview with Manfred Clynes." In *The Cyborg Handbook*, ed. Chris Hables Gray, Heidi J. Figueroa-Sarriera, and Steven Mentor, 43–53. New York: Routledge, 1995.
Gray, Chris Hables, and Steven Mentor. "The Cyborg Body Politic and the New World Order." In *Prosthetic Territories: Politics and Hypertechnologies*, ed. Gabriel Brahm, Jr., and Mark Driscoll, 219–47. Boulder, CO: Westview, 1995.
Gray, Chris Hables, Steven Mentor, and Heidi J. Figueroa-Sarriera, eds. *The Cyborg Handbook*. New York: Routledge, 1995.
———. "Cyborgology: Constructing the Knowledge of Cybernetic Organisms." In *The Cyborg Handbook*, ed. Chris Hables Gray, Heidi J. Figueroa-Sarriera, and Steven Mentor, 1–14. New York: Routledge, 1995.
Greely, Henry T. "Health Insurance, Employment Discrimination, and the Genetics Revolution." In *The Code of Codes: Scientific and Social Issues in the Human Genome Project*, ed. Daniel J. Kevles and Leroy Hood, 264–80. Cambridge, MA: Harvard University Press, 1992.
Groce, Nora Ellen. *Everyone Here Spoke Sign Language: Hereditary Deafness on Martha's Vineyard*. Cambridge, MA: Harvard University Press, 1985.
Groce, Nora Ellen, and Jonathan Marks. "The Great Ape Project and Disability Rights: Ominous Undercurrents of Eugenics in Action." *American Anthropologist* 102, no. 4 (2001): 818–22.
Grodin, Michael, and Harlan Lane. "Ethical Issues in Cochlear Implant Surgery: An Exploration into Disease, Disability, and the Best Interests of the Child." *Kennedy Institute of Ethics Journal* 7, no. 3 (1997): 231–51.
Grossmann, John. "Expanding the Palette." *National Parks,* Summer 2010. http://www.npca.org/magazine/2010/summer/expanding-the-palette.html.
Gunther, D. F., and D. S. Diekema. "Attenuating Growth in Children with Profound Developmental Disability: A New Approach to an Old Dilemma." *Archives of Pediatrics and Adolescent Medicine* 160, no. 10 (2006): 1013–17.
———. Letter in reply to Carole Marcus, "Only Half of the Story." *Archives of Pediatrics and Adolescent Medicine* 161 (June 2007): 616.
Gupte, Pranay. "Tranquilizing Held a Factor in Deaths of Mental Patient." *New York Times.* July 17, 1978.
Gutiérrez, Elena R. *Fertile Matters: The Politics of Mexican-Origin Women's Reproduction.* Austin: University of Texas Press, 2008.
Hakim, Danny. "At State-Run Homes, Abuse, and Impunity." *New York Times.* March 12, 2011.
Halberstam, Judith. *In a Queer Time and Place: Transgender Bodies, Subcultural Lives.* New York: New York University Press, 2005.
Halperin, David M. *Saint Foucault: Toward a Gay Hagiography.* New York: Oxford University Press, 1995.
Hamilton, Sheryl N. "The Cyborg, Eleven Years Later: The Not-So-Surprising Half-Life of the Cyborg Manifesto." *Convergence* 3, no. 2 (1997): 104–20.
Haraway, Donna J. "The Actors Are Cyborg, Nature Is Coyote, and the Geography Is Elsewhere: Postscript to 'Cyborgs at Large.'" In *Technoculture*, ed. Constance Penley and Andrew Ross, 21–26. Minneapolis: University of Minnesota Press, 1991.
———. "Cyborgs, Coyotes, and Dogs: A Kinship of Feminist Figurations: An Interview with Nina Lykke, Randi Markussen, and Finn Olesen." In *The Haraway Reader*, ed. Donna Haraway, 321–42. New York: Routledge, 2004.

———. "Cyborgs and Symbionts: Living Together in the New World Order." In *The Cyborg Handbook*, ed. Chris Hables Gray, Steven Mentor, and Heidi J. Figueroa-Sarriera, xi–xx. New York: Routledge, 1995.

———. *How Like a Leaf: An Interview with Thyrza Nichols Goodeve*. New York: Routledge, 2000.

———. "Introduction: A Kinship of Feminist Figurations." In *The Haraway Reader*, ed. Donna Haraway, 1–6. New York: Routledge, 2004.

———. "A Manifesto for Cyborgs: Science, Technology, and Socialist Feminism in the 1980s." *Socialist Review*, no. 80 (1985): 65–108.

———. *Modest_Witness@Second_Millennium.FemaleMan©_Meets_OncoMouse™: Feminism and Technoscience*. New York: Routledge, 1997.

———. "The Promises of Monsters: A Regenerative Politics for Inappropriate/d Others." In *Cultural Studies*, ed. Lawrence Grossberg, Cary Nelson, and Paula A. Treichler, 295–337. New York: Routledge, 1992.

———. *Simians, Cyborgs, and Women: The Reinvention of Nature*. New York: Routledge, 1991.

Harmon, Kristen. "Deaf Matters: Compulsory Hearing and Ability Trouble." In *Deaf and Disability Studies: Interdisciplinary Perspectives*, ed. Susan Burch and Alison Kafer, 31–47. Washington, DC: Gallaudet University Press, 2010.

Hart, George. "'Enough Defined': Disability, Ecopoetics, and Larry Eigner." *Contemporary Literature* 51, no. 1 (2010): 152–79.

Hasian, Marouf Arif, Jr. *The Rhetoric of Eugenics in Anglo-American Thought*. Athens: University of Georgia, 1996.

Hayles, N. Katherine. "The Life Cycle of Cyborgs: Writing the Posthuman." In *The Cyborg Handbook*, ed. Chris Hables Gray, Steven Mentor, and Heidi J. Figueroa-Sarriera, 321–35. New York: Routledge, 1995.

Heller, Chaia. "For the Love of Nature: Ecology and the Cult of the Romantic." In *Ecofeminism: Women, Animals, Nature*, ed. Greta Gaard, 219–42. Philadelphia: Temple University Press, 1993.

"Herded Like Cattle." *Time*. December 20, 1948. http://www.time.com/time/magazine/article/0,9171,799558-1,00.html.

Herndl, Diane Price. "Reconstructing the Posthuman Body Twenty Years after Audre Lorde's *Cancer Journals*." In *Disability Studies: Enabling the Humanities*, ed. Sharon L. Snyder, Brenda Jo Brueggemann, and Rosemarie Garland-Thomson, 144–55. New York: Modern Language Association, 2002.

Hershey, Laura. "Choosing Disability." *Ms.* July/August 1994, 26–32.

———. "Crip Commentary." http://www.cripcommentary.com/LewisVsDisabilityRights.html.

———. "Disabled Woman's Lawsuit Exposes Prejudices." *The Ragged Edge*. Accessed from http://www.raggededgemagazine.com/extra/hersheychamberstrial.html.

———. "From Poster Child to Protestor." *Spectacle* (Spring/Summer 1997). The Independent Living Institute. http://www.independentliving.org/docs4/hershey93.html.

———. *Just Help*. Unpublished manuscript, last modified September 24, 2009. Microsoft Word file.

———. "Stunting Ashley." *off our backs* 37, no. 1 (2007): 8–11.

Higgins, A. J. "Canoe Launch Divides Environmentalists, Disabled." *Boston Globe*. June 4, 2000, C1.

Hoffmeister, Robert. "Border Crossings by Hearing Children of Deaf Parents: The Lost History of Codas." In *Open Your Eyes: Deaf Studies Talking*, ed. H-Dirksen L. Bauman, 189–215. Minneapolis: University of Minnesota Press, 2008.

Hood, Leroy. "Biology and Medicine in the Twenty-First Century." In *The Code of Codes: Scientific and Social Issues in the Human Genome Project*, ed. Daniel J. Kevles and Leroy Hood, 136–163. Cambridge, MA: Harvard University Press, 1992.

Horton, Sarah, and Judith C. Barker. "'Stains' on Their Self-Discipline: Public Health, Hygeine, and the Disciplining of Undocumented Immigrant Parents in the Nation's Borderlands." *American Ethnologist* 36, no. 4 (2009): 784–98.

Hubbard, Ruth. "Abortion and Disability: Who Should and Who Should Not Inhabit the World?" In *The Disability Studies Reader*, ed. Lennard J. Davis, 93–103. New York: Routledge, 2006.

Huber, Joe. "Accessibility vs. Wilderness Preservation—Maine's Allagash Wilderness Waterway." *Palaestra: Forum of Sport, Physical Education, and Recreation for Those with Disabilities* 16, no. 4 (2000): 23–29.

———. "Trailblazing in a Wheelchair: An Oxymoron?" *Palaestra: Forum of Sport, Physical Education, and Recreation for Those with Disabilities* 17, no. 4 (2001): 52.

Huckle, Patricia. "Women in Utopias." In *The Utopian Vision: Seven Essays on the Quincentennial of Sir Thomas More*, ed. E. D. S. Sullivan, 115–36. San Diego: San Diego State University Press, 1983.

Hughes, Jim. "Blind Woman Sues Fertility Clinic: Englewood Facility Halted Treatments after Questions about Her Fitness as a Parent." *Denver Post*. November 7, 2003.

Human Sterilization. Pasadena, CA: Human Betterment Foundation, 1933. Cold Spring Harbor Eugenics Archive. http://www.dnalc.org/view/11671--Human-Sterilization-Human-Betterment-Foundation-3-.html.

Hutchins, Loraine. "Trouble and Mediation at Yosemite." *off our backs* 11, no. 10 (1981): 12–13, 25.

Imrie, Rob, and Huw Thomas. "The Interrelationships between Environment and Disability." *Local Environment* 13, no. 6 (2008): 477–83.

Jain, Sarah Lochlann. "Living in Prognosis: Toward an Elegiac Politics." *Representations* 98 (Spring 2007): 77–92.

Jesudason, Sujatha Anbuselvi. "In the Hot Tub: The Praxis of Building New Alliances for Reprogenetics." *Signs: Journal of Women in Culture and Society* 34, no. 4 (2009): 901–24.

Johnson, Harriet McBryde. "The Disability Gulag." *New York Times Magazine*. November 23, 2003. http://www.nytimes.com/2003/11/23/magazine/the-disability-gulag.html.

———. "Unspeakable Conversations." *New York Times Magazine*. February 16, 2003. http://www.nytimes.com/2003/02/16/magazine/unspeakable-conversations.html.

Johnson, Mary. *Make Them Go Away: Clint Eastwood, Christopher Reeve, and the Case against Disability Rights*. Louisville, KY: Advocado Press, 2003.

Johnson, Merri Lisa. "Crip Drag Swan Queen: Two Readings of Darren Aronofsky's *Black Swan*." National Women's Studies Association Conference, Atlanta, GA. November 2011.

Johnson, Valerie Ann. "Bringing Together Feminist Disability Studies and Environmental Justice." *Barbara Faye Waxman Fiduccia Papers on Women and Girls with Disabilities*. Center for Women Policy Studies. February 2011, 5. http://www.centerwomenpolicy.org/programs/waxmanfiduccia/BFWFP_BringingTogetherFeministDisabilityStudiesandEnvironmentalJustice_ValerieAnnJohnso.pdf.

Jordan, John W. "Reshaping the 'Pillow Angel': Plastic Bodies and the Rhetoric of Normal Surgical Solutions." *Quarterly Journal of Speech* 95, no. 1 (February 2009): 20–42.

Kafer, Alison. "Compulsory Bodies: Reflections on Heterosexuality and Able-bodiedness." *Journal of Women's History* 15, no. 3 (2003): 77–89.

———. "Cyborg." In *Encyclopedia of U.S. Disability History*, ed. Susan Burch, 223–24. New York: Facts on File, 2009.

———. "Seeing Animals." Exhibition essay for *Animal*. Sunaura Taylor, solo exhibition at Rowan Morrison Gallery, Oakland, CA. October 2009. http://www.sunaurataylor.org/portfolio/animal/.

Kafka, Bob. "Disability Rights vs. Workers Rights: A Different Perspective." *Znet*. November 14, 2003. http://www.zcommunications.org/disability-rights-vs-workers-rights-a-different-perspective-by-bob-kafka.

Keller, Evelyn Fox. "Nature, Nurture, and the Human Genome Project." In *The Code of Codes: Scientific and Social Issues in the Human Genome Project*, ed. Daniel J. Kevles and Leroy Hood, 281–99. Cambridge, MA: Harvard University Press, 1992.

Kelly, John B. "Incontinence." *Ragged Edge*, no. 1 (2002). http://www.ragged-edge-mag.com/0102/0102ft3.htm.

———. "Inspiration." *Ragged Edge Online*. January/February 2003. http://www.ragged-edgemagazine.com/0103/0103ft1.html.

———. "'It Could Have Been Worse:' Quadriplegic Athletes and the Ideology of Ability.'" Society for Disability Studies Annual Meeting, Chicago, June 2000.

Kelly, Tim. "Cyborg Waiting List." *Forbes*. September 3, 2007. http://www.forbes.com/forbes/2007/0903/038.html.

———. "Rise of the Cyborg." *Forbes*. October 4, 2006. http://www.forbes.com/forbes/2006/0904/090.html.

Kenney, Colleen. "Lincoln Receives Several Messages of Hope from up Above." *Lincoln Journal Star*. February 5, 2004.

Kent, Deborah. "Somewhere a Mockingbird." In *Prenatal Testing and Disability Rights*, ed. Erik Parens and Adrienne Asch, 57–63. Washington, DC: Georgetown University Press, 2000.

Kent, Le'a. "Fighting Abjection: Representing Fat Women." In *Bodies Out of Bounds: Fatness and Transgression*, ed. Jana Evans Braziel and Kathleen LeBesco, 130–50. Berkeley: University of California Press, 2001.

Kerr, Anne, and Tom Shakespeare. *Genetic Politics: From Eugenics to Genome*. Cheltenham, England: New Clarion Press, 2002.

Kevles, Daniel J. "Out of Eugenics: The Historical Politics of the Human Genome." In *The Code of Codes: Scientific and Social Issues in the Human Genome Project*, ed. Daniel J. Kevles and Leroy Hood, 3–36. Cambridge, MA: Harvard University Press, 1992.

Kevles, Daniel J., and Leroy Hood, eds. *The Code of Codes: Scientific and Social Issues in the Human Genome Project*. Cambridge, MA: Harvard University Press, 1992.

———. "Reflections." In *The Code of Codes: Scientific and Social Issues in the Human Genome Project*, ed. Daniel J. Kevles and Leroy Hood, 300–328. Cambridge, MA: Harvard University Press, 1992.

Kirchner, Corinne, and Liat Ben-Moshe. "Language and Terminology." In *Encyclopedia of U.S. Disability History*, ed. Susan Burch, 546–50. New York: Facts on File, 2009.

Kirkland, Anna. "When Transgendered People Sue and Win: Feminist Reflections on Straegy, Activism, and the Legal Process." In *The Fire This Time: Young Activists and the New Feminism*, ed. Vivien Labaton and Dawn Lundy Martin, 181–219. New York: Anchor, 2004.

Kirkup, Gill, Linda Janes, Kath Woodward, and Fiona Hovenden, eds. *The Gendered Cyborg: A Reader*. London: Routledge, 2000.

———. Introduction to *The Gendered Cyborg: A Reader*, ed. Gill Kirkup, Linda Janes, Kath Woodward, and Fiona Hovenden, xiii–xiv. London: Routledge, 2000.

Kiss and Tell Collective. *Her Tongue on My Theory*. Vancouver: Press Gang, 1994.

Kitchin, Rob, and Robin Law. "The Socio-spatial Construction of (In)accessible Public Toilets." *Urban Studies* 38, no. 2 (2001): 287–98.

Kittay, Eva Feder. "Discrimination against Children with Cognitive Impairments?" *Hastings Center Report* 40, no. 6 (2010): 32.

Kittay, Eva, and Jeffrey Kittay. "Whose Convenience? Whose Truth?" *Hastings Center Bioethics Forum*. February 28, 2007. Accessed from http://www.thehastingscenter.org/Bioethicsforum/Post.aspx?id=350&blogid=140.

Kleege, Georgina. *Blind Rage: Letters to Helen Keller*. Washington, DC: Gallaudet University Press, 2006.

———. *Sight Unseen*. New Haven: Yale University Press, 1999.

Kline, Wendy. *Building a Better Race: Gender, Sexuality, and Eugenics from the Turn of the Century to the Baby Boom*. Berkeley: University of California Press, 2001.

Klugman, Craig M. "From Cyborg Fiction to Medical Reality." *Literature and Medicine* 20, no. 1 (Spring 2001): 39–54.

Kolko, Beth E., Lisa Nakamura, and Gilbert B. Rodman. Introduction to *Race in Cyberspace*, ed. Beth E. Kolko, Lisa Nakamura, and Gilbert B. Rodman, 1–13. New York: Routledge, 2000.

Kostir, Mary Storer. "The Family of Sam Sixty." In *White Trash: The Eugenic Family Studies, 1877–1919*, ed. Nicole Hahn Rafter, 185–209. Boston: Northeastern University Press, 1988.

Koshy, Kavitha. "Feels Like Carving Bone: (Re)Creating the Activist-Self, (Re)Articulating Transnational Journeys, while Sifting Through Anzaldúan Thought." In *Bridging: How Gloria Anzaldúa's Life and Work Transformed Our Own*, ed. Analouise Keating and Gloria González-López, 197–203. Austin: University of Texas Press, 2011.

Kraut, Alan M. *Silent Travelers: Germs, Genes, and the "Immigrant Menace."* New York: Basic Books, 1994.

Kroll-Smith, Steve, Phil Brown, and Valerie J. Gunter. "Introduction: Environments and Diseases in a Postnatural World." In *Illness and the Environment: A Reader in Contested Medicine*, ed. Steve Kroll-Smith, Phil Brown, and Valerie J. Gunter, 1–6. New York: New York University Press, 2000.

Kudlick, Catherine J. "Disability History: Why We Need Another 'Other.'" *American Historical Review* 108, no. 3 (2003): 763–93.

———. "A History Profession for Every Body." *Journal of Women's History* 18, no. 1 (2006): 163–67.

Kumbier, Alana. "Hanky Pancreas: Insulin Pump Accessories and Cyborg Embodiment." *Threadbared*. June 1, 2010. Accessed June 22, 2010, http://iheartthreadbared.wordpress.com/2010/06/01/hanky-pancreas-insulin-pump-accessories-and-cyborg-embodiment/.

Kunzru, Hari. "You Are Cyborg." *Wired* 5, no. 2 (1997). Accessed from http://www.wired.com/wired/archive/5.02/ffharaway_pr.html.

Kuppers, Petra. "Addenda, Phenomenology, Embodiment: Cyborgs and Disability Performance." In *Performance and Technology: Practices of Virtual Embodiment and Interactivity*, ed. Susan Broadhurst and Josephine Machon, 169–80. New York: Palgrave Macmillan, 2006.

———. "Disability and Language: Introduction." *Profession* (2010): 107–11.

Kurzman, Steven L. "Presence and Prosthesis: A Response to Nelson and Wright." *Cultural Anthropology* 16, no. 3 (2001): 374–87.

Kusters, Annelies. "Deaf Utopias? Reviewing the Sociocultural Literature on the World's 'Martha's Vineyard Situations.'" *Journal of Deaf Studies and Deaf Education* 15, no. 1 (2010): 3–16.

LaFleur, Jennifer. "Nursing Homes Get Old for Many with Disabilities." *ProPublica*. June 21, 2009. http://www.propublica.org/article/nursing-homes-get-old-for-many-with-disabilities-621.

Lamm, Nomy. "Private Dancer: Evolution of a Freak." In *Restricted Access: Lesbians on Disability*, ed. Victoria A. Brownworth and Susan Raffo, 152–61. Seattle: Seal Press, 1999.

Lane, Harlan. "Constructions of Deafness." In *The Disability Studies Reader*, ed. Lennard J. Davis, 154–71. New York: Routledge, 1997.

Lantos, John. "It's Not the Growth Attenuation, It's the Sterilization!" *American Journal of Bioethics* 10, no. 1 (2010): 45–46.

Lee, Joyce. "Tall Girls: The Social Shaping of a Medical Therapy." *Archives of Pediatrics and Adolescent Medicine* 160 (October 2006): 1035–39.

"Let Disabled Katie Thorpe's Mother Decide." *Telegraph* (UK). October 8, 2007. http://www.telegraph.co.uk/comment/3643172/Let-disabled-Katie-Thorpes-mother-decide.html.

Levi, Jennifer, and Bennett Klein. "Pursuing Protection for Transgender People through Disability Laws." In *Transgender Rights*, ed. Paisley Currah, Richard M. Juang, and Shannon Price Minter, 74–92. Minneapolis: University of Minnesota Press, 2006.

Levy, N. "Deafness, Culture, and Choice." *Journal of Medical Ethics* 28 (2002): 284–85.

Levy-Navarro, Elena. "Fattening Queer History: Where Does Fat History Go from Here?" In *The Fat Studies Reader*, ed. Esther Rothblum and Sondra Solovay, 15–22. New York: New York University Press, 2009.

Lewis, Bradley. *Moving Beyond Prozac, DSM, and the New Psychiatry: The Birth of Postpsychiatry*. Ann Arbor: University of Michigan Press, 2006.

Linton, Simi. *Claiming Disability: Knowledge and Identity*. New York: New York University Press, 1998.

Lippman, Abby. "The Genetic Construction of Prenatal Testing: Choice, Consent, or Conformity for Women?" In *Women and Prenatal Testing: Facing the Challenges of Genetic Technology*, ed. Karen H. Rothenberg and Elizabeth J. Thomson, 9–34. Columbus: Ohio State University Press, 1994.

———. "Mother Matters: A Fresh Look at Prenatal Genetic Testing." *Issues in Reproductive and Genetic Engineering* 5, no. 2 (1992): 141–54.

Litwinowicz, Jo. "In My Mind's Eye: I." In *Bigger than the Sky: Disabled Women on Parenting*, ed. Michele Wates and Rowen Jade, 29–33. London: Women's Press, 1999.

Livingston, Julie. "Insights from an African History of Disability." *Radical History Review* 94 (Winter 2006): 111–26.

Lombardo, Paul. *Three Generations, No Imbeciles: Eugenics, the Supreme Court, and* Buck v. Bell. Baltimore, MD: The Johns Hopkins University Press, 2008.

Lorde, Audre. *The Cancer Journals: Special Edition*. San Francisco: Aunt Lute, 1997.

Love, Heather. *Feeling Backward: Loss and the Politics of Queer History*. Cambridge, MA: Harvard University Press, 2007.

———. "Wedding Crashers." *GLQ: A Journal of Lesbian and Gay Studies* 13, no. 1 (2007): 125–39.

Lurie, Samuel. "Loving You Loving Me: Tranny/Crip/Queer Love and Overcoming Shame in Relationship." Paper presented at the Queer Disability Conference, San Francisco State University, San Francisco, June 3, 2002.

MacDonald, V. "Abort Babies with Gay Genes, Says Nobel Winner." *Telegraph* (UK). February 16, 1997.

Mairs, Nancy. *Plaintext: Essays.* Tucson: University of Arizona Press, 1992.

———. *Waist-High in the World: A Life among the Nondisabled.* Boston: Beacon Press, 1996.

Mak, Cayden. "Cyborg Theory, Cyborg Practice." *The Outlet.* May 11, 2010. http://tinyurl.com/2wm7vag.

Mamo, Laura. *Queering Reproduction: Achieving Pregnancy in the Age of Technoscience.* Durham, NC: Duke University Press, 2007.

Marshall, Jessica. "Hysterectomy on Disabled US Girl Was Illegal." *New Scientist.* May 9, 2007. http://www.newscientist.com/article/dn11809-hysterectomy-on-disabled-us-girl-was-illegal.html.

Martin, Biddy. "Success and Its Failures." In *Women's Studies on the Edge*, ed. Joan Wallach Scott, 169–97. Durham, NC: Duke University Press, 2008.

Mason, Carol. "Terminating Bodies: Toward a Cyborg History of Abortion." In *Posthuman Bodies*, ed. Judith Halberstam and Ira Livingston, 225–43. Bloomington: Indiana University Press, 1995.

Masters, Cristina. "Bodies of Technology: Cyborg Soldiers and Militarized Masculinities." *International Feminist Journal of Politics* 7, no. 1 (2005): 112–32.

Mathers, A. R. "Hidden Voices: The Participation of People with Learning Disabilities in the Experience of Public Open Space." *Local Environment* 13, no. 6 (2008): 515–29.

Mauldin, Laura. "Cultural Commentary: Trig or Treat? The 2008 Election, Sarah Palin, and Teaching." *Disability Studies Quarterly* 28, no. 4 (2008). http://dsq-sds.org/

McCreery, Patrick. "Save Our Children/Let Us Marry: Gay Activists Appropriate the Rhetoric of Child Protectionism." *Radical History Review* 2008, no. 100 (2008): 186–207.

McDonald, Anne. "The Other Story from a 'Pillow Angel.'" *Seattle Post-Intelligencer.* June 16, 2007. http://www.seattlepi.com/opinion/319702_noangel17.html.

McGee, Glenn. *The Perfect Baby: Parenthood in the New World of Cloning and Genetics.* Lanham, MD: Rowman and Littlefield, 2000.

McGuire, Cathleen, and Colleen McGuire, "Grassroots Ecofeminism: Activating Utopia." In *Ecofeminist Literary Criticism: Theory, Interpretation, Pedagogy*, ed. Greta Gaard and Patrick D. Murphy, 186–203. Urbana: University of Illinois Press, 1998.

McKenna, Erin. *The Task of Utopia.* Lanham, MD: Rowman and Littlefield, 2001.

McNeil, Donald, Jr. "Broad Racial Disparities Seen in Americans' Ills." *New York Times.* January 14, 2011.

McRuer, Robert. "As Good as It Gets: Queer Theory and Critical Disability." *GLQ: A Journal of Lesbian and Gay Studies* 9, nos. 1–2 (2003): 79–105.

———. "Compulsory Able-Bodiedness and Queer/Disabled Existence." In *Disability Studies: Enabling the Humanities*, ed. Sharon L. Snyder, Brenda Jo Brueggemann, and Rosemarie Garland-Thomson, 88–99. New York: Modern Language Association, 2002.

———. *Crip Theory: Cultural Signs of Queerness and Disability.* New York: New York University Press, 2006.

———. "Critical Investments: AIDS, Christopher Reeve, and Queer/Disability Studies." *Journal of Medical Humanities* 23, nos. 3–4 (2002): 221–37.

———. "Disability Nationalism in Crip Times." *Journal of Literary and Cultural Disability Studies* 4, no. 2 (2010): 163–78.

———. "Taking It to the Bank: Independence and Inclusion on the World Market." *Journal of Literary Disability* 1, no. 2 (2007): 5–14.

McRuer, Robert, and Abby L. Wilkerson. Introduction to "Desiring Disability: Queer Theory Meets Disability Studies." Special issue. *GLQ: A Journal of Lesbian and Gay Studies* 9, nos. 1–2 (2003): 1–23.

McVeigh, Karen. "The 'Ashley Treatment': Erica's Story." *Guardian* (UK). March 16, 2012. http://www.guardian.co.uk/society/2012/mar/16/ashley-treatment-ericas-story.

McWhorter, Ladelle. "Foreword." In *Foucault and the Government of Disability*, ed. Shelley Tremain, xiii–xvii. Ann Arbor: University of Michigan Press, 2005.

Medgyesi, Victoria. "Crip Caste: Owning Up to the Pecking Order and Prejudice within the Disability Community." *New Mobility.* November 1997. Accessed September 18, 2004, http://newmobility.com.

Meekosha, Helen. "Superchicks, Clones, Cyborgs, and Cripples: Cinema and Messages of Bodily Transformations." *Social Alternatives* 18, no. 1 (1999): 24–28.

Michalko, Rod. *The Two in One: Walking with Smokie, Walking with Blindness.* Philadelphia: Temple University Press, 1999.

Milbern, Stacey. "Thoughts on National Coming Out Day." *Cripchick.* October 11, 2010. Accessed from http://blog.cripchick.com/archives/8359.

Mingus, Mia, Leah Lakshmi Piepzna-Samarasinha, and Ellery Russian. "Crip Sex, Crip Lust, and the Lust of Recognition." *Leaving Evidence.* May 25, 2010. Accessed from http://leavingevidence.wordpress.com/2010/05/25/video-crip-sex-crip-lust-and-the-lust-of-recognition/.

Miserandino, Christine. "The Spoon Theory." *But You Don't Look Sick.* 2003. Accessed from http://www.butyoudontlooksick.com.

Mitchell, David T. "The Frontier that Never Ends." *Electric Edge.* January/February 1997.

Mitchell, David T., and Sharon L. Snyder. "Introduction: Disability Studies and the Double Bind of Representation." In *The Body and Physical Difference: Discourses of Disability*, ed. David Mitchell and Sharon Snyder, 1–31. Ann Arbor: University of Michigan Press, 1999.

———. "Introduction: Exploring Foundations: Languages of Disability, Identity, and Culture." *DSQ: Disability Studies Quarterly* 17, no. 4 (1997): 241–47.

———. *Narrative Prosthesis: Disability and the Dependencies of Discourse.* Ann Arbor: University of Michigan Press, 2000.

Mog, Ashley, and Amanda Lock Swarr. "Threads of Commonality in Transgender and Disability Studies." *Disability Studies Quarterly* 28, no. 4 (2008). Accessed from www.dsq-sds.org.

Mohanty, Chandra Talpede. *Feminism without Borders: Decolonizing Theory, Practicing Solidarity.* Durham, NC: Duke University Press, 2003.

Mohanty, Chandra Talpede, and Biddy Martin. "What's Home Got to Do with It?" In *Feminism Without Borders: Decolonizing Theory, Practicing Solidarity,* 86–105. Durham, NC: Duke University Press, 2003.

Molina, Natalia. "Constructing Mexicans as Deportable Immigrants: Race, Disease, and the Meaning of 'Public Charge.'" *Identities: Global Studies in Culture and Power* 17 (2010): 641–66.

———. "Medicalizing the Mexican: Immigration, Race, and Disability in the Early-Twentieth-Century United States." *Radical History Review* 94 (2006): 22–37.

Mollow, Anna. "Identity Politics and Disability Studies: A Critique of Recent Theory." *Michigan Quarterly Review* 43, no. 2 (2004): 269–96.

———. "No Safe Place." *WSQ: Women's Studies Quarterly* 39, nos. 1–2 (2011): 188–99.

———. "'When *Black* Women Start Going on Prozac': Race, Gender, and Mental Illness in Meri Nana-Ama Danquah's *Willow Weep for Me.*" *MELUS* 31, no. 3 (2006): 67–99.

Mollow, Anna, and Robert McRuer. Introduction to *Sex and Disability*, ed. Robert McRuer and Anna Mollow, 1–34. Durham, NC: Duke University Press, 2012.

Molotch, Harvey. "Learning from the Loo." Introduction to *Toilet: Public Restrooms and the Politics of Sharing*, ed. Harvey Molotch and Laura Norén, 1–20. New York: New York University Press, 2010.

Molotch, Harvey, and Laura Norén, eds. *Toilet: Public Restrooms and the Politics of Sharing.* New York: New York University Press, 2010.

Montgomery, Cal. "A Hard Look at Invisible Disability." *Ragged Edge Online* 2 (2001). http://www.ragged-edge-mag.com/0301/0301ft1.htm.

Mortimer-Sandilands, Catriona. "Unnatural Passions: Notes Toward a Queer Ecology." *Invisible Culture*, no. 9 (2005). http://www.rochester.edu/in_visible_culture/Issue_9/sandilands.html.

Mortimer-Sandilands, Catriona, and Bruce Erickson, eds. "Introduction: A Genealogy of Queer Ecologies." In *Queer Ecologies: Sex, Nature, Politics, Desire*, ed. Catriona Mortimer-Sandilands and Bruce Erickson, 1–47. Bloomington: Indiana University Press, 2010.

———. *Queer Ecologies: Sex, Nature, Politics, Desire.* Bloomington: Indiana University Press, 2010.

Mouffe, Chantal. "Feminism, Citizenship, and Radical Democratic Politics." In *Feminists Theorize the Political*, ed. Judith Butler and Joan W. Scott, 369–84. New York: Routledge, 1992.

———. *The Return of the Political.* London: Verso, 1993.

Mundy, Liza. "A World of Their Own." *Washington Post Magazine.* March 31, 2002.

Muñoz, José Esteban. *Cruising Utopia: The Then and There of Queer Futurity.* New York: New York University Press, 2009.

Munson, Peggy. "Fringe Dweller: Toward an Ecofeminist Politic of Femme." In *Visible: A Femmethology*, vol. 2., ed. Jennifer Clarke Burke, 28–36. Ypsilanti, MI: Homofactus Press, 2009.

Munt, Sally R. "The Butch Body." In *Contested Bodies*, ed. Ruth Holliday and John Hassard, 95–106. London: Routledge, 2001.

Murillo, Sandra. "Caregiver Is Charged in Beating Death of Disabled Girl in Pedley." *Los Angeles Times.* May 13, 2004, B1.

Murphy, Caryle. "Gay Parents Find More Acceptance." *Washington Post.* June 14, 1999. http://www.washingtonpost.com/wp-srv/local/daily/june99/gays14.htm.

Nakamura, Lisa. "After/Images of Identity: Gender, Technology, and Identity Politics." In *Reload: Rethinking Women + Cyberculture*, ed. Mary Flanagan and Austin Booth, 321–31. Cambridge, MA: MIT Press, 2002.

———. *Cybertypes: Race, Ethnicity, and Identity on the Internet.* New York: Routledge, 2002.

Navarro, Mireya. "National Parks Reach Out to Blacks Who Aren't Visiting." *New York Times.* November 2, 2010.

Nelkin, Dorothy. "The Social Power of Genetic Information." In *The Code of Codes: Scientific and Social Issues in the Human Genome Project*, ed. Daniel J. Kevles and Leroy Hood, 177–90. Cambridge, MA: Harvard University Press, 1992.

Nelson, Jennifer. *Women of Color and the Reproductive Rights Movement.* New York: New York University Press, 2003.

Nicki, Andrea. "The Abused Mind: Feminist Theory, Psychiatric Disability, and Trauma." *Hypatia* 16, no. 4 (2001): 80–104.

Niles, Maria. "Am I Too Cynical for a Better Life?" *BlogHer*. June 7, 2008. http://www.blogher. com/am-i-too-cynical-better-life.

Nishime, LeiLani. "The Mulatto Cyborg: Imagining a Multiracial Future." *Cinema Journal* 44, no. 2 (Winter 2005): 34–49.

Norén, Laura. "Only Dogs Are Free to Pee: New York Cabbies' Search for Civility." In *Toilet: Public Restrooms and the Politics of Sharing*, ed. Harvey Molotch and Laura Norén, 93–114. New York: New York University Press, 2010.

Nosek, Margaret A. "Sexual Abuse of Women with Physical Disabilities." *Physical Medicine and Rehabilitation: State of the Art Reviews* 9, no. 2 (1995): 487–502.

Oaks, Laury. "What Are Pro-Life Feminists Doing on Campus?" *NWSA Journal* 21, no. 1 (2009): 178–203.

O'Brien, Michelle. "Tracing This Body: Transsexuality, Pharmaceuticals, and Capitalism." *deadletters: scattered notes toward the remembering of a misplaced present* (Summer 2003): 1–14. Accessed from http://www.deadletters.biz/body.html.

O'Brien, Ruth. *Crippled Justice: The History of Modern Disability Policy in the Workplace*. Chicago: University of Chicago Press, 2001.

Ordover, Nancy. *American Eugenics: Race, Queer Anatomy, and the Science of Nationalism*. Minneapolis: University of Minnesota Press, 2003.

Orr, Jackie. *Panic Diaries: A Genealogy of Panic Disorder*. Durham, NC: Duke University Press, 2006.

Ortega, Mariana. "Being Lovingly, Knowingly Ignorant: White Feminism and Women of Color." *Hypatia* 21, no. 3 (Summer 2006): 56–74.

Osgood, Robert L. *The History of Special Education: A Struggle for Equality in American Public Schools*. Westport, CT: Praeger, 2007.

Ostrander, R. Noam. "When Identities Collide: Masculinity, Disability, and Race." *Disability and Society* 23, no. 6 (2008): 585–97.

Ostrom, Carol M. "Child's Hysterectomy Illegal, Hospital Agrees." *Seattle Times*. May 9, 2007. http://community.seattletimes.nwsource.com/archive/?date=20070509&slug=childrens 09m.

O'Toole, Corbett Joan. "Dale Dahl and Judy Heumann: Deaf Man, Disabled Woman—Allies in 1970s Berkeley." In *Deaf and Disability Studies: Interdisciplinary Perspectives*, ed. Susan Burch and Alison Kafer, 162–87. Washington, DC: Gallaudet University Press, 2010.

———. "The Sexist Inheritance of the Disability Movement." In *Gendering Disability*, ed. Bonnie G. Smith and Beth Hutchison, 294–300. New Brunswick, NJ: Rutgers University Press, 2004.

———. "The View from Below: Developing a Knowledge Base about an Unknown Population." *Sexuality and Disability* 18, no. 3 (2000): 207–24.

Ott, Katherine. "The Sum of Its Parts: An Introduction to Modern Histories of Prosthetics." In *Artificial Parts, Practical Lives: Modern Histories of Prosthetics*, ed. Katherine Ott, David Serlin, and Stephen Mihm, 1–42. New York: New York University Press, 2002.

Overall, Christine. "Public Toilets: Sex Segregation Revisited." *Ethics and the Environment* 12, no. 2 (2007): 71–91.

Padden, Carol, and Tom Humphries. *Deaf in America: Voices from a Culture*. Cambridge, MA: Harvard University Press, 1988.

Page, Lewis. "Cyborg-Style 'iLimb' Hand a Big Hit with Iraq Veterans." *Register.* July 18, 2007. http://www.theregister.co.uk/2007/07/18/robo_hand_gets_big_hand.

Parens, Erik, and Adrienne Asch, eds. *Prenatal Testing and Disability Rights.* Washington, DC: Georgetown University Press, 2000.

Paul, Diane B. *Controlling Human Heredity: 1865 to the Present.* Atlantic Highlands, NJ: Humanities Press, 1995.

Paul, Gregory S., and Earl D. Cox. *Beyond Humanity: CyberEvolution and Future Minds.* Rockland, MA: Charles River Media, 1996.

Panzarino, Connie. "Camping with a Ventilator." In *That Takes Ovaries! Bold Females and Their Brazen Acts,* ed. Rivka Solomon, 139–42. New York: Three Rivers Press, 2002.

———. *The Me in the Mirror.* Seattle: Seal Press, 1994.

Peace, William. "Ashley and Me." *Bioethics Forum.* June 22, 2010. Accessed from http://www.thehastingscenter.org/Bioethicsforum/Post.aspx?id=4742&blogid=140.

Penley, Constance, and Andrew Ross. "Cyborgs at Large: An Interview with Donna Haraway." In *Technoculture,* ed. Constance Penley and Andrew Ross, 1–20. Minneapolis: University of Minnesota Press, 1991.

Penna, David, and Vickie D'Andrea-Penna. "Developmental Disability." In *Encyclopedia of U.S. Disability History,* ed. Susan Burch, 261–62. New York: Facts on File, 2009.

Perez, Hiram. "You Can Have My Brown Body and Eat It, Too!" *Social Text* 84–85, vol. 23, nos. 3–4 (2005): 171–91.

Perillo, Lucia. *I've Heard the Vultures Singing: Field Notes on Poetry, Illness, and Nature.* San Antonio, TX: Trinity University Press, 2007.

Pernick, Martin S. *The Black Stork: Eugenics and the Death of "Defective" Babies in American Medicine and Motion Pictures since 1915.* New York: Oxford University Press, 1996.

Piercy, Marge. *Woman on the Edge of Time.* New York: Fawcett Crest, 1976.

Pilkington, Ed. "Frozen in Time: The Disabled Nine-Year-Old Girl Who Will Remain a Child All Her Life." *Guardian.* January 4, 2007. http://www.guardian.co.uk/world/2007/jan/04/health.topstories3.

Pilkington, Ed, and Karen McVeigh. "'Ashley Treatment' On the Rise amid Concerns from Disability Rights Groups." *Guardian* (UK). March 15, 2012. http://www.guardian.co.uk/society/2012/mar/15/ashley-treatment-rise-amid-concerns.

Pitcher, Ben, and Henriette Gunkel. "Q&A with Jasbir Puar." *darkmatter Journal.* May 2, 2008. Accessed from http://www.darkmatter101.org/site/2008/05/02/qa-with-jasbir-puar/.

Plaskow, Judith. "Embodiment, Elimination, and the Role of Toilets in Struggles for Social Justice." *Cross Currents* (Spring 2008): 51–64.

Plotz, David. "The 'Genius Babies' and How They Grew." *Slate.* February 8, 2001. http://www.slate.msn.com.

Potts, Annie. "Cyborg Masculinity in the Viagra Era." *Sexualities, Evolution and Gender* 7, no. 1 (2005): 3–16.

Pratt, Minnie Bruce. *Rebellion: Essays, 1980–1991.* Ann Arbor, MI: Firebrand, 1991.

Price, Janet, and Margrit Shildrick. "Uncertain Thoughts on the Dis/abled Body." In *Vital Signs: Feminist Reconfigurations of the Bio/logical Body,* ed. Margrit Shildrick and Janet Price, 224–49. Edinburgh: Edinburgh University Press, 1998.

Price, Margaret. "Access Imagined: The Construction of Disability in Conference Policy Documents." *DSQ: Disability Studies Quarterly* 29, no. 1 (2009). Accessed from http://www.dsq-sds.org/article/view/174/174.

———. "'Her Pronouns Wax and Wane': Psychosocial Disability, Autobiography, and Counter-Diagnosis." *Journal of Literary and Cultural Disability Studies* 3, no. 1 (2009): 11–33.

———. *Mad at School: Rhetorics of Mental Disability and Academic Life*. Ann Arbor: University of Michigan Press, 2010.

Priestley, Mark. *Disability: A Life Course Approach*. Cambridge: Polity Press, 2003.

"Psychiatric Aide Accused of Rape." *New York Times*. November 26, 1979.

Puar, Jasbir K. "Prognosis Time: Toward a Geopolitics of Affect, Debility and Capacity." *Women and Performance: A Journal of Feminist Theory* 19, no. 2 (2009): 161–72.

———. *Terrorist Assemblages: Homonationalism in Queer Times*. Durham, NC: Duke University Press, 2007.

Quinlan, Margaret, and Benjamin Bates. "*Bionic Woman* (2007): Gender, Disability, and Cyborgs," *Journal of Research in Special Educational Needs* 9, no. 1 (2009): 48–58.

Rabin, Roni Caryn. "Disparities: Illness More Prevalent among Older Gay Adults." *New York Times*. April 1, 2011.

Rafter, Nicole Hahn, ed. *White Trash: The Eugenic Family Studies, 1877–1919*. Boston: Northeastern University Press, 1988.

Rapp, Rayna. *Testing Women, Testing the Fetus: The Social Impact of Amniocentesis in America*. New York: Routledge, 1999.

Ray, Sarah Jaquette. "Risking Bodies in the Wild: The 'Corporeal Unconscious' of American Adventure Culture." *Journal of Sport and Social Issues* 33, no. 3 (2009): 257–84.

Razack, Sherene. "From Pity to Respect." In *Looking White People in the Eye: Gender, Race, and Culture in Courtrooms and Classrooms*, 130–56. Toronto: University of Toronto Press, 1998.

Reagan, Leslie J. *Dangerous Pregnancies: Mothers, Disabilities, and Abortion in Modern America*. Berkeley: University of California Press, 2010.

Reagon, Bernice Johnson. "Coalition Politics: Turning the Century." In *Home Girls: A Black Feminist Anthology*, ed. Barbara Smith, 356–68. New York: Kitchen Table Press, 1983.

Reeve, Christopher. *Nothing Is Impossible: Reflections on a New Life*. New York: Random House, 2002.

Reeve, Donna. "Cyborgs and Cripples: What Can Haraway Offer Disability Studies?" In *Disability and Social Theory: New Developments and Directions*, ed. Dan Goodley, Bill Hughes, and Lennard Davis. New York: Palgrave Macmillan, forthcoming.

Reilly, Philip R. *The Surgical Solution: A History of Involuntary Sterilization in the United States*. Baltimore: Johns Hopkins University Press, 1991.

Rembis, Michael A. *Defining Deviance: Sex, Science, and Delinquent Girls, 1890–1960*. Champaign: University of Illinois Press, 2011.

Report of Committee on Classification of Feeble-Minded. In *Mental Retardation in America: A Historical Reader*, ed. Steven Noll and James W. Trent, Jr., 87–88. New York: New York University Press, 2004.

Rich, Adrienne. "Notes Toward a Politics of Location." In *Blood, Bread, and Poetry: Selected Prose, 1979–1985*, 210–31. New York: W. W. Norton, 1986.

Richardson, Mattie Udora. "No More Secrets, No More Lies: African-American History and Compulsory Heterosexuality." *Journal of Women's History* 15, no. 3 (2003): 63–76.

Roberts, Dorothy. *Fatal Invention: How Science, Politics, and Big Business Re-create Race in the Twenty-first Century*. New York: The New Press, 2011.

———. *Killing the Black Body: Race, Reproduction, and the Meaning of Liberty*. New York: Vintage, 1999.

———. "Race, Gender, and Genetic Technologies: A New Reproductive Dystopia?" *Signs: Journal of Women in Culture and Society* 34, no. 4 (2009): 783–804.

Roberts, Geneviève. "Brain-damaged Girl Is Frozen in Time by Parents to Keep Her Alive." *Independent*. January 4, 2007. http://www.independent.co.uk/news/world/americas/braindamaged-girl-is-frozen-in-time-by-parents-to-keep-her-alive-430734.html.

Rodríguez, Juana María. *Queer Latinidad: Identity Practices, Discursive Spaces.* New York: New York University Press, 2003.

Rohrer, Judy. "Toward a Full-Inclusion Feminism: A Feminist Deployment of Disability Analysis." *Feminist Studies* 31, no. 1 (Spring 2005): 34–63.

Rothenberg, Karen H., and Elizabeth J. Thomson, eds. *Women and Prenatal Testing: Facing the Challenges of Genetic Technology.* Columbus: Ohio State University Press, 1994.

Ruiz, Jason. "The Violence of Assimilation: An Interview with Mattilda aka Matt Bernstein Sycamore." *Radical History Review* 100 (Winter 2008): 237–47.

Russell, Julia Scofield. "The Evolution of an Ecofeminist." In *Reweaving the World: The Emergence of Ecofeminism*, ed. Irene Diamond and Gloria Feman Orenstein, 223–30. San Francisco: Sierra Club Books, 1990.

Russo, Mary. *The Female Grotesque: Risk, Excess, and Modernity.* New York: Routledge, 1994.

Ryan, Sean. "Cyborgs in the Woods." *Leisure Studies* 21 (2002): 265–84.

Sack, Kevin. "Research Finds Wide Disparities in Health Care by Race and Region." *New York Times.* June 5, 2008. http://www.nytimes.com/2008/06/05/health/research/05disparities.html.

Salleh, Anna. "Cyborg Rights 'Need Debating Now.'" *ABC Science Online.* June 5, 2010. http://www.abc.net.au/news/stories/2010/06/05/2918723.htm.

Samantrai, Ranu. *AlterNatives: Black Feminism in the Postimperial Nation.* Stanford, CA: Stanford University Press, 2002.

Samuels, Ellen. "Bodies in Trouble." In *Restricted Access: Lesbians on Disability*, ed. Victoria A. Brownworth, 192–200. Seattle: Seal Press, 1999.

———. "Critical Divides: Judith Butler's Body Theory and the Question of Disability." *NWSA Journal* 14, no. 3 (2002): 58–76.

———. "My Body, My Closet: Invisible Disability and the Limits of Coming-Out Discourse." *GLQ: A Journal of Lesbian and Gay Studies* 9, nos. 1–2 (2003): 233–55.

———. "Normative Time: How Queerness, Disability, and Parenthood Impact Academic Labor." Paper presented at the Modern Languages Association Annual Meeting, December 2006.

Sandahl, Carrie. "Ahhhh, Freak Out! Metaphors of Disability and Femaleness in Performance." *Theatre Topics* 9, no. 1 (March 1999): 11–30.

———. "Anarcha Anti-Archive: Depends®." *Liminalities: A Journal of Performance Studies* 4, no. 2 (2008). http://liminalities.net/4-2/anarcha.

———. "Performing Metaphors: AIDS, Disability, and Technology." *Contemporary Theatre Review* 11, nos. 3–4 (2001): 49–60.

———. "Queering the Crip or Cripping the Queer? Intersections of Queer and Crip Identities in Solo Autobiographical Performance." *GLQ: A Journal of Lesbian and Gay Studies* 9, nos. 1–2 (2003): 25–56.

Sandilands, Catriona. "Eco Homo: Queering the Ecological Body Politic." *Social Philosophy Today* 19 (2004): 17–39.

———. "From Unnatural Passions to Queer Nature." *Alternatives Journal* 27, no. 3 (Summer 2001): 30–35.

———. *The Good-Natured Feminist: Ecofeminism and the Quest for Democracy.* Minneapolis: University of Minnesota Press, 1999.

Sandoval, Chela. "New Sciences: Cyborg Feminism and the Methodology of the Oppressed." In *The Cyborg Handbook*, ed. Chris Hables Gray, Steven Mentor, and Heidi J. Figueroa-Sarriera, 407–21. New York: Routledge, 1995.

Sasaki, Betty. "Toward a Pedagogy of Coalition." In *Twenty-First-Century Feminist Classrooms: Pedagogies of Identity and Difference*, ed. Amie A. MacDonald and Susan Sánchez-Casal, 31–57. New York: Palgrave, 2002.

Savoy, Lauret. "The Future of Environmental Essay: A Discourse." *Terrain* (Summer/Fall 2008). Accessed from terrain.org.

Saxton, Marsha. "Disability Rights and Selective Abortion." In *Abortion Wars: A Half-Century of Struggle, 1950–2000*, ed. Rickie Solinger, 374–93. Berkeley: University of California Press, 1998.

Schoen, Johanna. *Choice and Coercion: Birth Control, Sterilization, and Abortion in Public Health and Welfare.* Chapel Hill: University of North Carolina Press, 2005.

Schriempf, Alexa. "Hearing Deafness: Subjectness, Articulateness and Communicability." *Subjectivity* 28 (2009): 279–96.

Schueller, Malini Johar. "Analogy and (White) Feminist Theory: Thinking Race and the Color of the Cyborg Body." *Signs* 31, no. 1 (Autumn 2005): 63–92.

Schweik, Susan M. *The Ugly Laws: Disability in Public.* New York: New York University Press, 2009.

"Scientists Test First Human Cyborg." *CNN.com.* March 22, 2002. http://archives.cnn.com/2002/TECH/science/03/22/human.cyborg/.

Scott, Catherine. "Time Out of Joint: The Narcotic Effect of Prolepsis in Christopher Reeve's *Still Me.*" *Biography* 29, no. 2 (2006): 307–28.

Scott, Joan W. "Cyborgian Socialists?" In *Coming to Terms: Feminism, Theory, Politics*, ed. Elizabeth Weed, 215–17. New York: Routledge, 1989.

———. "'Experience.'" In *Feminists Theorize the Political*, ed. Judith Butler and Joan W. Scott, 22–40. New York: Routledge, 1992.

Sedgwick, Eve Kosofsky. *Tendencies.* Durham, NC: Duke University Press, 1994.

Selden, Steven. *Inheriting Shame: The Story of Eugenics and Racism in America.* New York: Teachers College Press, 1999.

Serlin, David. "Pissing without Pity: Disability, Gender, and the Public Toilet." In *Toilet: Public Restrooms and the Politics of Sharing*, ed. Harvey Molotch and Laura Norén, 167–85. New York: New York University Press, 2010.

Shabot, Sara Cohen. "Grotesque Bodies: A Response to Disembodied Cyborgs." *Journal of Gender Studies* 15, no. 3 (2006): 223–35.

Shakespeare, Tom. "Arguing about Genetics and Disability." *Interaction* 13, no. 3 (2000): 11–14.

———. *Disability Rights and Wrongs.* New York: Routledge, 2006.

———. "The Social Model of Disability." In *The Disability Studies Reader,* 2nd ed., ed. Lennard J. Davis, 197–204. New York: Routledge, 2006.

Shands, Kerstin W. *The Repair of the World: The Novels of Marge Piercy.* Westport, CT: Greenwood Press, 1994.

Shannon, Sarah E., and Teresa A. Savage. "The Ashley Treatment: Two Viewpoints." *Pediatric Nursing* 32, no. 2 (2007): 175–78.

Shapiro, Joseph. *No Pity: People with Disabilities Forging a New Civil Rights Movement.* New York: Three Rivers Press, 1994.

Sherry, Mark. *Disability Hate Crimes: Does Anyone Really Hate Disabled People?* Burlington, VT: Ashgate, 2010.

Shildrick, Margrit. *Dangerous Discourses of Disability, Subjectivity, and Sexuality.* New York: Palgrave Macmillan, 2009.

———. *Embodying the Monster: Encounters with the Vulnerable Self.* London: Sage, 2002.

———. *Leaky Bodies and Boundaries: Feminism, Postmodernism, and (Bio)Ethics.* London: Routledge, 1997.

Shiva, Vandana. "The Impoverishment of the Environment: Women and Children Last." In *Ecofeminism*, ed. Vandana Shiva and Maria Mies, 81–82. London: Zed, 1993.

Siebers, Tobin. "Disability in Theory: From Social Constructionism to the New Social Realism of the Body." *American Literary History* (2001): 737–54.

———. *Disability Theory.* Ann Arbor, MI: University of Michigan Press, 2008.

Sieck, Ann. "Preservation and Disability Access." *Sierra Club Yodeler: The Newspaper of the San Francisco Bay Chapter.* July/August 2004. Accessed August 28, 2004, http://sanfran-ciscobay.sierraclub.org/yodeler/html/2004/7/feature10.htm.

Signorello, L. B., et al. "Comparing Diabetes Prevalence between African Americans and Whites of Similar Socioeconomic Status." *American Journal of Public Health* 97, no. 12 (2007): 2260–67.

Silliman, Jael, Marlene Gerber Fried, Loretta Ross, and Elena R. Gutiérrez. *Undivided Rights: Women of Color Organize for Reproductive Justice.* Boston: South End Press, 2004.

Skotko, Brian. "Prenatally Diagnosed Down Syndrome: Mothers Who Continued Their Pregnancies Evaluate Their Health Care Providers." *American Journal of Obstetrics and Gynecology* 192 (2005): 670–77.

Smith, Andrea. "Beyond Pro-Choice versus Pro-Life: Women of Color and Reproductive Justice." *NWSA Journal* 17, no. 1 (2005): 119–40.

Smith, J. David. *Minds Made Feeble: The Myth and Legacy of the Kallikaks.* Rockville, MD: Aspen Systems, 1985.

Smith, Marquard, and Joanne Morra, eds. *The Prosthetic Impulse: From a Posthuman Present to a Biocultural Future.* Cambridge, MA: MIT Press, 2006.

Snyder, Sharon, Brenda Brueggemann, and Rosemarie Garland-Thomson. "Introduction: Integrating Disability in Theory and Scholarship." In *Disability Studies: Enabling the Humanities*, ed. Sharon Snyder, Brenda Brueggemann, and Rosemarie Garland-Thomson, 1–12. New York: The Modern Language Association of America, 2002.

Snyder, Sharon L., and David T. Mitchell. *Cultural Locations of Disability.* Chicago: University of Chicago Press, 2006.

Sobchack, Vivian. "A Leg to Stand On: Prosthetics, Metaphor, and Materiality." In *The Prosthetic Impulse: From a Posthuman Present to a Biocultural Future*, ed. Marquard Smith and Joanne Morra, 17–41. Cambridge, MA: MIT Press, 2006.

Sobsey, Dick, D. Wells, R. Lucardie, and S. Mansell, eds. *Violence and Disability: An Annotated Bibliography.* Baltimore, MD: Paul H. Brookes Publishing Company, 1995.

Sofoulis, Zoë. "Cyberquake: Haraway's Manifesto." In *Prefiguring Cyberculture: An Intellectual History*, ed. Darren Tofts, Annemarie Jonson, and Allesio Cavallaro, 84–103. Cambridge, MA: MIT Press, 2002.

Solinger, Rickie. *Beggars and Choosers: How the Politics of Choice Shapes Adoption, Abortion, and Welfare in the United States.* New York: Hill and Wang, 2001.

———. *Pregnancy and Power: A Short History of Reproductive Politics in America.* New York: New York University Press, 2005.

Spade, Dean. "Resisting Medicine, Re/modeling Gender." *Berkeley Women's Law Journal* 18 (2003): 15–37.

———. *Toilet Training: Companion Guide for Activists and Educators.* Sylvia Rivera Law Project. New York: Urban Justice Center, 2004.

Spelman, Elizabeth V. *Inessential Woman: Problems of Exclusion in Feminist Thought.* Boston: Beacon Press, 1988.

Spillers, Hortense. "Mama's Baby, Papa's Maybe: An American Grammar Book." *Diacritics* 17, no. 2 (1987): 64–81.

Spretnak, Charlene. "Toward an Ecofeminist Spirituality." In *Healing the Wounds: The Promise of Ecofeminism,* ed. Judith Plant, 127–32. Philadelphia, PA: New Society Publishers, 1989.

Springer, Claudia. "The Pleasure of the Interface." In *Sex/Machine: Readings in Culture, Gender, and Technology,* ed. Patrick D. Hopkins, 484–500. Bloomington: Indiana University Press, 1998.

Squier, Susan Merrill. *Babies in Bottles: Twentieth-century Visions of Reproductive Technology.* New Brunswick, NJ: Rutgers University Press, 1994.

———. *Liminal Lives: Imagining the Human at the Frontiers of Biomedicine* Durham, NC: Duke University Press, 2004.

Stabile, Carol A. *Feminism and the Technological Fix.* Manchester: Manchester University Press, 1994.

Stacey, Meg. "The New Genetics: A Feminist View." In *The Troubled Helix: Social and Psychological Implications of the New Human Genetics,* ed. Theresa Marteau and Martin Richards, 331–49. Cambridge: Cambridge University Press, 1996.

Stewart, Jean, and Marta Russell. "Disablement, Prison, and Historical Segregation." *Monthly Review* 53, no. 3 (2001): 61–75. Accessed from http://monthlyreview.org/2001/07/01/disablement-prison-and-historical-segregation.

Stolen, Jeremy David. "Big Money behind 'Inspirational' Billboard Campaign." http://www.theportlandalliance.org/2002/april/billboard.html.

———. "Foundation for a Better Life." Portland Independent Media Center. http://portlandindymedia.org/2002/02/7617.shtml.

Stryker, Susan, and Stephen Whittle, eds. *The Transgender Studies Reader.* New York: Routledge, 2006.

Stubblefield, Anna. "Beyond the Pale: Tainted Whiteness, Cognitive Disability, and Eugenic Sterilization." *Hypatia* 22, no. 2 (2007): 162–81.

Sturgeon, Noël. *Ecofeminist Natures: Race, Gender, Feminist Theory, and Political Action.* New York: Routledge, 1997.

———. *Environmentalism in Popular Culture: Gender, Race, Sexuality, and the Politics of the Natural.* Tucson: University of Arizona Press, 2009.

Sturken, Marita, and Lisa Cartwright. "Consumer Culture and the Manufacturing of Desire." In *Practices of Looking: An Introduction to Visual Culture,* 189–236. New York: Oxford University Press, 2001.

Sullivan, Ronald. "Panel Rejects Charges that Tranquilizer Use Led to Patient Deaths." *New York Times.* March 27, 1979.

Swan, Jim. "Disabilities, Bodies, Voices." In *Disability Studies: Enabling the Humanities,* ed. Sharon L. Snyder, Brenda Jo Brueggemann, and Rosemarie Garland-Thomson, 283–95. New York: Modern Languages Association, 2002.

Swartz, Leslie, and Brian Watermeyer. "Cyborg Anxiety: Oscar Pistorius and the Boundaries of What It Means to be Human." *Disability and Society* 23, no. 2 (2008): 187–90.

Tarzian, Anita J. "Disability and Slippery Slopes." *Hastings Center Report* 37, no. 5 (2007): c3.

Taylor, Janelle. *The Public Life of the Fetal Sonogram: Technology, Consumption, and the Politics of Reproduction.* New Brunswick, NJ: Rutgers University Press, 2008.

Taylor, Sunaura. *Animal.* Solo exhibition at Rowan Morrison Gallery, Oakland, CA. October 2009. http://www.sunaurataylor.org/portfolio/animal/.

———. "Beasts of Burden: Disability Studies and Animal Rights." *Qui Parle: Critical Humanities and Social Sciences* 19, no. 2 (2011): 191–222.

Teather, David. "Lesbian Couple Have Deaf Baby by Choice." *Guardian* (UK). April 8, 2002. http://www.guardian.co.uk/world/2002/apr/08/davidteather.

Terry, Jennifer. "'Unnatural Acts' in Nature: The Scientific Fascination with Queer Animals." *GLQ: A Journal of Lesbian and Gay Studies* 6, no. 2 (2000): 151–93.

Thompson, Becky. *A Promise and a Way of Life: White Antiracist Activism.* Minneapolis: University of Minnesota Press, 2001.

Thompson, Sandra. "Billboards Marketing Virtues We Can Use Now." *St. Petersburg Times.* February 2, 2002.

Titchkosky, Tanya. "'To Pee or Not to Pee?': Ordinary Talk about Extraordinary Exclusions in a University Environment." *Canadian Journal of Sociology/Cahiers Canadiens de Sociologie* 33, no. 1 (2008): 37–60.

"Trailblazing in a Wheelchair: An Oxymoron?" *Palaestra: Forum of Sport, Physical Education, and Recreation for Those with Disabilities* 17, no. 4 (2001): 52.

Tregaskis, Claire. "Applying the Social Model in Practice: Some Lessons from Countryside Recreation." *Disability and Society* 19, no. 6 (2004): 601–11.

Tremain, Shelley. "On the Subject of Impairment." In *Disability/Postmodernity: Embodying Political Theory*, ed. Mairian Corker and Tom Shakespeare, 32–47. New York: Continuum, 2002.

———. "Reproductive Freedom, Self-Regulation, and the Government of Impairment in Utero." *Hypatia* 21, no. 1 (2006): 35–53.

Trent, James W. *Inventing the Feeble Mind: A History of Mental Retardation in the United States.* Berkeley: University of California Press, 1994.

Twine, Richard T. "Ma(r)king Essence: Ecofeminism and Embodiment." *Ethics and the Environment* 6, no. 2 (2001): 31–57.

Vance, Linda. "Ecofeminism and the Politics of Reality." In *Ecofeminism: Women, Animals, and Nature*, ed. Greta Gaard, 118–45. Philadelphia: Temple University Press, 1993.

———. "Ecofeminism and Wilderness." *NWSA Journal* 9, no. 3 (Fall 1997): 60–76.

Van Cleve, John Vickrey, and Barry Crouch. *A Place of Their Own: Creating the Deaf Community in America.* Washington, DC: Gallaudet University Press, 1989.

Van Dijck, José. *Imagenation: Popular Images of Genetics.* New York: New York University Press, 1998.

Vidali, Amy. "Seeing What We Know: Disability and Theories of Metaphor." *Journal of Literary and Cultural Disability Studies* 4, no. 1 (2010): 33–54.

Vincent, Norah. "Enabling Disabled Scholarship." *Salon.* August 18, 1999. Accessed from http://www.salon.com/books/it/1999/08/18/disability/index.html.

von Schrader, S., W. A. Erickson, and C. G. Lee. *Disability Statistics from the Current Population Survey.* Ithaca, NY: Cornell University Rehabilitation Research and Training Center on Disability Demographics and Statistics, 2010. www.disabilitystatistics.org.

Warner, Michael. *The Trouble with Normal: Sex, Politics, and the Ethics of Queer Life.* New York: Free Press, 1999.

Warren, Karen J. *Ecofeminist Philosophy: A Western Perspective on What It Is and Why It Matters.* Lanham, MD: Rowman and Littlefield, 2000.

———. "Ecological Feminist Philosophies: An Overview." In *Ecological Feminist Philosophies,* ed. Karen J. Warren, ix–xxvi. Indianapolis: Indiana University Press, 1996.

———. "The Power and the Promise of Ecological Feminism." In *Ecological Feminist Philosophies,* ed. Karen J. Warren, 19–41. Indianapolis: Indiana University Press, 1996.

Washington Protection and Advocacy System. "Executive Summary—Investigative Report Regarding the 'Ashley Treatment.'" October 1, 2010. Accessed from http://www.disabilityrightswa.org/home/Executive_Summary_InvestigativeReportRegardingtheAshley-Treatment.pdf/view?searchterm=ashley.

———. Exhibit L. "Special CHRMC Ethics Committee Meeting/Consultation." *Investigative Report Regarding the "Ashley Treatment."* May 4, 2004. Accessed from http://www.disabilityrightswa.org/home/Exhibits_K_T_InvestigativeReportRegardingtheAshleyTreatment.pdf.

———. Exhibit O. "Letter from Larry Jones." *Investigative Report Regarding the "Ashley Treatment."* June 10, 2004. Accessed from http://www.disabilityrightswa.org/home/Exhibits_K_T_InvestigativeReportRegardingtheAshleyTreatment.pdf.

———. Exhibit R. "Hospital Billing Report." *Investigative Report Regarding the "Ashley Treatment."* March 28, 2007. Accessed from http://www.disabilityrightswa.org/home/Exhibits_K_T_InvestigativeReportRegardingtheAshleyTreatment.pdf.

———. Exhibit T. "Agreement Between Children's Hospital and Regional Medical Center and the Washington Protection and Advocacy System (Disability Rights Washington) Promoting Protection of Individuals with Developmental Disabilities." *Investigative Report Regarding the "Ashley Treatment."* May 1, 2007. http://www.disabilityrightswa.org/home/Exhibits_K_T_InvestigativeReportRegardingtheAshleyTreatment.pdf.

———. "Press Release—Investigative Report Regarding the 'Ashley Treatment.'" May 8, 2007. Accessed from http://www.disabilityrightswa.org/home/Press_Release_WPASFinds HospitalThatPerformedAshleyTreatmentViolatedLawByNo.pdf.

Weheliye, Alexander G. "'Feenin': Posthuman Voices in Contemporary Black Popular Music." *Social Text 71* vol. 20, no. 2 (2002): 21–47.

Weihenmayer, Erik. *Touch the Top of the World: A Blind Man's Journey to Climb Farther than the Eye Can See.* New York: Plume, 2002.

Weil, Elizabeth. "Breeder Reaction." *Mother Jones* 31, no. 4 (2006): 33–37.

———. "A Wrongful Birth?" *New York Times Magazine.* March 12, 2006.

Weise, Jillian. "Going Cyborg." *New York Times Magazine.* January 10, 2010, 50.

Wekker, Gloria. "The Arena of Disciplines: Gloria Anzaldúa and Interdisciplinarity." In *Doing Gender in Media, Art and Culture,* ed. Rosemarie Buikema and Iris van der Tuin, 54–69. New York: Routledge, 2007.

Wendell, Susan. *The Rejected Body: Feminist Philosophical Reflections on Disability.* New York: Routledge, 1996.

———. "Unhealthy Disabled: Treating Chronic Illnesses as Disabilities." *Hypatia: A Journal of Feminist Philosophy* 16, no. 4 (2001): 17–33.

White, Evelyn C. "Black Women and the Wilderness." In *The Stories That Shape Us: Contemporary Women Write about the West,* ed. Teresa Jordan and James Hepworth, 376–83. New York: W. W. Norton, 1995.

Wilfond, Benjamin S., Paul Steven Miller, Carolyn Korfatis, Douglas S. Diekema, Denise M. Dudzinski, Sara Goering, and the Seattle Growth Attenuation and Ethics Working

Group. "Navigating Growth Attenuation in Children with Profound Disabilities: Children's Interests, Family Decision-Making, and Community Concerns." *Hastings Center Report* 40, no. 6 (2010): 27–40.

Wilkerson, Abby. "Ending at the Skin: Sexuality and Race in Feminist Theorizing." *Hypatia* 12, no. 3 (1997): 164–73.

Williams, Patricia J. "Judge Not?" *Nation* (New York). March 26, 2007, 9.

Williams, Zoe. "Abortion and Euthanasia: Was Virginia Ironside Right?" *Guardian*. October 5, 2010. http://www.guardian.co.uk/world/2010/oct/04/virginia-ironside-tv-euthanasia-abortion.

Wilson, Daniel J. "Fighting Polio Like a Man: Intersections of Masculinity, Disability, and Aging." In *Gendering Disability*, ed. Bonnie G. Smith and Beth Hutchison, 119–33. New Brunswick, NJ: Rutgers University Press, 2004.

Wilson, Elizabeth A. "Organic Empathy: Feminism, Psychopharmaceuticals, and the Embodiment of Depression." In *Material Feminisms*, ed. Stacy Alaimo and Susan Hekman, 373–99. Bloomington: Indiana University Press, 2008.

Winnubst, Shannon. *Queering Freedom*. Bloomington: Indiana University Press, 2006.

———. "Temporality in Queer Theory and Continental Philosophy." *Philosophy Compass* 5, no. 2 (2010): 136–46.

———. "Vampires, Anxieties, and Dreams: Race and Sex in the Contemporary United States." *Hypatia* 18, no. 3 (2003): 1–20.

Winterson, Jeanette. "How Would We Feel If Blind Women Claimed the Right to a Blind Baby?" *Guardian* (UK). April 9, 2002. Features section, 9.

Winzer, Margret. *The History of Special Education: From Isolation to Integration*. Washington, DC: Gallaudet University Press, 1993.

Wolfe, Cary. "Learning from Temple Grandin, or, Animal Studies, Disability Studies, and Who Comes After the Subject." *New Formations* 64 (2008): 110–23.

Wong, Sophia Isako. "At Home with Down Syndrome and Gender." *Hypatia* 17, no. 3 (2002): 89–117.

Young, Iris Marion. *Justice and the Politics of Difference*. Princeton, NJ: Princeton University Press, 1990.

Young, Mary Ellen, Margaret A. Nosek, Carol Howland, Gail Chanpong, and Diana H. Rintala. "Prevalence of Abuse of Women with Physical Disabilities." *Archives of Physical Medicine and Rehabilitation* 78, no. 12 (1997): supplement 5, S34–38.

Yuval-Davis, Nira. "Beyond Difference: Women and Coalition Politics." In *Making Connections: Women's Studies, Women's Movements, Women's Lives*, ed. Mary Kennedy, Cathy Lubelska, and Val Walsh, 2–9. London: Taylor and Francis, 1993.

Zola, Irving Kenneth. "The Language of Disability: Problems of Politics and Practice." *Australian Disability Review*. 1988. Accessed from http://www.disabilitymuseum.org/lib/docs/813.card.htm.

Zwillinger, Rhonda. *The Dispossessed: Living with Multiple Chemical Sensitivities*. Paulden, AZ: The Dispossessed Outreach Project, 1999.

Index

Abbey, Edward, 132, 134, 135, 214n11, 214n18

Abel, Elizabeth, 154

able-bodiedness/able-mindedness, 8, 17, 19, 43, 130, 153; able-bodiedness, 16, 23, 102, 106, 116, 132–35, 184n54; able-mindedness, 16, 101, 184n54

abled/disabled binary, 10–11, 13, 19, 25, 108, 111, 186n13; as mutually constitutive, 6, 8

ableism, 10, 32, 67, 69–70, 77, 82, 89–90, 125, 134, 153, 166, 184n63; anti-ableism, 23–24, 118, 120, 126; as internalized, 4, 75, 79, 143

abortion, 28, 157–68, 224n72; access to, 161, 164, 178, 179n2, 223n71; disability as justification for, 84, 163, 165–68, 178, 223n71; as selective, 23, 29, 162–66, 177–78, 179n2, 186n22, 197n1, 221n61, 223n63

access, 3, 18, 20, 27, 152–53, 154, 156, 161, 220n38; activism regarding, 9, 101, 154–57, 161, 171–76, 218n15, 218n19; as alternative formats, 136, 215n27; and architecture, 6–7, 154, 172–73, 174; and disability, 154–57, 172–73; and gender, 155–57, 172–73, 174, 219n27; to nature, 129–30, 135–36, 136–39, 140, 142, 215n27, 216n33; as scent-free spaces, 161, 171, 175–76, 190n66, 221n49. See also restrooms

activism, 3, 9, 14–15, 100–101, 120–24, 171–78; telethon protests, 123, 212n101. See also access

ADAPT, 100–101, 205n34

agility, 210n76

AIDS, 11, 124, 189n54. See also queer time

Alaimo, Stacy, 23, 158, 160, 211n88, 214n9, 217n9, 221n47

animal rights movements, 216n51

Anschutz, Philip, 92, 94, 97, 203n10, 204n20

Asch, Adrienne, 61, 64, 166, 167, 197n83

Ashley Treatment, the, 21, 47–48, 49, 51–52, 192n4, 192n6, 192n8; controversy over, 48, 50–51, 58, 61; and growth attenuation, 50–52, 55, 61, 192n7, 192n11, 193n14, 193n24, 197n83; and mastectomy (breast bud removal), 52, 55–56, 65, 192n7, 193n14, 194n30, 194n32, 195n51; and privatization, 60–62; as template, 48, 50–51, 52, 57–60, 67, 195n60, 196n64; and sterilization (hysterectomy), 49–50, 51–52, 55–57, 192n7, 195n57; Washington Protection and Advocacy System (WPAS) report on, 49–51, 60, 193n12. See also Seattle Children's Hospital; Seattle Growth Attenuation and Ethics Working Group

Ashley Treatment, The (blog), 51, 52, 58, 61, 195n60; photos on, 194n34

Ashley X, 21, 47, 49, 197n86; asynchrony of, 48, 49, 53–55, 57, 63, 66, 68, 192n7; and futurity, 47–48; and gender, 49, 55–57, 58, 65, 195n56; as grotesque, 49, 55, 57, 61, 68; as noncommunicative, 63–65; as pillow angel, 52–53, 54–55; and pleasure, 65, 68; quality of life of, 47–48, 51–52, 63–65, 66, 193n14, 197n83; and whiteness, 66

Asian Communities for Reproductive Justice, 222n60

asthma, 12, 14, 153

attendant care, 8, 30, 38–39, 40, 61–62, 169, 224n85

autism, 144–45

Baggs, A. M., 144–45

Baker, Sherry, 107, 108, 208n37

Balsamo, Anne, 22, 106

Bauman, H-Dirksen L., 84

Baynton, Douglas, 149

Bell, Chris, 12, 183n53

Ben-Moshe, Liat, 168, 191n91

Berlant, Lauren, 28, 96–97, 204n18

Berrier, Justin, 97

Bérubé, Michael, 181n21, 185n3

Bienvenu, MJ, 200n19

blindness, 4–5, 80, 102, 201n26, 210n76, 220n30

Boellstorff, Tom, 36

Breast Cancer Action (BCA), 160

Brueggemann, Brenda Jo, 26, 42, 211n85

Buck v. Bell, 30

Butler, Judith, 16, 46, 98

Butler, Octavia, 116, 209n62, 209n64

cancer, 7, 11, 33; breast, 159–60, 217n9

Cangemi, Phyllis, 216n33

capitalism, 39–40, 190n72, 224n85

Carlson, Licia, 54, 223n71

Cavanaugh, Sheila, 219n22

Chambers, Kijuana, 80–82, 202n41

Chandler, Eliza, 36

Charo, Alta, 82–83

Chen, Mel Y., 38, 44, 161

Child, the, 20, 28–29, 31–34, 96–97, 204n18

Children of Deaf Adults (CODAs), 13

253

ALISON KAFER is Associate Professor and Chair of the Feminist Studies program at Southwestern University. Her work on gender, sexuality, and disability has appeared in anthologies including *Sex and Disability, Feminist Disability Studies* (IUP, 2011), and *Gendering Disability*, as well as in the *Journal of Women's History*. She coedited *Deaf and Disability Studies: Interdisciplinary Approaches*.

Printed in the USA
CPSIA information can be obtained
at www.ICGtesting.com
LVHW010415220924
791621LV00034B/600